Between Flesh *and* Steel

Also by Richard A. Gabriel

Man and Wound in the Ancient World: A History of Military Medicine from Sumer to the Fall of Constantinople
Hannibal: The Military Biography of Rome's Greatest Enemy
Philip II of Macedonia: Greater than Alexander
Thutmose III: A Military Biography of Egypt's Greatest Warrior King
Scipio Africanus: Rome's Greatest General
The Battle Atlas of Ancient Military History
The Warrior's Way: A Treatise on Military Ethics
Muhammad: Islam's First Great General
Soldiers' Lives Through History: The Ancient World
Jesus the Egyptian: The Origins of Christianity and the Psychology of Christ
Empires at War: A Chronological Encyclopedia
Subotai the Valiant: Genghis Khan's Greatest General
The Military History of Ancient Israel
The Great Armies of Antiquity
Sebastian's Cross
Gods of Our Fathers: The Memory of Egypt in Judaism and Christianity
Warrior Pharaoh: A Chronicle of the Life and Deeds of Thutmose III, Great Lion of Egypt, Told in His Own Words to Thaneni the Scribe
Great Captains of Antiquity
The Culture of War: Invention and Early Development
The Painful Field: Psychiatric Dimensions of Modern War
No More Heroes: Madness and Psychiatry in War
Military Incompetence: Why the American Military Doesn't Win
To Serve with Honor: A Treatise on Military Ethics and the Way of the Soldier

With Donald W. Boose Jr.

Great Battles of Antiquity: A Strategic and Tactical Guide to Great Battles That Shaped the Development of War

With Karen S. Metz

A Short History of War: The Evolution of Warfare and Weapons
History of Military Medicine, Vol. 1: From Ancient Times to the Middle Ages
History of Military Medicine, Vol. 2: From the Renaissance Through Modern Times
From Sumer to Rome: The Military Capabilities of Ancient Armies

Between Flesh *and* Steel

A HISTORY *of* MILITARY MEDICINE
from the MIDDLE AGES
to the WAR *in* AFGHANISTAN

RICHARD A. GABRIEL

Potomac Books
An imprint of the University of Nebraska Press

An earlier version of this book was published as A *History of Military Medicine: From the Renaissance through Modern Times*, by Richard A. Gabriel and Karen S. Metz, by Praeger, an imprint of ABC-CLIO, LLC, Santa Barbara, CA. Copyright 1992 by the authors. Used by arrangement with ABC-CLIO, LLC, Santa Barbara, CA. All rights reserved.

First Nebraska paperback printing: 2016.

Manufactured in the United States of America.

♾

Cover: This Civil War cartoon depicts the military surgeon in his most-feared role as the amputator of limbs. The term "sawbones" to describe a surgeon dates from this period when the most common military surgical procedure was amputation. Original artwork by James Dunn; color rendition by Daniel Pearlmutter.

Library of Congress Cataloging-in-Publication Data
Names: Gabriel, Richard A.
Title: Between flesh and steel: a history of military medicine
from the Middle Ages to the war in Afghanistan / Richard A. Gabriel.
Description: Potomac Books, an imprint of the University of Nebraska Press, 2016. |
Originally published: c2013. | "First Nebraska paperback printing: 2016." |
Includes bibliographical references and index.
Identifiers: LCCN 2015038639 | ISBN 9781612348223 (pbk.: alk. paper)
Subjects: LCSH: Medicine, Military—History. | Weapons—History.
Classification: LCC RC971 .G33 2016 | DDC 616.9/8023— dc23
LC record available at http://lccn.loc.gov/2015038639

for Jude Alfred Nurik and the
miracle of life

and

for Suzi, my beloved wife, whose
pretty blue eyes warm my soul

CONTENTS

ILLUSTRATIONS

FIGURES

TABLES

1

THE EMERGENCE OF MODERN WARFARE

1453 to the Twenty-First Century

Death came quickly to soldiers wounded on the battlefields of antiquity. The muscle-powered weapons that tore at their flesh inflicted death suddenly. Bodies pierced by spears or hacked by swords lingered in agony for only a short time until the loss of blood brought on shock and the merciful unconsciousness that precedes death. The lethality of the ancient soldier's weapons and the primitive condition of military medical care, where it existed at all, ensured that death could not be protracted. The stricken soldier did not suffer long before slipping away.

With the appearance of gunpowder, wounding took on a more terrible character. Bullets drove fragments of clothing deep into the body, broke the long bones, and caused tracking wounds that, unless extensively incised and cleansed of loose tissue, became seats of infection. Gunpowder-driven projectiles instantly amputated arms and legs, grossly disfigured the face, laid open the skull to expose the brain, and caused multiple penetrations of the intestines. The new weapons caused terrible wounds that stimulated the search for medical techniques to deal with them. But medical innovation was unable to keep pace, and its treatments served mostly to prolong the suffering of the wounded without ultimately preventing their death from shock, blood loss, or infection. The wounded now simply took longer to die. The Middle Ages brought with it the introduction of new medical techniques that held out the promise, mostly unfulfilled, of saving the soldier's life. But this progress was only a glimpse into the medical future and the beginning of the long road to effective military medical care.

The armies of the Middle Ages were a reflection of the political, social, and economic decentralization of the larger feudal social order. Most wars in this period were fought not by nation states but by rival monarchs that raised armies by levying requirements for soldiers and arms upon their vassals. Centralized arms industries, permanent standing armies, and logistical organizations or trained armies did not exist.[1] Military doctrine and tactics of the day were almost nonexistent, and battles revealed the low sophistication of armed scuffles among groups of mounted men. It was, as has been remarked, "a period of squalid butchery."[2] The knights returned home under the command of their local lords, and the armies disbanded after each battle. Tax collections for military purposes were sporadic, usually taken in-kind, and left to local military commanders, who were also the political officials of the realm. As the fourteenth century dawned, Europe found itself in a period of political, economic, social, and military transition between feudalism and the rise of the embryonic nation state.

The decentralization of feudalism placed the armored knight at the pinnacle of the socio-military order, and the form of individual mounted combat at which the knight excelled had swept infantry from the field almost a thousand years earlier. The last time Europe had seen a disciplined infantry force command the battlefield was under the Roman Empire. At the start of the Hundred Years' War (1337–1457), the supremacy of the mounted knight remained unchallenged. When this series of dynastic wars ended, new military forms were emerging that signaled that supremacy's decline.

To counter the power of the mounted knight, the infantry had to be able either to withstand the shock of a mounted assault or to deliver sufficient missiles from a distance great enough to inflict casualties on the mounted formation and prevent it from closing with the infantry. At the Battle of Laupen (1339) Swiss infantry annihilated a force of mounted French knights by reinventing the Macedonian phalanx, complete with eighteen-foot-long pikes similar to the *sarissae* that Alexander the Great's infantry had used sixteen hundred years earlier.[3] Comprising sturdy and disciplined citizen soldiers, the Swiss infantry stood its ground against the mounted charge, stopping the French cavalry with their pikes. With the cavalry halted before the wall of pikes, Swiss halberdsmen and ax throwers attacked, chopping off the legs of the horses and butchering the fallen knights as they lay helpless on the ground. At Crécy (1346) the English reinvented the second solution for confronting a cavalry charge and destroyed a force of French knights with hails of metal-tipped arrows fired from longbows.[4] In both instances, the solutions represented the rediscovery and reapplication of long-forgotten techniques that Alexander and the Romans once had used for defeating cavalry. For the first time in more than a thousand years, disciplined infantry forces again began to appear on the battlefields of Europe.

The Hundred Years' War witnessed the beginning of national identity and loyalty as a series of dynastic wars crystallized national identities. The need for large military forces, including mercenary contingents, gave rise to the replacement of in-kind taxes with regular tax collections of specie. This effort required developing a centralized governmental mechanism, and the embryonic nation states began to build governmental infrastructures under the national monarchs' control. Both during the war and for more than a hundred years afterward, bands of demobilized ex-soldiers who fought for pay and constantly switched sides plagued Europe. The rulers' problem was how to bring these military bands under the authority of a national army. Their solution was to offer permanent pay, to build regular garrisons, to enforce strict codes of military discipline, and to establish military rank and administrative structures. By the 1600s, for the first time since the collapse of Rome, Europe began to develop stable, permanent armed forces directed by central national authorities and supported by taxation.

The emergence of national authorities spurred the organizational, tactical, and technological development of armies during this period and set the pattern for the next four centuries. A standing army of professionals could be disciplined, schooled in new battle tactics, and trained to utilize the new firearms with great effect. This preparation, in turn, helped stabilize the new role of infantry, whose musket and pike tactics permitted thinner linear formations of infantry on the battlefield. The appearance and evolution of the firearm increased the demand for a disciplined soldier, and this requirement ushered in a permanent and articulated rank and administrative structure to train and lead the soldier. Permanent rank and military organization reappeared, and by the time of the Thirty Years' War (1618–1648), all the major elements of the modern army were in place.

THE GUNPOWDER REVOLUTION

The most significant invention in weaponry of the Hundred Years' War was gunpowder, which when coupled with new techniques for casting metal produced the primitive cannon. Siege mortars used to batter down castle walls quickly came into widespread use. In 1453, the Ottoman armies used cannon to destroy the walls of Constantinople, bringing the Byzantine Empire to an end. Mobile siege guns played a leading role in several battles of the Hundred Years' War,[5] which also saw the first effective use of field artillery in Europe. True field artillery appeared in the final decade of the fifteenth century when the French mounted light cast bronze cannon on two-wheeled, horse-drawn carriages. The introduction of the trunnion—a device for raising and lowering the gun independently of the carriage—increased the soldier's ability to aim these guns with greater accuracy. By the seventeenth century, gun manufacture had progressed to where the range, power, and types of guns would change little for the next two centuries.

During the fifteenth and sixteenth centuries, gunpowder was revolutionizing the battlefield. The appearance of the musketeer, the forerunner of the modern rifleman, and his firelock musket made it possible for the first time for tightly packed infantry formations to stop cavalry without engaging in close combat. The slow rate of fire of these early weapons, however, required that musketeers be protected from the hostile advance, a problem that led to mixing musketeer formations with those of pikemen. Although the mix of pike to musket changed considerably over the next three hundred years, the mixed infantry formation remained the basic infantry formation during that time.

The cavalry most immediately felt the effect of portable firearms on the battlefield. The invention of the wheel lock allowed the soldier to aim and fire the pistol with one hand. As the introduction of pike and musket to the infantry reduced the shock effect of cavalry, the cavalry armed itself with saber and pistol and began to rely more on mobility and firepower than on shock.[6] After more than a thousand-year interregnum, infantry again became the arm of decision on the battlefield. Leaders now used the cavalry, no longer decisive, to pin the flanks of infantry formations so that they could rake them with artillery and musket fire. At the same time, the siege mortar gave way to the smoothbore cannon that could function as genuine field artillery. By the seventeenth century, genuine horse artillery had replaced horse-drawn artillery, and all members of artillery units rode into battle. This development greatly increased the flexibility and mobility of field artillery, making it a full partner in the newly emerging maneuver warfare.[7]

By the sixteenth century, the feudal order was creaking toward its demise, and in its place arose the nation state governed by the absolute monarch in command of a permanent standing army. The professional army was the instrument of creating and protecting the nation state. Whereas feudal armies had attempted to capture the enemy's strong points, the new armies engaged in wars of attrition with the primary goal of destroying the enemy's armed force. The time was right for the ideology of nationalism and dynastic rivalry to propel a new round of national conflicts, which, in turn, would spawn yet another generation of new and more destructive weapons.

The Thirty Years' War was the most destructive of these conflicts. What began as a clash of feudal armies ended by setting the stage for the emergence of modern war. During this period, the musket revolutionized the role of infantry. The original musket was a firelock, itself a great improvement on the earlier matchlock, which had required a forked stand to hold its long barrel. The rifleman had to ignite the powder in the touchhole with a hand-held burning wick, conditions that made the weapon impossible to aim or fire quickly. The firelock used a trigger attached to a rod that moved a serpentine burning wick to the touchhole, thereby allowing the rifleman to hold the weapon with both hands and aim. The lighter, more reliable, and more mobile firelock could fire a round every two to three minutes. For the first time the infantry had a relatively reliable and accurate weapon.

The firelock was later replaced by the wheel lock, in which a rotating geared wheel powered by a cocked spring caused a flint to ignite the powder in the flash pan. A century later, the wheel lock was replaced by the flintlock, in which a spring-loaded hammer struck a flint to ignite the charge. By the 1800s, the percussion cap, a truly reliable system, had replaced the former mechanism. With each development, the rifle became more certain to fire on cue and the rate of fire increased.

Corned gunpowder was another significant innovation of this period. Early gunpowder for rifles and cannon tended to separate into its component materials when the powder was stored for long periods or when moved in the logistics train. The separation made it unlikely that the powder would explode evenly in the rifle barrel, increasing misfires and propelling the bullet at much lower velocity. Corned powder was made of component materials shaped into little nuggets that reduced settling and made the powder more certain to fire evenly, maintaining the projectile's velocity. This configuration resulted in longer range and deadlier firearms and cannon.[8]

In the sixteenth century, the rifleman carried his powder and ball, ranging from .44- to .51-caliber lead shot, in small leather bags. In rainy weather, the weapons often would not fire because of damp powder. In the Thirty Years' War King Gustavus Adolphus of Sweden (1594–1632) invented the paper cartridge, which protected the powder from dampness and greatly improved the rifle's reliability. Musketeers could now fire two rounds a minute instead of a single round every two or three minutes. By the end of the American Civil War (1861–1865), the completely self-contained modern cartridge with powder and bullet in a single metal container made its appearance. By the Franco-Prussian War of 1870–1871, the breech-loading rifle had become standard issue for European armies. Two decades later, the clip- and magazine-fed infantry rifle revolutionized infantry tactics. The breech-loading, clip-fed, bolt or lever action rifle made it unnecessary for the rifleman to stand or kneel to reload. This freedom of action made the introduction of modern dispersed infantry tactics possible and further increased the infantry's ability to fire and maneuver.[9]

Regardless of the type of firing mechanism, the musket remained an inaccurate weapon with limited range and a slow rate of fire until the American Civil War. The smoothbore musket was usually ineffective beyond 100 yards. By the early 1700s, the British Brown Bess could hit a man at 80 yards with some regularity. The Americans truly revolutionized riflery when they invented the first reliable rifled barrel, the famed Kentucky rifle. The invention of rifling made it possible to hit a target reliably at 180 yards, increasing the range and accuracy of infantry rifle fire by a factor of three.[10]

The rifle changed the tactical battlefield. In feudal armies, infantry was packed into dense squares to maximize firepower and to resist shock from cavalry attack. As the rifle became more reliable and firepower became deadlier at longer range, it became possible to thin out the packed masses of infantry into lines while still providing sufficient firepower and defense against cavalry. Gustavus Adolphus was the first to deploy his infantry in lines four men deep, alternating pikemen with musketeers. This innovation represented the birth of linear tactics, a tactical arrangement that remained unchanged in its essentials until almost the twentieth century. Linear tactics provided the infantry with yet more mobility without sacrificing firepower or defense, opening the way for more sophisticated battlefield maneuvers and tactical deployments. No longer the primary striking force, the pikeman had the task of protecting the musketeers from cavalry attack. As muskets became more reliable, powerful, and accurate, thinner and thinner infantry formations could be used without sacrificing killing power until, finally, the pikeman disappeared from the field altogether.

The legacy of the pikeman remained, however, in the form of the bayonet, which is still standard issue in modern armies. The first one, a plug bayonet, was inserted into the rifle's muzzle. Because it made the firearm inoperable, the musketeer had to rely heavily upon the pikeman for protection. By the end of the seventeenth century, the ring bayonet made its appearance. Attached to a plug below the rifle barrel, this apparatus allowed the rifle to fire while the bayonet was in place, but the attachment was clumsy and unreliable. The standard barrel bayonet attached to a permanent stud welded to the rifle barrel appeared shortly afterward, and within a decade it became standard issue in all European armies.[11] The musketeer had now become his own pikeman. Musket infantry was expected to protect itself from cavalry attack and, when closing with the enemy, to fight hand to hand with the bayonet. By combining the functions of the musketeer with the pikeman, all infantry could now be armed with firearms, greatly increasing the killing power of the infantry. In 1746, the British infantry first used the fluted bayonet at the Battle of Culloden Moor, and it has remained a basic close combat tool of the infantryman ever since.[12]

Still other advances increased the power of infantry. In the mid-1700s, the Prussians introduced a standard-size iron ramrod to replace the nonstandard wooden rod. When coupled with proper training of the soldier, it doubled the musket's rate of fire.[13] At the same time, the infantry began to diversify its weapons' capability with a primitive hand grenade. The first hand grenades were hollow iron balls packed with black powder ignited by a burning wick. Within a decade, the infantry grenadier had become a standard feature of European infantry formations.

The most significant advances in firepower and range came in artillery.[14] At the beginning of the Thirty Years' War, individual craftsmen still cast artillery by hand, so no two guns or barrels were exactly alike. The weight of these artillery pieces was too great to make them mobile enough for effective use against troop formations, although they served well in sieges. Gustavus Adolphus standardized not only the size of cannon and shot, producing the first lightweight artillery guns, but also infantry barrels and musket shot. Adopted almost universally, this system of millimeter caliber measurement is still used by most modern armies.[15] Adolphus standardized artillery firing procedure as well, and his artillery gunners could fire eight rounds from a single gun in the time it took a musketeer with a firelock to load and fire a single round.[16]

Over the next century, the French introduced a number of innovations in artillery, including mounting the gun on wheeled carriages and introducing the trunnion to improve aiming. Until this time, horses usually pulled the artillery guns, while the artillery crews walked behind. This arrangement slowed the artillery's mobility, and it was common practice never to move the guns once deployed on the battlefield. Frederick the Great of Prussia (1712–1786) introduced the idea of mounting the guns and gun crews on horseback and wagons, so that guns, crews, and ammunition could all move together. The invention of horse artillery greatly increased the mobility of field artillery, and commanders could routinely move the guns around and change deployments for maximum effect.[17] At the same time, their guns were becoming lighter and equipped with more accurate aiming mechanisms. The result was the emergence of a deadly combat arm, field artillery, that over time would be responsible for more casualties than any other weapon.

The range of artillery gradually increased as well, and by the Napoleonic era, cannon fire could reach three hundred yards, or about the range of a Roman ballista. Until the Crimean War (1853–1856), 70 percent of all cannon shot was solid ball shot. But as early as the 1740s, artillery gunners had various types of artillery rounds at their disposal. Howitzers primarily used heavy rounds that exploded on contact, and artillery guns with a flatter trajectory of fire used canister, chain, and grapeshot against cavalry and infantry formations. Later, these rounds were coupled with exploding charges that made it possible to burst artillery rounds over the enemy's heads, considerably increasing lethality and casualties. During the American Civil War, rifled cannon came into its own, with a corresponding increase in range and accuracy. Later, advances in breech loading, gas canister sealing, and recoil mechanisms vastly improved rates of fire.

The killing power of infantry and artillery drove cavalry from the field as a major killing arm. Horse cavalry gradually became lighter, and being armed with pistols, carbines, and sabers, it was relegated to filling the gaps in the line, performing reconnaissance, conducting raids, and protecting the flanks of the infantry. Cavalry did not return as a major battlefield player until the end of World War I, when the internal combustion engine made possible the first primitive tanks.[18]

THE BEGINNINGS OF MODERN WARFARE

The period between the fifteenth and seventeenth centuries witnessed the emergence and consolidation of the nation state as the primary form of sociopolitical organization and as the most dynamic actor in international affairs. With the collapse of feudalism, the new dynastic social orders of the West developed different forms of social, political, economic, and military organization, all of which eventually influenced the course of weapons development and the conduct of war. At the beginning of the period, monarchy was the most common form of domestic political organization of the nation state. By the seventeenth century, national monarchs had gradually subdued or destroyed all competing centers of political power and parochial loyalty within their national borders. The age of absolutism, when national monarchs wielded absolute power over their politico-social orders, had begun. Consequently, various monarchs declared war upon one another at will, often over trivial and personal concerns, for almost a hundred years.

During the seventeenth century, however, other centers of domestic power, some of them arising as a consequence of the changing economic structure, gradually circumscribed the national monarchs' power. Expanding domestic and international economies brought into existence new classes of domestic political claimants that demanded a share in the power of the political establishment. By the nineteenth century, the empowerment of new societal segments culminated in the rise of representative legislatures that gave these new classes some participation in public policy. The increased influence of these new domestic political actors, however, was in proportion to how valuable they were to the national authorities in conducting their war and foreign policies.

To ensure the king's control over his domestic realm, he built the armies of the new nation states. Control of these military forces became central to establishing and expanding monarchical power, and the new standing professional armies became the chief means of suppressing domestic dissent and protecting the monarchy from foreign threats. The early bureaucracies that were set up to achieve the monarch's directives in the domestic realm became the prototypes of those modern civil and military bureaucracies deemed necessary to govern the modern state.

As the social and economic structures of the new states became more complex, they gave rise to merchant and financial classes that began to challenge the monarchical order and demand a greater share in the political process. The new financial instruments—hard currencies, banking systems, letters of credit, international trade, and cross-national financing and manufacturing—used to cope with a developing international economy forced the national monarchs to depend upon the new classes more heavily to raise armies and fight wars. By the seventeenth century, national monarchs could no longer maintain armies or fight wars without the support of the merchant and financial classes.

The development of a complex international economy made the support of the new classes indispensable. Resources available for war varied greatly from state to state, and the ability to sustain one's position in the international arena required that economic resources remain securely tied to national aspirations and interests. Economic concerns began to drive military ambitions in equal measure with political and military concerns. The internationalization of economic affairs made it impossible for any one state to secure solely for itself the resources for war and to gain military dominance over all other states or even a coalition of states for long. In military adventures any one state could hope only to achieve marginal gains at the expense of other states. Under these circumstances, a constantly shifting balance of power among many national states came to characterize the international order.

The economic costs of weapons and warfare increased enormously, and wars of this period often produced the near or actual financial collapse of the participants. Professional armies and weapons were expensive, and the resources required to produce and maintain a large military force led a number a states into bankruptcy.[19] The loss or transfer of manpower from industry and agriculture to military service, the high costs of borrowing on domestic and international markets, and the disruption of domestic and international trade caused by national conflicts resulted in destruction and economic dislocation that often served to make even a successful war a near financial disaster. These circumstances gradually forced the national monarchs to share power with the new merchant classes that controlled the sinews of war and had the most to lose or gain economically by war.

By the early 1800s, the transition from the old feudal orders to the modern national era was complete insofar as weaponry, tactics, and military organization were concerned. The old political order hung on for yet another century but more in form than substance. Militarily, the pike disappeared from the battlefield, and the new musket infantry came of age while fighting in disciplined linear combat formations, a form that lingered into the twentieth century. Mobile artillery also came into its own and became a major killing combat arm used in coordination with cavalry and infantry. The standing army had come into being, with organization, logistics trains, and command structures comparable to those of modern armies.

Napoleon Bonaparte introduced yet a new element into this equation and, in doing so, revolutionized the conduct of war. Until the French Revolution, armies remained professional forces whose manpower was drawn from the least socially and economically useful elements of the population. Most soldiers came from the ranks of the urban poor or the excess rural population that had no land. Even the officer corps was drawn from the second and third sons of the nobility, leaving the first son to manage the family's estates and business interests. These professional military forces' loyalty was based largely upon regular pay. Napoleon instituted the mass citizen army based on conscription and developed an officer corps with men who were selected for their talent rather than their social origins. A number of industrial and agricultural innovations allowed him to extract ever larger groups of manpower from the economic base without serious disruption. Still, the size of the Napoleonic armies was impossible to maintain unless the entire social and economic resources of the state were mobilized for war. The age of modern war had dawned.

The Napoleonic armies replaced the old enticements of loyalty to the king and regular pay with loyalty based on national patriotism fired by the ideal of social revolution. This appeal made it possible for Napoleon to raise mass armies. The idea of a "nation in arms" based on national patriotic fervor and sacrifice to ideals meant that all segments of the population were expected to contribute to the war effort. Entire national economies were now marshaled to support war, and private control of the resources of war passed to the control of the state. The state's economic structures were required to produce the sinews of war upon command, even to the detriment of other aspects of economic and social activity if necessary. Thus the most significant contribution of the Napoleonic era was the invention of a new national model for war, the nation in arms.

Historians sometimes call the American Civil War the first truly modern war, for it was the first conflict not only to take maximum advantage of the new efficiencies of production that the Industrial Revolution fostered but also to involve the *entire* populations of each combatant. Large conscript armies, larger than the world had ever seen, required a monumental industrial base to feed, clothe, and supply them for combat. The Industrial Revolution, the factory system, and machine mass production, along with technological innovations in metallurgy, chemistry, and machine tools, created an explosion in military technology. The great reduction in time between developing new ideas and manufacturing their prototypes was among the most important consequence. New concepts were quickly translated to mechanical drawings, then to models, then to prototypes, and finally to full-scale implementation, all within a very short time. The widespread introduction of technical journals accelerated the time it took for innovations in one discipline to have an impact on a related field. The result was a rapid increase in information transfer.

Overall these circumstances led to new technologies being rapidly applied to warfare at a historically unprecedented pace, and correspondingly weapons became more lethal than ever. As new means of economic organization and impressive increases in productivity freed large numbers of men for military service without causing serious economic dislocation in the national wartime economy, the civilian population that manned the war machine's productive base became at least as important as the war machine itself. For the first time, the production base and the civilian industrial manpower pool became legitimate and necessary military targets to achieve victory.

The Crimean War witnessed the British Army first wielding both rifled and breech-loading artillery. Both of these improvements already had been used as early as the sixteenth century, if only as prototypes. Technical problems in barrel casting and breech sealing had prevented their operation on a widespread basis. Half the Union artillery in the Civil War comprised rifled and breech-loading guns. Rifling increased the speed of the projectiles up the barrel, enabling cannon to fire at much longer ranges and with greater accuracy. Rifled cannon also packed more penetrating power, a considerable advantage against fixed fortifications. Originally made of bronze, and later cast iron with steel reinforcing bands, the rifled breech-loading cannon could also deliver a much faster rate of fire. Improved black powder added to the shell's velocity and range. Near the end of the war, the first primitive recoil mechanisms further increased the rate of fire and accuracy of the rifled field artillery cannon.[20]

The musket had acquired rifling long before the Crimean War, and rifled muskets had been produced as prototypes in the sixteenth century. The most important innovation to Civil War musketry was the introduction of the conoidal bullet. Shaped like a small egg, the conoidal bullet had a hollow "basket" behind its penetrating head. Cast in one piece of soft lead, the "basket" expanded upon firing as the hot combustion gases filled the rear of the bullet. The soft lead expanded outward, forcing the raised spirals on the basket into the rifled grooves in the barrel. The result was a greater sealing of the propulsive gases and a tighter grasp of the rifling by the bullet. Both range and accuracy vastly improved. A rifled Civil War musket could easily kill at a thousand yards and was accurate at six hundred yards.[21]

The infantry's firepower was increasing exponentially. The Spencer carbine, a .56-caliber repeating rifle with a seven-shot capacity, appeared near the end of the war. In the hands of a competent rifleman, it could expend all seven rounds in the time it took a musket rifleman to load and fire a single round. Manufacturers also improved handguns, long the mainstay of the cavalry. Able to fire six shots of .44-caliber ball before requiring reloading, these new weapons were so effective that John Singleton Mosby, the famous Gray Ghost of the Confederacy, required each of his cavalrymen to strap six pistols to both sides of his horse's neck. Mosby's cavalrymen also carried two spare carbines in addition to the carbine and pistol they usually had.

Infantry firepower continued to increase with the introduction of the Gatling gun, the first primitive machine gun. This mechanized contraption was a multibarreled gun that rotated each barrel into firing position in succession by means of a cast gear as the firing handle was turned. The Gatling gun was capable of a sustained rate of fire of a hundred rounds a minute, equal to the rate of fire from forty infantrymen. In 1870, the French deployed a highly reliable, if somewhat cumbersome, twenty-five-barrel machine gun capable of firing 125 rounds a minute and accurate at two thousand yards. In 1870, the Prussian Dreyse needlegun introduced a modern firing pin system for the rifle that again increased rates of fire. The introduction of the magazine-fed (British Lee-Enfield) and clip-fed (German Mauser) bolt-action rifles at the time of the Boer Wars increased the infantry's firepower and mobility yet again. In the 1880s, an American named Hiram Maxim invented a truly modern machine gun capable of a sustained rate of fire of six hundred rounds a minute. The Maxim gun was so effective that all the major armies of the world produced it under license. It became the definitive weapon of World War I, the conflict that came to be called "the machine gun war."

The military capitalized on numerous other inventions of the Industrial Revolution. Probably most important for its impact on military operations was the railroad. Industrial nations lived by rail transport, and armies soon discovered that the railways allowed them to move large numbers of men and matériel over great distances very rapidly.[22] Mobility of deployment increased dramatically, as did the ability to sustain large forces in the field over vast distances by supplying them by rail. It is important to remember that until the railway, no army could move faster than men or horses would carry it. Tinned food, although Napoleon first used it in small amounts, became common and contributed to logistical capability, as did the introduction of condensed food.[23] The telegraph for the first time enabled corps- and army-level commanders to exercise relative tactical control over their subordinate units across long distances. When the telegraph was used in conjunction with the railway, units could achieve both strategic and tactical surprise at force levels never witnessed before. The ironclad steam-powered ship signaled the end of the era of wood and sail, and the use of the balloon for military purposes presaged the function that the airplane would fulfill in the next century.

Behind these military applications lay many other innovations of the Industrial Revolution. Among the most important were the factory system, mass production, and the use of machines to make weapons and military equipment. The factory system represented an entirely new form of social organization for work because for the first time larger numbers of workers directed at a specific task could gather at one workplace. Mass production, especially Eli Whitney's championing of the idea of the interchangeability of parts, made possible previously unimagined levels of weapons production. Making goods by machine increased rates of production to unprecedented levels as implements of all types could be manufactured at a faster unit production rate. And because machines do not require rest, production schedules could be extended around the clock. During the Civil War, factories routinely ran on twenty-four-hour schedules.

The lesson that European powers took from the American Civil War was that military might required a sufficient industrial base and a supply of manpower that, except for the brief period under Napoleon, had never before been placed under arms. None of the European military establishments, however, seemed to appreciate that the Industrial Revolution had brought about a qualitative change in the nature of combat killing power. As European armies adopted each new weapon, they retained the traditional unit formations and battlefield tactics that the increased range and firepower of the new infantry and artillery weapons had made fatally obsolete. When the British adopted the machine gun to their infantry formations, for instance, they assigned only one gun per battalion, relying upon the traditional rifleman to provide the firepower for defense. Not a single European power recognized that the qualitative change in killing power had now made offensive infantry operations a deadly practice. The battlefield advantage had swung completely to the defense.

The armed forces of Europe began to expand their standing armies to record size. They also created larger reserve forces that could be mobilized in one large-scale and almost irreversible deployment maneuver on short notice and transported along military rail nets to augment the standing forces. The railway officer, who could plan and implement deployment schedules, became the most valuable officer on the newly created and professionalized military staffs. In Germany, retired army sergeants, still under military obligation as reserve forces, staffed almost the entire civilian railway service.

As one innovation after another developed during the Industrial Revolution, military forces found more and more applications for them. The armies of the early twentieth century had at their disposal a killing and destructive capacity greater than anything the world had ever seen. The fatal flaw was that they did not know it.

In the half century between the end of the Civil War and the advent of World War I, no fewer than six military conflicts involving one or more of the major powers took place. Almost a score of smaller colonial wars were fought in the same period.

These frequent, if short, wars provided laboratories to test the new implements of destruction.

Among the more important developments of this period was the replacement of muzzle-loading smoothbore cannon with rifled breechloaders. By 1890, every major army in the West was equipped with this new type of cannon. Time fuses were developed in France around 1877 and served to make overhead burst artillery more lethal than ever. The French also developed the first smokeless powder, more stable and potent than black powder, in 1884, and in 1891 the British synthesized cordite, a new shell explosive that became the standard artillery explosive by 1914. In 1888, long-recoil hydraulic cylinders were introduced to stabilize artillery, an improvement that tripled the rate of fire and accuracy of artillery guns. The rifled breech-loading artillery gun now operated with "fixed ammunition," or brass and steel shells in which powder, fuse, and projectile were one piece. The introduction of shrapnel shells added even more destructive power to artillery. In 1896, wire-wound heavy guns were introduced, making gun barrels much stronger than cast barrels. A short time later, frettage—a method of manufacture in which hot steel tubes were shrunk one into another to make gun barrels—made its appearance, resulting in more durable and much higher-caliber guns. Improved breeches and gas-sealing systems completed the development of artillery in this period. In 1897, the French introduced the 75mm field gun, which incorporated all of these improvements. This new French gun's maximum rate of fire was twenty-five rounds per minute. In the 1880s, massive siege cannon, often mounted on railway cars, began to make their appearance. The Krupp "Big Bertha" howitzer could raise an eighteen-hundred-pound shell three miles into the air and hit a target ten thousand yards away.[24]

The Russo-Turkish War of 1877–1878 was the first war in which infantry was universally equipped with modern repeating rifles and artillery with breech-loading rifled cannon. By the outbreak of the Russo-Japanese War (1904–1905), the use of indirect heavy artillery fire was standard practice. The invention of improved panoramic sights, goniometers for measuring angles, the observation balloon for directing fire, and the field telephone allowed forward artillery observers to direct artillery fire on targets that gunners could not see. Advances in fire control enabled an entire artillery corps to mass its fire upon a single target for the first time.[25]

Measured against these advances, the development of naval weapons between the fifteenth and eighteenth centuries was hardly perceptible. Ships remained mostly platforms for transporting infantry and, later, for serving as basic gun platforms.

Sail and wood construction limited the ship's role and sharply reduced the number and caliber of guns that could be placed aboard them. In the early 1800s, the steam engine began to change the ship's military role. The first steam-powered naval ships were produced in the 1820s, but the need for side paddlewheels and huge engines still limited the ship's role as gun platforms. By 1850, the first screw propeller made the side-wheeler obsolete and freed up the necessary deck space to carry sufficient guns. The modern artillery shell had already made the wooden-hulled vessel obsolete, but in 1855 the French introduced iron plating along the wooden hull for increased protection. The weight of heavy guns and large steam engines placed too much strain on wooden-hulled ships, and in 1860 the British launched HMS *Warrior*, the world's first iron-hulled warship.

The armored turret was first used on major ships in 1868, and gradually the advances in artillery weapons were applied to naval guns. Ships began to mount multiple turrets, first with one gun per turret and, by 1900, a standard four guns per turret. The caliber of these guns grew from twelve inches in1908 to a standard fifteen inches by 1914. The last decade of the nineteenth century saw the introduction of steel construction for naval vessels. By 1913, naval vessels were powered by oil instead of coal boilers, greatly increasing their propulsive power while reducing space. In less than a hundred years, these advances culminated in the production of the first modern battleship, the HMS *Dreadnought*. Launched in 1906, this battleship was 527 feet long, 82 feet at the beam, and displaced 17,900 tons. It carried ten 12-inch guns, twenty-seven 12-pounders, and five 18-inch torpedo tubes. Powered by engines generating 23,000 horsepower, the ship could make twenty-one knots. In less than a decade, however, it was already obsolete.

The invention and improvements in mines and, later, the guided torpedo made even the largest ships vulnerable. The Americans in 1843 developed the controlled mine, which was detonated by electric current from wires leading to the shore. Chemically triggered contact mines were in use as early as 1862, and by World War I the mine had become a potent defensive weapon capable of sinking the largest ships. The torpedo—called the "locomotive torpedo" because it proceeded under its own power and did not have to be towed as earlier models did—made its first appearance in 1866. Developed by the Austrians, the first models had a range of 370 yards at six knots and carried an eighteen-pound explosive warhead. By 1877, the contra-rotating propeller was fitted to a torpedo, an innovation that kept the missile steady on course. Soon the torpedo was fitted with a horizontal rudder to keep it at a constant depth as it ran to its target. In 1895, the invention of the gyroscope improved the torpedo's accuracy, and by the turn of the century a torpedo could carry a three-hundred-pound warhead to a thousand-yard range at thirty knots.[26] These developments called into existence a new class of cheap, fast, and destructive naval vessels, the torpedo boat.

The most revolutionary naval advance of the period, however, was the submarine. By 1900, the use of steel hulls, a safe method of propulsion in the internal combustion engine, the accumulator battery, the gyroscope, and the gyrocompass combined to make the submarine possible. At the same time the development of the reliable torpedo provided the submarine with an excellent weapon of attack. In 1900, the six major navies of the world had only ten submarines among them. In 1905, the American submarine *USS Holland* became the prototype for other navies to copy. Displacing 105 tons, the *Holland* had three separate watertight compartments housing its engine, control, and torpedo rooms. Its second lower deck housed the tanks and battery engines. The *Holland* could make almost nine knots while submerged. A few years later, the British introduced the conning tower and the periscope, and the Germans in 1906 contributed the development of double hulls and twin screws for propulsion and stability. By 1914, the six major naval powers of the world put 249 submarines to sea.

In 1903, Orville Wright (1871–1948) made the first sustained—twelve seconds—flight in a heavier-than-air flying machine powered by the internal combustion engine. In only two years, Orville and his brother Wilbur (1867–1912) had improved the Wright Flyer so that it could stay airborne for forty minutes at a speed of forty miles per hour. In 1907 the pusher biplane flew, and by 1908 the Wright airplane was staying in the air for two and a half hours. The invention of the aileron to control an aircraft around its roll axis greatly increased the plane's maneuverability.[27] For the most part, however, military men of the time saw the airplane as performing only the limited functions of the old balloon—namely, observation and reconnaissance.

Others, however, had more important uses in mind. In November 1910 an American, Eugene Ely (1886–1911), took off in an airplane from a platform erected on the deck of a naval cruiser. Two months later it was proven possible to land the aircraft back on the flight deck. In 1911 another American, Glenn Curtiss (1878–1930), became the first man to conduct a practice bombing run against a naval ship, touching off a fierce debate about the vulnerability of ships to air attack. That same year, two-way radio communication from an airplane to the ground was accomplished, making possible aerial artillery observation and fire direction; Curtiss manufactured the first seaplane, foreseeing its use as a weapon against the submarine; the U.S. Army dropped the first bombs from an airplane; and the first machine gun was mounted on an aircraft, the French Nieuport fighter. A year later, monocoque construction was introduced, a method of arranging stress points in aircraft construction that allowed greater loads on airplane structures. In that same year an airplane flew at speeds more than a hundred miles per hour. And in April 1912, the British Royal Flying Corps became the first official air force. Later that year, the first parachute descent from an airplane was made.

In 1913, people set speed (127 mph), distance (635 miles), and altitude (20,079 feet) records as they began to prove the airplane's capability as a weapon of war. The Russians introduced the world's first heavy bomber, the Sikorsky Bolshoi, with a wingspan of more than ninety feet. During the Turco-Italian War (1911–1912) in Libya, the world witnessed the first use of the airplane in war when the Italians employed the airplane for artillery observation, for aerial photography, and for dropping bombs against an enemy force in combat. The age of the modern strike and bomber airplane as major implements of war was under way.

THE TWENTIETH CENTURY

By the early 1900s, the social, political, and economic context in which armies were raised and wars fought had changed considerably since the American Civil War. The political structures of the European nation states were under attack from new ideologies of the left and center that greatly weakened the power of the national executives while increasing the influence of the legislatures. The ruling nobility was replaced or had to share power with elected leaders, while the monarchies, though retained in form, lost most of their substantive power. Needing to sustain their new electoral bases, leaders cast national conflicts in moral and ideological terms. Wars became crusades, which made them easier to start and more difficult to resolve, short of total victory.

The search for national economic self-sufficiency led the major powers to engage in competition for colonial possessions that could provide stable sources of raw materials and secure markets for manufactured goods.[28] The competition for economic advantage threatened the relative security of all states. These conditions, coupled with the rapid development of military technology, led to a continuous armaments race that provoked a spate of alliances between the major powers with the fragmented states of eastern Europe. The stage was set to draw the larger states into direct conflict when these smaller states challenged one another. Inevitably, clashes in peripheral colonial areas also embroiled the major powers in collisions on the rim of Europe itself until, finally, they engulfed the entire European heartland in a world war.

The standing armies of the day grew enormously to take advantage of the new military technologies. The destructiveness of modern weapons required that large numbers of fighting men be readily available for war in anticipation of huge casualties. Propelled by the contemporary strategic doctrine that the side mobilizing the quickest would have the opportunity of striking a lethal blow, nations established large reserve forces that could be mobilized and deployed within days. Once mobilization plans were set in motion, however, they could not be easily stopped without conceding a significant advantage to one's opponent. Once war broke out, the nation's entire economy and productive capacity had to be marshaled for war. While Napoleon had created the new reality of a nation in arms, World War I, following the model of the American Civil War, gave birth to the idea of a nation at war.

On the eve of World War I, Europe was a tinderbox waiting for a spark. National economies were pre-positioned for war, with large standing armies facing one another across disputed boundaries and civilian populations able to be put into uniform within days of mobilization. The major powers were caught in a series of entangling alliances with small, unstable states whose local conflicts could quickly escalate into war, and while an arms race fed the growing fear, the strategic doctrine of the day required that one strike first. Superimposed upon it all was a political process that produced weak political leadership that was forced to sustain itself by appearing uncompromising on national security issues driven by ideological and moral perspectives that, in turn, made compromise almost impossible. When pistol shots were fired in the narrow streets of Sarajevo in June 1914, they produced a world war.

World War I became known as the "machine gun war," with the machine gun causing an estimated 80 percent of all British casualties.[29] In a war of fixed positions, artillery guns grew larger, firing ever bigger shells in concentrated barrages for days at a time. The siege mortar reached almost forty-two inches in diameter, and railway guns fired 210mm rounds eighty-two miles. Trench mortars reached 170mm caliber and could fire mustard and chlorine gas shells. Poison gas released from canisters made its appearance in 1915, and as the combatants used it throughout the war, the gas mask became standard military equipment. The pack howitzer for the mountain infantry's use made its battlefield debut, as did the first antiaircraft guns.

The first operational battle tank was a revolutionary development. Early tanks were terribly unreliable. Engines and suspensions frequently broke down, and temperatures in the crew compartments often reached a hundred degrees from the heat of the engine. By 1917, the British introduced a much improved Mark IV tank at the Battle of Cambrai and waged history's first massed tank attack involving more than 476 tanks. In the spring of 1918, the French introduced the lighter and faster Renault FT, the first tank equipped with a revolving turret. By the end of the war, the Allies had built and deployed more than 6,000 battle tanks. The age of armor had begun.

The war at sea, meanwhile, remained deadlocked. The British countered the German submarine threat by inventing the ship convoy. Of the 16,070 ships that sailed in British convoys, only 96 were lost to submarine attack. In 1915, the first use of the hydrophone made it possible to detect submarines by sound. A year later, another deadly invention, the depth charge, was first used successfully to destroy a submarine. By that time, naval forces routinely used the seaplane, and in 1917 HMS *Furious* added the world's first flight deck to its forward superstructure. In the same year, HMS *Argus* became the first naval vessel built with both a takeoff and landing deck. With the incorporation of the deck catapult and arresting gear, the prototype of the modern aircraft carrier was born.

The war quickened the development of the first aircraft designed for military use. The interrupter gear made machine guns mounted on aircraft more effective by allowing the guns to fire through a turning propeller. Improvements in design, materials, and structure of aircraft manufacture made it possible for aircraft to fly 140 miles per hour at altitudes of twenty thousand feet. The first bombers capable of two-thousand-pound bomb loads appeared. For the most part, however, antagonists used their aircraft for reconnaissance, fire direction, trench strafing, and fighting one another.

Europe emerged from World War I almost bankrupt. While research and development into new and improved weapons continued, it did so on a much smaller scale than before the war. Overall expenditures on military equipment and manpower declined as the nations of Europe tried to find the money to repair their devastated domestic infrastructures. The war's lingering effects left the political and social institutions of the European powers badly shaken. The war produced a revolution in Russia, leading to the establishment of a Soviet state. Benito Mussolini (1883–1945) deposed the Italian monarchy and produced the first fascist state in Italy. A weak republican government replaced Germany's monarchy but proved unable to handle the increasing social and economic instability. Both the Left and the Right attacked France's republican institutions from within, sapping the national political will of the citizenry. In England, an assault mounted from the Left weakened the hold of the traditional ruling classes. Only America, which had suffered light losses and no material damage in the war, seemed immune from the its social, political, and economic aftershocks.

Most of the European powers could no longer sustain large military establishments. In 1918, the dictate of the victorious powers at Versailles reduced the military forces of Germany, which spent almost nothing on military development until 1932. England reduced its air and ground forces significantly. By 1939, the British Navy was a shell of its former self. France reduced its expenditures as well, choosing to concentrate on ground forces and leaving its naval, air, and armor forces too small to counter the German threat. The U.S. government rescinded military conscription and reduced military expenditures across the board. U.S. ground forces shrunk to fewer than 200,000 men, armor was nonexistent, and the air force could deploy only a handful of obsolete machines. Famine, political terror, and civil war crippled any Soviet attempts at military growth. Although by the early 1930s the Red Army had the largest artillery and tank forces in the world, in 1937 Joseph Stalin purged the Red Army's officer corps, killing more than 90 percent of its members. The army disbanded its new tank units and assigned the vehicles as adjuncts to infantry formations. When the Soviets came to blows with tiny Finland in 1939, they were barely able to achieve victory.

Only in Japan and Italy did military expenditures and weapons development increase significantly in the interwar years, but after 1932 Germany also embarked on a major rearmament program under the Nazis. Japan's need to build an industrial base sufficient to maintain a modern military establishment led to its creation of a military society whose every effort went toward increasing the state's military power. The Japanese reliance on overseas sources for critical raw materials forced it to wage wars of conquest in Asia to gain control of oil fields, steel deposits, and other raw materials needed for the sinews of war. Mussolini's attempt to make Italy a great power foundered on the insufficient resource base of Italy itself, as he never obtained sufficient coal, steel, and oil supplies required for a first-rate military machine. By 1939, when Italian military prestige was at its highest and Italian airplanes, ships, and small arms were among the best quality in the world, the fact remained that Italy's industrial base was never adequate to sustain a large military for very long.

Meanwhile, weapons development continued apace. The tank design improved with the appearance of the low-profile hull, the revolving turret, better gun sights, and better tracks and suspension. By the 1930s, the Russians had developed the famed T-34, the best tank of its day. Tank cannon grew to 90 millimeters, and new propellants and shot—particularly the sabot round—made them even more accurate and deadlier. The tank called into existence the first antitank guns. The German Gerlich gun fired a 28mm round of tungsten carbide at four thousand feet per second that was capable of penetrating any known tank armor. A later German invention, the 88mm gun, was originally developed as an antitank weapon but doubled as both an antiaircraft and direct fire gun. The "eighty-eight" is generally adjudged the best weapon of its kind in World War II.

Developments in aircraft design—the stressed metal skin and the monoplane—made the introduction of the modern fighter aircraft possible. Engines producing more than a thousand horsepower made speeds greater than 350 miles per hour commonplace. Companies developed the long-range bomber, capable of flying at altitudes of more than forty thousand feet and at ranges of five thousand miles. For the navies, the light and fast destroyer was built to protect the larger battleships at sea. Submarines could remain at sea for sixty days at a time. The Japanese developed a new torpedo, the Type 93 Long Lance, that was propelled by oxygen, left no track, and had a range of twenty-five miles at thirty-six knots. Torpedoes typically carried warheads of four hundred pounds of high explosive. During this period the aircraft carrier also came into its own. The Japanese carrier *Kaga*, built in the 1920s, carried sixty aircraft and displaced thirty-nine thousand tons. The American carrier USS *Lexington*, of World War II fame, displaced thirty-six thousand tons and carried ninety aircraft. The integration of naval and air forces was almost complete.

The destructive power of infantry, armor, and artillery forces highly increased in World War II. Armed in large numbers with the new, all-metal submachine gun, infantry delivered firepower at rates five times greater than the World War I infantryman could. Infantry carried its own antitank weapons in the form of the American 3.5-inch bazooka rocket launcher or the German Panzerfaust. Dependable motorized transport, such as the Jeep, the "deuce and a half" truck, and the armored personnel carrier—fully tracked, half-tracked, or pneumatic tire vehicles—increased infantry mobility twenty-fold and enabled it to keep pace with the rapid armor advance that characterized combat in World War II.

The tank saw a remarkable increase in its combat capability, and for the first time in almost seven hundred years, cavalry again dominated the battlefield. The Russian

T-34, originally produced in 1935, proved the best battle tank of the war. Mounting an 85mm gun with a new muzzle-brake to reduce recoil, the T-34 could travel at 32 miles per hour with a range of 180 miles. It introduced the sloped armored glacis in front to deflect antitank rounds and had a ground pressure of only ten pounds per square inch, and on its Christie suspension, it could traverse terrain that most other Allied or Axis tanks found impassable. The American Sherman tank introduced cast armor to replace welded armor, the volute spring bogie suspension, and rubber block treads that increased track life by 500 percent. The Sherman also used a revolutionary hydroelectric gun stabilizing system and improved triangle sights. As their engines grew more powerful and more reliable, tanks quickly became the centerpiece of the striking forces for all armies except that of the Japanese.

Responding to the need to defend itself against armor and air attack, artillery's developments resulted in the self-propelled artillery gun. These 8-inch, or 122mm caliber, guns were mobile artillery mounted on tank chassis. Self-propelled artillery came in two forms—the assault gun, which was designed for firepower, and the light assault gun, designed for mobility. The appearance of the dive-bomber and the ground attack fighter required improvements in antiaircraft guns. The Bofors 40mm cannon was capable of firing two rounds per second over a slant range of four miles. The American M-2 90mm gun fired twenty-five rounds per minute to a height of nine miles. The introduction of reliable electronic fire control systems coupled with radar detectors and trackers linked to primitive computers provided great advances in the accuracy and lethality of these guns.

The U.S. 90mm gun and the German eighty-eight were the best antitank guns of the war. Unguided rocket artillery, which the Chinese first used a thousand years earlier, reappeared in the form of the German 15cm Nebelwerfer ("fog thrower" rocket launcher) that could fire six seventy-pound rocket rounds in less than three seconds. The Soviet Katyusha, first at 90 millimeters and then at 122 millimeters, fired more than forty rockets at once while the American T34 Calliope fired sixty rockets at a time. Used as area saturation weapons, these rockets caused large numbers of psychiatric as well as physical casualties.[30] The variable timed fuse, which the U.S. Navy used against attacking planes in January 1943, significantly increased the lethality of artillery fire against ground troops. Each shell contained a tiny radio transceiver that could be set so that the round exploded at a precise distance above the ground. This innovation increased the killing power of artillery by a factor of ten over shells fitted with conventional fuses.

The war at sea saw the final demise of the battleship as it became increasingly vulnerable to air and undersea attack. The aircraft carrier became the major naval weapon. Carriers of the Essex and Midway class were 820 feet long with beams of 147 feet, moved at speeds of thirty-two knots, and carried more than a hundred strike aircraft. Carrier-based aircraft carried two thousand pounds of bombs; flew at 350 miles per hour; attacked with rockets, torpedoes, and machine guns; and ranged more than three hundred miles. Although submarines operated with new electric motors to make them increasingly difficult to detect, antisubmarine technology improved markedly. Radar and radio sets allowed antisubmarine aircraft to detect submarines at night, for instance, and new depth charges provided surface vessels with another means of submarine destruction. By 1944, the submarine was no longer a significant naval threat.

The air war saw the emergence of tremendously improved strike aircraft. The British Spitfire, among other fighter aircraft on both sides, could range outward for a thousand miles at speeds greater than four hundred miles per hour. These aircraft were equipped with 20mm and 37mm cannon, heavy machine guns, and two thousand pounds of bombs. Ground support tactics developed rapidly as strike aircraft made heavy firepower at close ranges available to advancing infantry. Meanwhile, the heavy strategic bomber appeared. The American B-24 Liberator carried 12,800 pounds of bombs at 290 miles per hour for a range of 2,100 miles, and the B-29 Superfortress carried 20,000 pounds of bombs for 3,250 miles at an altitude of 31,850 feet. By war's end the Germans (Messerschmitt Me-262), the British (Vampire), and the Americans (P-59 Aircomet) had produced prototypes of jet-powered aircraft. In August 1945, the United States unveiled the most awesome weapon of war yet invented by man, the atomic bomb, and devastated the civilian population centers of Hiroshima and Nagasaki.

WORLD WAR II TO THE TWENTY-FIRST CENTURY

The debut of nuclear weapons at the end of World War II made it necessary to distinguish clearly between nuclear and conventional weapons. Only eight years after the attack on Hiroshima nuclear artillery shells made their appearance, and three years later nuclear artillery shells were small enough to be fired from a 155mm howitzer. By 1970, U.S. and Soviet navies had deployed nuclear torpedoes capable of sinking the largest aircraft carriers with a single shot. Nuclear bombs, which in the 1950s weighed many tons and were in the thirty-five-megaton range, became much smaller so that by the 1980s they could be placed on air-breathing cruise missiles or carried under the wings of fighter aircraft. In the 1950s, the U.S. Navy used nuclear reactors for the first time to power a strike carrier, the USS *Forrestal.* Within a decade, nuclear-powered guided-missile frigates and cruisers appeared. Nuclear missiles mounted on nuclear-powered submarines capable of staying submerged for months were developed by the 1960s. The USS *George Washington* was the first nuclear submarine that could fire its missiles while still submerged. It soon became possible to place several multiple independent reentry vehicles or warheads on a single missile. By 1985, the Trident II submarine carried twenty-four missiles, each mounting twenty separate warheads of almost a half megaton each. Firing submerged, the Trident's missiles have a range of more than eight thousand miles, while land-based strategic missiles are capable of destroying cities from ten thousand miles away. By 1980, the United States and the Soviet Union had acquired enough nuclear weapons and delivery systems of various kinds to destroy each other several hundred times.

While nuclear weapons were increasing the firepower of war, conventional weapons were undergoing similar developments. From the perspective of military medicine, the advances in conventional weapons are much more important because conventional weapons are far more likely to be used in combat than nuclear weapons are. It is quite pointless to talk of military medicine in a nuclear environment. The scope of destruction would be so enormous as to make any attempts at medical treatment ridiculous in the extreme. Tactical nuclear weapons would almost completely destroy the units struck by them and render the area of impact so contaminated that providing medical care to the few survivors would be militarily useless. Current U.S. medical doctrine is to make no attempt at treating the survivors, leaving them to self-treatment until the battle area is stabilized to the point where medical units can reach the wounded. Even then, treating the severely contaminated or burned would be a low priority. This approach does not pertain to conventional weapons. While killing significant numbers of combatants, conventional weapons still leave multitudes of injured than can reasonably be salvaged with prompt medical intervention.

Napoleon remarked that quantity conveys a quality all its own. The increase in destructive capacities of conventional weapons in the modern era has been so huge that in any other age these quantitative changes would have been regarded as qualitative revolutions in the nature of war. In the modern age, nuclear weapons provide the baseline from which weapons' effects are measured. It does not seem so horrendous, for example, that a single artillery barrage from new artillery weapons can exterminate whole battalions when entire cities can be eradicated in the time it takes a camera flash to occur. Even the destructive effects of war have become grotesquely relative. In 1980, the U.S. Army estimated that modern nonnuclear conventional war had become between 400 to 700 percent more lethal and intense than it had been in World War II.[31] At Fort Irwin, California, where the U.S. Army routinely exercises its troops in realistic battle maneuvers, achieving simulated casualty rates that exceed 90 percent for both the offensive and defensive forces utilizing only conventional weapons is not uncommon. The increases in killing power have been enormous and far greater than in any other period in man's history.

For example, the artillery firepower of a maneuver battalion has doubled since World War II, while the "casualty effect" of modern artillery guns has increased by 400 percent. Range has increased by 60 percent and the "zone of destruction" of battalion artillery by 350 percent.[32] Advances in metallurgy and the replacement of TNT with new chemical compounds have increased the explosive power of basic caliber artillery by many times. A single round from an eight-inch gun has the same explosive power of a World War II–era 250-pound bomb. Modern artillery is lighter, stronger, and more mobile than ever before. Computerized fire direction centers can range guns on target in only a few seconds compared to the six minutes required in World War II. Additionally, the rates of fire of these guns are three times what they used to be. The new artillery guns are so durable that they can routinely fire five hundred rounds over a four-hour period without damaging the barrel. Range has increased to the point where the M-110 gun can fire a 203mm shell twenty-five miles. The self-propelled gun has a travel range of 220 miles at a speed of thirty-five miles per hour. Area saturation artillery, in its infancy in World War II, has also become terribly lethal. A single Soviet artillery battalion firing eighteen BM-21 multiple rocket launchers can place thirty-five tons of explosive rockets on a target seventeen miles away in only thirty seconds. The American multiple rocket launching system is a totally mobile, self-contained artillery system that can place eight thousand M-77 explosive rounds on a target the size of six football fields eighty miles away in less than forty-five seconds. Air defense guns also have developed to where a single M-163 Vulcan cannon can fire three thousand rounds of explosives or armor-piercing 20mm shot per minute with 100 percent accuracy within two miles of the gun's position. During World War II, air defense guns could command the airspace only one mile around their position. Modern antiaircraft cannon command thirty-six times that space.[33]

Tanks have also improved in speed, reliability, and firepower. Modern tanks can travel forty miles per hour over a three-hundred-mile range, or three times that of earlier tanks. A tank equipped with modern gun sights and a cannon stabilization system has a probability of 98 percent of scoring a first-round hit, or thirteen times greater than that of World War II tanks. Modern battle tanks can also fire while on the move, with their probability of hitting the target being almost ten times greater than the probability of a World War II tank firing from a standing position. New propellants and ammunition design have increased the modern tank cannon's lethality as well. The armor-piercing discarding-sabot round leaves the gun muzzle at 5,467 feet per second and can pierce 9.5 inches of armor plate. Tank gun sights now feature lasers connected to computers that can locate a target at three thousand yards in the dark, smoke, rain, or snow.[34]

Conventional strike aircraft can deliver ordnance at rates undreamed of in World War II. The A-10 carries sixteen thousand pounds of bombs and mounts a 30mm rotating GAU-8 cannon in its nose that fires 4,200 rounds of 20mm ammunition per minute. A two-second burst, for example, places 135 rounds of armor-piercing bullets into a tank target. The AC-130H Spectre gunship is equipped with four 20mm Vulcan cannon with rates of fire of six thousand rounds per minute per gun. The Spectre also carries four 7.62mm multibarreled Honeywell guns with rates of fire of ten thousand rounds per minute. Also aboard this aerial attack platform is a 40mm Bofors cannon capable of firing two thousand rounds per minute and an automatic howitzer that can fire fifteen rounds per minute of 105mm artillery rounds. All of these weapons are linked to a sophisticated infrared sensing system tied to computers that allow the aircraft to detect ground targets while simultaneously directing fire upon them. A one-minute burst from the Spectre's armament systems is capable of reducing an entire city block to rubble.[35]

The modern combat helicopter has wrought a revolution in tank- and armor-killing power available to the combat commander. These weapons can be configured to kill either troops (Soviet Hind, or Mi-24) or tanks (AH-64 Apache) and are awesome weapons. The Apache carries sixteen Hellfire antitank missiles that need no further direction after they are fired and automatically home in on the target. The Apache also mounts nineteen 2.75-inch rockets and a Hughes 30mm chain gun linked to electronic computers and killer sights. The helicopter has added new mobility and stealth to the battlefield, permitting a division commander to strike with troops or antitank weapons sixty miles to his front, or four times the range possible in World War II.

The infantry, too, has increased its range, mobility, and firepower with new armored personnel carriers and infantry fighting vehicles like the Bradley M2. Infantry can bring to bear shoulder-fired antiaircraft missiles, back-carried antitank missiles, and Jeep- and Hummer-mounted tube-launched, optically tracked, wire-guided antitank missiles with devastating results.[36] The lethality of the infantry has been increased exponentially by its ability to discover and target enemy units and emplacements with great accuracy. Orbiting bombers can now deliver their munitions (guided bombs, missiles, cluster munitions, and so on) with pinpoint accuracy upon targets that individual infantrymen can illuminate with hand-carried lasers. Satellites have revolutionized communications with artillery and air resources, and graphics processing devices used to guide missiles, bombs, and even individual artillery shells have vastly increased their accuracy. Infantry, including irregular forces engaged in insurgencies, are routinely armed with automatic weapons that can deliver an intensity of fire that was formerly reserved for machine guns. Paradoxically automatic weapons do not result in more casualties or lethality when compared to earlier semiautomatic weapons (such as the M-1, M14, and FN rifle) whose larger-caliber rounds and greater accuracy, along with more disciplined training of the infantryman to aim before shooting, were much more lethal and produced a bigger percentage of hits on the target.

To place the increased intensity of the modern nonnuclear conventional battlefield in perspective, one need only remember that in World War II heavy combat was defined as two to four "combat pulses" a day. Modern combat divisions are configured to routinely deliver twelve to fourteen combat pulses a day and to fight around the clock by conducting night operations. A modern U.S. or Soviet division could deliver three times as much firepower at ten times the rate of fire as they could in World War II. By any historical standard, even conventional weapons have become quite unconventional in their casualty effects.[37]

CASUALTIES AND LETHALITY

Lethality in war is always the sum of a number of factors that go beyond the inherent death-dealing capabilities of military technology. Before a new weapon can reach its killing potential, military commanders must discover new fighting methods to use the new weapon in a manner that maximizes its lethality. Once the weapon's killing power is exposed for all to see, however, one's opponent adopts passive and active countermeasures to limit its most deadly effects. This turn requires the commander to change tactics and combat formations in an attempt to preserve the killing power of the new technology. Inevitably, this dynamic balance of behavior and technology usually results in the lethality of the new weapon remaining somewhat higher than that of the weapon it replaced, but not greatly so. It cannot be stressed too strongly in calculating the killing power of weaponry that any failure to adapt either weapons or tactics to new circumstances can be catastrophic. For example, the armies of World War I failed to alter their battle tactics in light of the machine gun's enormous rates of fire, resulting in horrendous casualties in the war's early days. The similar refusal of British commanders at the Somme to change their practice of massed infantry attacks against entrenched positions led to sixty thousand men being killed, wounded, or captured in less than eight hours.

Analysts have determined the effects of changes in numerous factors—such as rates of fire, number of potential targets per strike, relative incapacitating consequences, effective range, muzzle velocity, reliability, battlefield mobility, radius of action, and vulnerability—on the killing power of various weapons in order to calculate a theoretical lethality index that specifies their deadliness.[38] When gauged against the single variable of dispersion, however, the objective factors change radically in their ability to produce casualties under actual battlefield conditions. Paradoxically, the measurable casualty effects of modern weapons when computed over time result in far fewer casualties when compared to the weapons of the past.

When measured against the non-gunpowder weapons of antiquity and the Middle Ages, modern conventional weapons have increased in lethality by a factor of two thousand. But while lethality was growing, the dispersion of forces on the battlefield increased by a factor of four thousand because of mechanization and the ability of fewer soldiers to deliver exponentially more firepower.[39] The result, as figure 1 demonstrates, is that since 1865 CE, wars have killed fewer soldiers as a percentage of the deployed combat force than was the case in previous wars. Except for the Napoleonic Wars (1800–1815), which utilized the tactical field formation of the packed marching column, every war since 1600 has resulted in fewer and fewer casualties as a percentage of the total forces that both the victor and vanquished committed.

The impact of force dispersion on this equation is evident from the data in figure 2. As weapons became more and more destructive, armies adjusted their tactics to increase the dispersion of their forces and to minimize the targets available to the new weapons. The overall result has been a decline in battle casualties even as the lethality of weapons increased.

Figure 1. Weapons Lethality and Dispersion over History

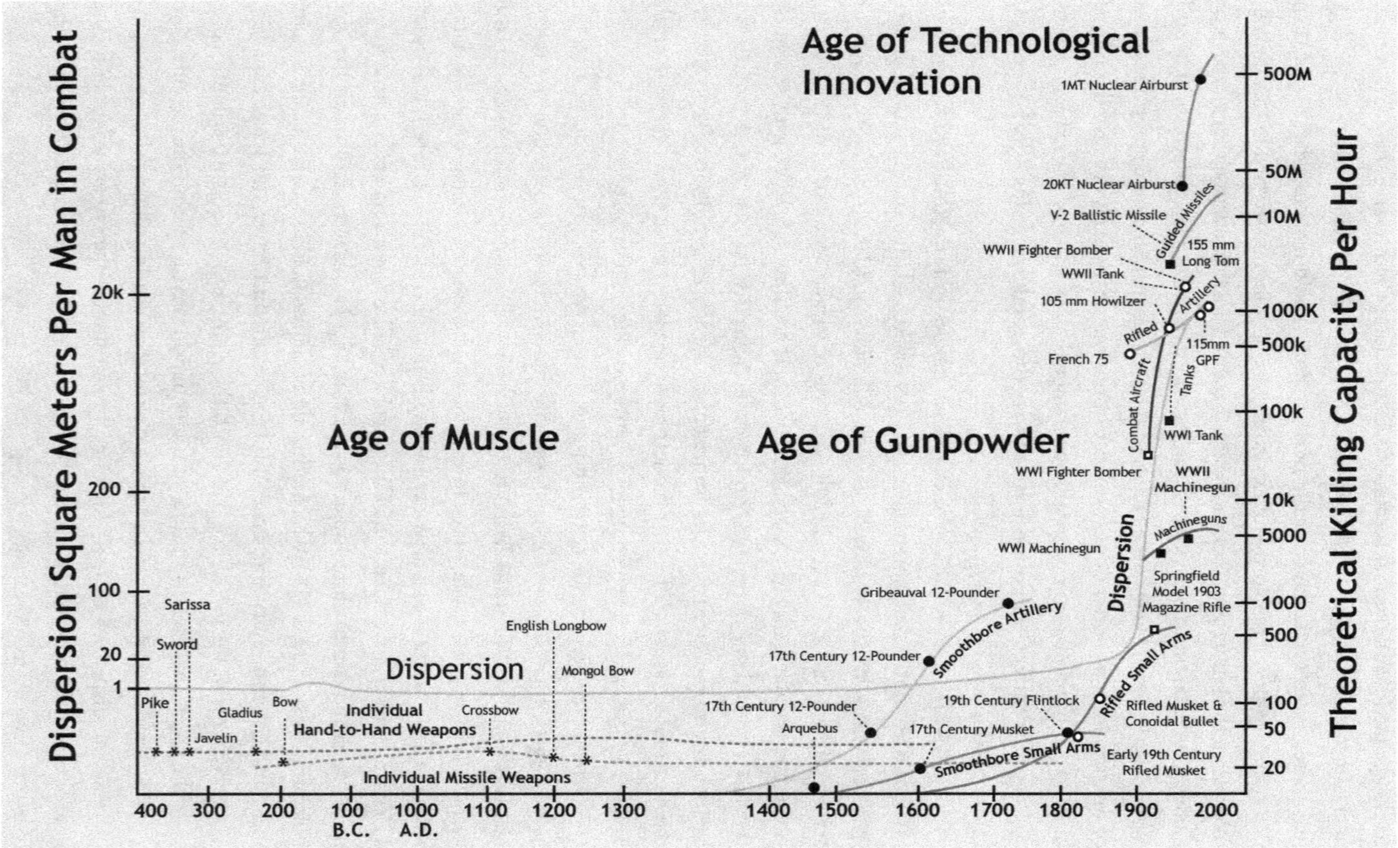

Source: T. N. Dupuy, *The Evolution of Weapons and Warfare* (New York: Bobbs-Merrill, 1980), 288.

Figure 2. Battle Casualties: 1600–1973 CE

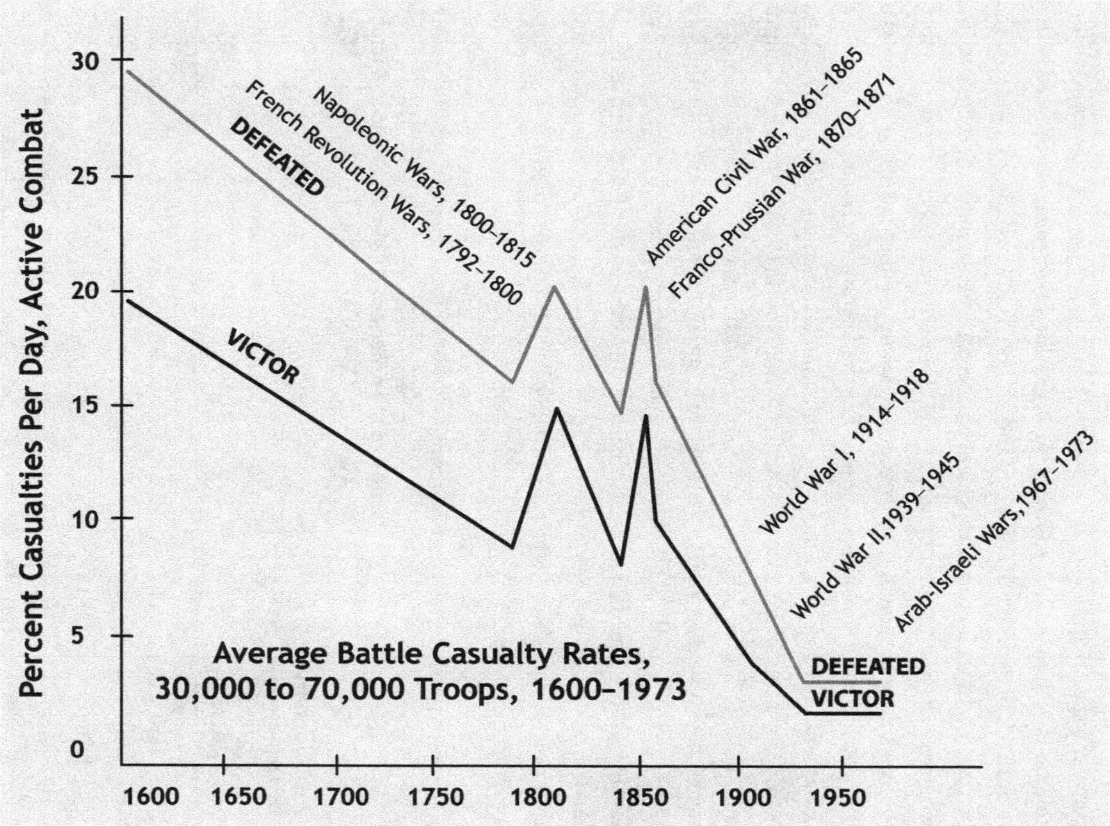

Source: T. N. Dupuy, *Evolution of Weapons and Warfare*, 314.

Some specific historical examples help clarify this point. Until the Napoleonic Wars, the proportion of casualties (killed and wounded) to total effective forces using the system of linear tactics had steadily declined from 19 percent for the victors to 28 percent for the losers in battles during the Thirty Years' War to about 9 and 16 percent, respectively, during the wars of the French Revolution.[40] Napoleon's use of column tactics forced him to *reduce* the dispersion of his forces when faced with the increased killing power of musketry and artillery,[41] and his casualty rates rose to 20 percent. By 1848, however, dispersion had begun once again to surge and continued with each war over the next hundred years. The result was a decline in the number of soldiers killed per thousand per year. In the Mexican-American War, U.S. forces lost 9.9 soldiers per thousand per annum. For the Spanish-American War (1898), the corresponding figure was 1.9; for the Philippine Insurrection (1899–1902), 2.2; for World War I (1914–1918), 12.0; and for World War II (1939–1945), 9.0. Only during the Civil War, which saw many battles with massed formations thrown against strong defensive positions (a violation of dispersion), did the rates for the North (21.3) and the South (23.0 estimated) again begin to approach those of the Napoleonic period.[42] The data show that barring incredible tactical stupidity, as lethal as modern weaponry had become and as intense as modern conventional wars can be, they generally produce fewer casualties per day of exposure than did the weapons and wars of the past.[43]

Table 1. Historical Army Dispersion Patterns for Units of 100,000 Troops

	Antiquity	Napoleonic Wars	American Civil War	World War I	World War II	October War
Area Occupied by Deployed Force, 100,000 Strong (sq km)	1.00	20.12	25.75	248	2.750	4.000
Front (km)	6.67	8.05	8.58	14	48	57
Depth (km)	0.15	2.50	3.0	17	57	70
Men per Sq Km	100.000	4.970	3.883	404	36	25
Square Meters/ Man	10.00	200	257.5	2.475	27.500	40.000

Source: T. N. Dupuy, *Evolution of Weapons and Warfare*, 312.

Studies of casualty rates from antiquity to the Korean War (1950–1953) reached the same conclusion regarding mortality rates.[44] Given that weapons and tactics changed little from the times of antiquity through the Middle Ages, the data provided for the Greek and Roman periods are assumed to be roughly similar to that for later periods of antiquity prior to the advent of gunpowder weapons. Table 2 presents mortality data for various wars at different periods in history. For the armies of antiquity, long-range weapons included slings, arrows, and the thrown spear, while in the modern period they were limited to rifles. Clearly for armies of antiquity, close-range weapons were the most lethal. Factoring in the weapons' lethality along the time dimension, the data demonstrate that although weapons became deadlier with each war, the mortality rates for each war tend to decline, with the highest found during wars of antiquity and the lowest rates in modern wars. Once again adjustments in tactics, mobility, and dispersion by and large offset the increased killing power of weaponry as far as their ability to generate casualties is concerned.

Table 2. Battle Mortality from Antiquity to the Korean War

Personnel Involved	Total	Died	% Mortality
"Iliad":			
All casualties	213	192	90.0
Close-range	147	138	93.0
Long-range	66	54	82.2
"Aeneid":			
All casualties	180	164	91.0
Close-range	120	115	96.0
Long-range	60	49	81.6
Crimea:			
British Army	26,803	5,498	21.5
World War I:			
Canadians	122,672	51,678	42.2
British Army	2,216,976	573,507	25.8
World War II:			
Australians	2,637	516	19.5
Normandy Troops	2,452	962	39.3
Korea:			
USA	142,091	30,928	21.7
Commonwealth	6,080	1,263	20.9
British			
all casualties	1,337	216	16.2
gunshot wounds	694	127	18.2

Source: P. B. Adamson, "A Comparison of Ancient and Modern Weapons in the Effectiveness of Producing Battle Casualties," *Journal of the Royal Army Medical Corps* 23 (1977): 97.

In Virgil's *Aeneid* (29 BCE–19 BCE), 96 percent of the wounds inflicted at short range by swords and spears were fatal. In Homer's *Iliad* (about 750 BCE), the corresponding number was 93.5 percent. In modern wars, however, the effectiveness of short-range weapons—bayonet, rifle butt, knife—lost much of their potential for lethality precisely because the rifle's range makes using these weapons with any frequency almost impossible. In World War II, for example, only 2.3 percent of the British Army's casualties came from close-range weapons.[45]

What is intriguing from the perspective of the military surgeon who must treat the wounded is the change in the types of wounds that modern weapons have caused. Table 3 presents data from the Crimean War to the Vietnam War (1959–1975) on the distribution of wounds that long-range infantry weapons inflicted on various areas of the body. The data demonstrate that most of the combat wounds inflicted by rifle fire are to the upper and lower limbs.

One reason for this outcome is simply that as J. D. Hardy and E. F. Dubois have calculated, the upper limbs comprise 19 percent of total body area and the lower limbs 39 percent, or a combined 58 percent of the body's area exposed to weapons' fire.[46] That these areas suffer the most wounds is hardly surprising; however, these rifle wounds are usually not fatal. In his study of combat casualties in the Crimean War, George H. B. MacLeod (1828–1892) shows that wounds to the upper limbs had a mortality rate of only 3.25 percent while wounds to the lower limbs produce an 8.05 percent mortality rate.[47] From the 1960s until 1998 in Northern Ireland, British forces incurred only 0.26 percent fatalities from wounds to the limbs.[48] Since Korea, body armor has become standard military equipment and has increased the rate of wounds to the unprotected limbs by reducing overall wounds to the trunk. Battle jackets reduce the rate of overall wounds by an estimated 30 percent.[49] This figure may be too high. In the Israeli–Palestine Liberation Organization war of 1983, a war that saw many close order battles, Israeli military doctors believed that the overall casualty rate would have been 28 percent higher had Israel Defense Force troops not been equipped with battle jackets.[50]

In analyzing weapons' lethality, clearly medical treatment makes a significant difference in lethality rates. Of course, a number of factors influence these rates, not the least of which is a modern army's ability to deliver high-quality medical care and rapidly to the soldier within the battle area. Moreover, these conditions have largely been extant for less than a hundred years. Tables 4 and 5 present data drawn from the mortality rates of those wounded in a number of wars who received treatment in

Table 3. Anatomical Distribution of Injuries from High-Explosive (HE) Fragments and Gunshot Wounds (GSW)

Campaign	Weapon	Head/ neck	Trunk	Upper limb	Lower Limb
Crimean War—Macleod (12). Tables 3–4	GSW	1816	1504	5023	
Hong Kong, 1941–1945—Crew (11). p. 31–34	GSW	112	117	208	247
Alamein, 1942—Crew (13)	GSW	57	67	294	
Sicily, 1943—Crew (15). Table 21	GSW	134	177	347	424
Normandy 1944—Crew (15). Table III	GSW	140	254	212	260
Vietnam War—Kovaric et al. (12)	GSW	112	277	282	422
Northern Ireland, 1971–1974—Moffat (12). p. 4–5	GSW	123	181	390	
Malta, 1940–1943—Crew (15). p. 630–1 Series 1 Series 2	 Bomb Bomb	 35 178	 10 111	 158 188	
Normandy, 1944—Crew (15). Table III	Shell Mortar Bomb	259 113 23	279 118 35	222 132 26	402 181 26
Vietnam War—Kovaric et al. (13)	HE	242	388	375	502

Source: Adamson, "A Comparison of Ancient and Modern Weapons," 99.

military hospitals for their injuries. Table 4, which covers the Crimean War until the Northern Ireland Troubles, includes the mortality rates of patients with gunshot or high-explosive fragment wounds to the head. Table 5 shows data for patients from various conflicts who suffered skull-penetrating injuries from the same projectiles. Despite the usual seriousness of these types of wounds, especially the latter, the data clearly demonstrate that the military medical services' ability to deal with these injuries has drastically reduced their associated mortality rate over the years, offering unequivocal proof of the value of prompt and adequate medical care on the battlefield. The data in table 6, which shows the lethality rates for Americans wounded in the

Table 4. Mortality from Head Injuries from GSW and HE Fragments

Group	Total	Deaths	% Mortality	Cause
Crimean War—Soldiers.	898	178	19.9	GSW all types
Macleod (17)	72	72	100.0	GSW penetrating
Boer War—Soldiers. Makins (17)	10	8	80.0	GSW all types
World War I—Soldiers. Cushing (17)				
Series 1	44	24	54.5	Mainly HE fragments
Series 2	44	28	40.9	Mainly HE fragments
Series 3	45	13	28.8	Mainly HE fragments
World War II—Soldiers. Eden (14)	258	37	14.4	Penetrating GSW and HE fragments
Normandy—Soldiers.	140	61	43.6	GSW
Crew 1962 (14)	414	89	21.6	HE fragments
Korean War—Soldiers, Hammon (44)	132	30	22.7	GSW
	1008	77	7.6	HE fragments
Civilians, Hammon (44)	54	16	29.6	GSW
	503	67	13.3	HE fragments
Northern Ireland—Soldiers				
Moffat (23)	87	46	53.0	GSW
Gordon (24)	93	53	56.0	GSW

Source: Adamson, "A Comparison of Ancient and Modern Weapons," 100.

Revolutionary War (1775–1783) to the wars in Iraq (2003–2011) and Afghanistan (from 2001 and ongoing, as of this writing), support the same conclusion.[51]

In the 350 years since the early prototypes of the gunpowder armies first emerged on the battlefields of the Thirty Years' War, the destructive power of weapons and the organizational sophistication of armies have proceeded at a developmental pace without historical precedent. These elements are the products of larger social and technological forces that have revolutionized the manner in which humans live their lives. For more than 5,500 years of human existence in organized societies, or since ancient Sumer, the means and methods by which humans destroyed each other in war had changed little. But in the last 350 years they have changed so drastically that they would be literally beyond the imaginations of the soldiers and commanders who have gone before us. The advent of modern weapons can only be seen as among humanity's most ingenious creations.

Table 5. Mortality from Penetrating Injuries of the Skull

Campaign	Reference	% Mortality	Comments
Trojan War	Homer "Iliad"	92.0	
Conquest of Italy	Virgil "Aeneid"	88.2	
Crimean War	Macleod (17)	100.0	GSW hospital cases only
American Civil War	Otis (25)	81.0	GSW and HE fragments
World War I	Cushing (17) Series 1 Series 2 Series 3 Jefferson (26)	 54.5 40.9 28.8 37.6	 Mainly HE Fragments hospitalized Mainly HE fragments
World War II	Eden (13) Crew 1962 (15)	23.6 27.2	GSW and HE fragments GSW and HE fragments
Vietnam War	Hammon (14) Kovaric et al. (28)	22.7 29.4	GSW hospital cases only Mainly HE fragments
Northern Ireland	Moffat (23) Byrnes et al. (27)	55.0 68.0 85.0	GSW only GSW traversing front to back of skull GSW traversing front to back of skull

Source: Adamson, "A Comparison of Ancient and Modern Weapons," 100.

Table 6. Lethality of War Wounds among U.S. Soldiers from the Revolution to the Afghan War

War	# Wounded	# Died	% Lethality
Revolutionary War (1775–1783)	10,633	4,435	42
War of 1812 (1812–1815)	6,675	2,260	33
Mexican War (1846–1848)	5,885	1,733	29
Civil War (Union: 1861–1865)	422,295	140,414	33
Spanish American War (1898)	2,047	385	19
World War I (1917–1918)	257,404	53,402	21
World War II (1941–1945)	963,403	291,557	30
Korea (1950–1953)	137,025	33,741	25
Vietnam (1961–1973)	200,727	47,424	24
Persian Gulf (1990–1991)	614	147	24
Iraq/Afghanistan (2001–2012)	10,369	1,004	10

Source: Atul Gawanda, "Casualties of War: Military Care for the Wounded from Iraq and Afghanistan," *New England Journal of Medicine* (December 9, 2004), 2471.

What has not changed are the death and pain that war has always inflicted upon its participants. The wounded soldier still bleeds, suffers, and worries that he or she will not survive his or her wounds. The psyche at the core of soldier's humanity must yet endure terrorizing fear. The same anxiety that drove the ancient soldier to psychiatric collapse afflicts the modern soldier to an equal degree once shot and shell begin to fly.[52] For most soldiers in combat, the risk of being driven mad by that fear remains the same as it was for those who stood at Marathon in 490 BCE. Humans remain as fragile as ever. Nowhere is this frailty more evident than in the hospital and surgical wards where, since earliest times, military surgeons have attempted to stem the tide of death and pain that has always accompanied war.

NOTES

1. See Robert Laffont, *The Ancient Art of Warfare* (London: Crescent Press, 1966), vol. 1, chapter 13, for an analysis of feudal armies as they related to the changing sociopolitical order.
2. R. Ernest Dupuy and Trevor N. Dupuy, *The Encyclopedia of Military History* (New York: Harper & Row, 1986), 168.
3. Richard A. Gabriel, *Philip II of Macedonia: Greater than Alexander* (Washington, DC: Potomac Books, 2010), 62–69, for an analysis of the Macedonian phalanx; and C. W. Oman, *The Art of War in the Middle Ages* (Ithaca, NY: Cornell University Press, 1982), chapter 5, for an examination of the Swiss infantry's innovations to defeat cavalry.
4. See Richard A. Gabriel, *Empires at War: A Chronological Encyclopedia* (Westport, CT: Greenwood Press, 2005), 3:957–63, for a detailed account of the Battle of Crécy.
5. T. N. Dupuy, *The Evolution of Weapons and Warfare* (New York: Bobbs-Merrill, 1980), 101.
6. Seigneur de Tavannes, writing in the sixteenth century, noted the impact of the pistol on cavalry when he wrote, "A cavalry battle which, in the past, would have lasted three or four hours and not killed ten men out of five hundred, has now become a murderous affair and the outcome of the battle is now decided in less than an hour." Quoted in Laffont, *The Ancient Art of Warfare*, 443.
7. The innovation of horse artillery as opposed to horse-drawn artillery is generally credited to the Prussian king Frederick the Great.
8. Dupuy and Dupuy, *Encyclopedia of Military History*, 295.
9. Richard A. Gabriel, "The History of Armaments," *Italian Encyclopedia of Social Sciences* (Rome: Marchesi Grafiche Editoriali, 1990), 352. This work traces the development of military technology from Rome to the modern era.
10. Ibid.
11. Dupuy, *Evolution of Weapons and Warfare*, 131.
12. The fluted bayonet had a channel depression running down the side called the "gutrunner" that made the bayonet easier to extract from the victim's body. The English seem to have been the first army to use this device in the battle at Culloden Moor, but the innovation's origins are obscure.
13. Although the standard iron ramrod could pack the powder down with fewer strokes without breaking, as often happened with the wooden version, much of the increased rate of

fire that resulted from the Prussian troops who first used this device was probably owed to their excellent discipline and training.

14. A good account of the development of artillery through the ages can be found in Albert Manucy, *Artillery through the Ages* (Washington, DC: U. S. Government Printing Office, 1985).
15. Gabriel, "History of Armaments," 8.
16. Ibid.
17. Before the increased mobility provided by horse artillery, it was common for one side or the other to overrun the opponent's gun positions. During battle, the forces ebbed and flowed over the same position several times. Special squads of "spikers" rendered the guns useless by driving a large iron spike into the touchhole of the cannon.
18. The idea that tanks are derivative from cavalry and to be used as such is an American and Western concept. In Russia, where artillery caused great casualties during World War I, tank design and tactics were derived from artillery doctrine, not cavalry. The Russians always mounted larger, longer-range guns on their tanks and used them in large numbers to bring the enemy under fire before the enemy's guns could engage the Russian and Soviet tanks. Right from the beginning, Russian and Soviet tanks mounted 85mm, then 120mm, and now 122mm guns, which are much larger and longer ranged than the common 105mm tank cannon used in the West.
19. A good work on the relationship of national economies to war in this period is Paul Kennedy's *The Rise and Fall of the Great Powers* (New York: Random House, 1987).
20. Gabriel, "History of Armaments," 8.
21. Dupuy, *Evolution of Weapons and Warfare*, 191.
22. The world's armies were quick to realize the potential of the railway. In the Italian War of 1859, the French moved 604,000 men and 129,000 horses by rail in three months. Dupuy, *Evolution of Weapons and Warfare*, 202.
23. Condensed milk was developed as a military ration that would not spoil in warm climates.
24. Gabriel, "History of Armaments," 12.
25. The process of massing artillery guns on target is called "sheaving," after the agricultural process of gathering individual stalks of wheat together in a single bundle. Modern firing computers now make what was once an important skill a common capability.
26. Gabriel, "History of Armaments," 13.
27. The aileron was not, however, an immediate success. In World War I, the famous German ace, Max Immelman, flew a Fokker Eindecker, a fighter aircraft that did not have ailerons. Immelman invented the complex maneuver that bears his name to this day, the Immelman turn.
28. Germany was the exception among the great powers and did not pursue colonial ambitions with any vigor. Setting German policy thirty years before, Chancellor Otto von Bismarck noted that colonies "were not worth the bones of a single Pomeranian grenadier."
29. Gabriel, "History of Armaments," 15.
30. These area saturation weapons inflicted most of the psychiatric casualties, as is the norm when troops in the defense are barraged with indirect fire. The Russian and German models had holes in the stabilizing fins of the rocket so that the round made an eerie, high-pitched sound as it flew toward its target.
31. Richard A. Gabriel, *No More Heroes: Madness and Psychiatry in War* (New York: Hill and Wang, 1987), 42.
32. Ibid., 22.

33. Ibid., 35.
34. Ibid., 27–29.
35. Ibid., 31–32.
36. Ibid.
37. Ibid., 42.
38. Dupuy, *Evolution of Weapons and Warfare*, 309–12. See also T. N. Dupuy, *Numbers, Predictions, and War* (New York: Bobbs-Merrill, 1979).
39. Dupuy, *Evolution of Weapons and Warfare*, 310.
40. Ibid., 170.
41. The time and expense involved in training a huge army of citizen soldiers in the sophisticated maneuver drills common to the professional soldiers of other armies largely led to Napoleon's use of the marching column as his primary tactical formation. Like Philip of Macedonia's early Macedonian phalanx, Napoleon's marching column formation made it possible to use large numbers of soldiers in combat with only minimal military training.
42. Dupuy, *Evolution of Weapons and Warfare*, 170.
43. The exception to this trend is the rate of psychological casualties, which have increased enormously as the tempo and lethality of war have increased. See Gabriel, *No More Heroes*, chapter 3.
44. P. B. Adamson, "A Comparison of Ancient and Modern Weapons in the Effectiveness of Producing Battle Casualties," *Journal of the Royal Army Medical Corps* 123 (1977): 93–103.
45. F. A. E. Crew, *History of the Second World War: The Army Medical Services*, vol. 2, *Campaigns* (London: Her Majesty's Stationery Office, 1957), 31–34, table 4.
46. J. D. Hardy and E. F. Du Bois, "The Technique of Measuring Radiation and Convection," *Journal of Nutrition* 15 (1938): 466.
47. G. H. B. Macleod, *Notes on the Surgery of the War in the Crimea, with Remarks on the Treatment of Gunshot Wounds* (London: J. Churchill, 1858), 46, table 1.
48. W. C. Moffat, "British Forces Casualties in Northern Ireland," *Journal of the Royal Army Medical Corps* 112 (1976): 3–8, table 6.
49. P. Meid and J. M. Yinling, *U.S. Marine Operations in Korea, 1950–1953*, vol. 5, *Operations in West Korea* (Washington, DC: Historical Division of the HQ US Marine Corps, 1958), 140.
50. Richard A. Gabriel, *Operation Peace for Galilee: The Israeli-PLO War in Lebanon* (New York: Hill and Wang, 1984), 179.
51. Atul Gawande, "Casualties of War: Military Care for the Wounded in Iraq and Afghanistan," *New England Journal of Medicine*, December 9, 2004, 2471–75.
52. Gabriel, *No More Heroes*, chapter 2. Psychiatric casualties are evident in every war for which we have a record from the earliest times.

2

THE RENAISSANCE AND THE REBIRTH OF THE EMPIRICAL SPIRIT

From a military perspective, the Renaissance can be conveniently dated from 1453—the year in which Constantinople fell to the Ottoman Turks, destroying forever the last major cultural center of the ancient world—to 1618, the beginning of the Thirty Years' War, when the use of contract armies, or the condottieri, and mercenary forces on a large scale was coming to an end as the emerging nation states became more organized and able to raise genuine national armies.[1] By 1618, European states were deploying national armies supported by regular taxation, stationed in permanent garrisons, sustained by regular pay, and directed by articulated administrative structures under the command of national sovereigns.

European culture underwent a genuine "revival of learning" during the Renaissance, a period when new methods of scientific inquiry arose. To attempt these new methods, especially with their emphasis on observation and incipient empiricism in science and medicine, and to explore new subjects, particularly those in medicine that the church and governmental edict had long forbidden or ignored as already answered by the scholastic methods of the Middle Ages, the old clerico-secular social order had to be weakened and its power to punish and censor diminished. As a prelude to change, the old alliance between secular and religious authority that for eight hundred years had sustained the feudal order and religious control of knowledge and inquiry had to be reduced.

A number of events came together to attenuate the old establishment's traditional hold on intellectual life. A major factor was the outbreak of the bubonic plague, which first occurred in 1348 and flared again several times in the same century.[2] The devastation it wrought was enormous. An estimated one in every three people in Europe died from the disease, a rate of death that sapped the physical and intellectual life of European culture. Within a century, a devastating outbreak of syphilis followed and became endemic to the European population for the next two centuries. In its wake a population already debilitated by the plague suffered an inevitable physical and mental deformation. The birth rate fell, and the population declined to where it had been a century earlier. Whole regions of Europe were almost completely depopulated. The weakened population became more susceptible to other diseases, and smallpox, influenza, measles, typhus, yellow fever, diphtheria, whooping cough, lead poisoning, and ergotism also became epidemics. Surviving records reveal that all these diseases reached pandemic proportions for the first time in European history.[3]

The effect of these conditions was to call into question the very basis of the clerico-secular society that had long been regarded as legitimate and ordained by god. The disease epidemics demonstrated the powerlessness of medical knowledge, and the medical profession lost status as society bristled with charlatans and quacks offering miraculous cures and amulets. The clerical elements of society were also revealed as powerless. The old doctrine that god visited death and disease as punishments for sin was hardly credible in an age when disease seemed to strike at random, when saint and sinner alike perished, and when large numbers of priests, monks, and even popes died.

The wave of epidemics also critically weakened the family's ability to socialize its young to the ideas and values of the old order. As diseases carried off parents, older brothers and sisters, aunts, and uncles—all vital mechanisms for transmitting and enforcing traditional social norms and values—new generations grew to adulthood removed from the familial and societal strictures that were enforced in the past. The randomness of death and the shortened life spans produced in these generations an attention to the present to a degree not seen in Europe for a thousand years. Concern for one's health provoked an emphasis on the physical body and material goods rather than on the spiritualism and eschatological views that underpinned the old clerico-secular order. The situation was not unlike those following social and military disasters in modern times. The defeats that Russia and Germany suffered in World War I produced a "lost generation" of youth that was no longer socialized to the beliefs and habits of the older Europeans who had suffered the defeats. The result in both cases was a revolution of new ideas, values, and behaviors that utterly destroyed the old orders.[4] The plagues and epidemics of the early Renaissance produced similar conditions and bred generations of unsocialized, rebellious, and materially concerned youth freed from the conventional intellectual, moral, and social strictures.

The declining size and quality of the general population made recruiting talent committed to traditional institutions very difficult. The Catholic Church could no longer sustain its monasteries without lowering its admission standards and reducing the harsher aspects of monastic life. Beginning in 1517, the Protestant Reformation produced the ultimate challenge to the old order's ability to control events. The idea of a single church exercising universal control was broken forever as Europe fragmented into scores of religious sects competing for the loyalty of a population frightened to death by death itself and desperately seeking answers to worldly concerns. The emergence of nation states encouraged secular authorities to take advantage of the religious strife by superimposing upon it an attempt to increase the scope of secular power. Religious issues became central to the dynastic wars of the period as the newly emergent national political authorities attempted to free themselves from the religious and secular power of the church. The resulting century of religious war and massacres further reduced the population and created yet more uncertainty in the world of the average citizen.

The aspirations of the new nation states' monarchs provoked frequent wars that also facilitated the destruction of the old order. In their efforts to establish effective control within their territorial realms, the monarchs of this period clashed repeatedly with ecclesiastical authorities in an attempt to reduce the power of the clergy in secular affairs and carve out a realm of political action independent of church oversight and censure. At the same time, the cost of these wars moved the monarchs to seize the material resources of the monasteries and churches within their national borders, further reducing ecclesiastical influence and control. The religious tenor of these dynastic wars was clear from the settlement that followed the Thirty Years' War in which national secular authorities were entitled to determine the religious loyalties of their respective subjects. That the religious loyalties of the national populations came to be regarded as a legitimate concern of the national kings was the clearest indication of the power of the new secular order.

The effect of waging more than a century of warfare further increased the uncertainty of life, forcing the individual back upon his or her own resources for survival. It was almost impossible to travel from one place to another without an armed guard. Bands of mercenaries and gangs roamed over the countryside, pillaging at will. Secular authority was often completely absent in the towns, and the citizenry was left to its own devices to secure its survival and livelihood. Sieges, attacks, and religious massacres were commonplace, and trouble in all social affairs was the order of the day. In many ways the situation was not unlike that which plagued Europe during the period of the tribal invasions that followed the breakdown of Roman authority in the sixth through eighth centuries. It was impossible for the old order to sustain its legitimacy. The time was ripe for new ideas.

Three events accelerated the search for new ideas: the Muslim armies' capture of Constantinople, the invention of printing, and the emergence of new perspectives on surgery precipitated by the frequent warfare during this period. The fall of Constantinople to the Ottoman Turks produced a flood of Byzantine scholars and physicians fleeing the Turkish sword. These refugees carried the intellectual legacy of Greece and Rome throughout Europe. Large numbers of them settled in Italy and France, where they became members of university faculties. These scholars and physicians then shared the cultural and empirical medical knowledge of Greece and Rome in its accurately preserved form.

The manuscripts and translations of the works of Greek and Roman medicine were available in their original versions only in Byzantium. While some of this knowledge had reached the West during the Middle Ages, much of the original empirical medical knowledge of the Greek and Roman texts had been lost or distorted over the centuries by Arab and Christian scholars, physicians, and clerical authorities who, in translation after translation, had edited and reedited the texts and removed information considered dangerous to the faith. Moreover, the scholastic approach to intellectual inquiry that characterized Western and Arabic medicine during the Middle Ages emphasized logical consistency and ratiocination to the extreme detriment of empirical observation and experimentation. The resulting medical profession was mired in medical questions and treatments in which empirical evidence was largely ignored. There is no more telling example of how corrupted the traditional empirical texts became than the fact that Galen (129–200 CE), the accepted medical authority of anatomy and medical practice in the Middle Ages, was regarded as the father of the doctrine of necessary suppuration of wounds when, instead, he clearly states pursuing the opposite course in the original text.

When the Byzantine refugee scholars reintroduced classical Greek and Roman medical texts to the West, they presented physicians with a new source of empirical medical knowledge that had been lost for more than a thousand years. Most of the texts were written in Greek, and their translation required a determined effort, especially in light of the opposition to the new knowledge that came from the traditional medical and ecclesiastical authorities. A group of courageous physicians and scholars, nonetheless, attempted the task. This group of translator-physicians is known to history as the medical humanists.[5] Their translations of the original classical medical texts from the Greek into Latin and then into the vernacular were directly responsible for providing Renaissance physicians with a new stock of empirical medical knowledge from which numerous further discoveries proceeded. Perhaps more important, the empirical methodology of the classical texts introduced to the Renaissance a new mode of reasoning and hypothesis testing that eventually became the new basis of medical diagnosis, treatment, and inquiry. After more than a millennium, Europe had rediscovered its empirical past.

Regaining this knowledge might have remained a useless enterprise were it not for the introduction of the printing press. Its invention in Europe has numerous claimants, but by 1454 the first printed work accomplished in any number was the Gutenberg Bible printed in Mainz, the center of European printing.[6] The guilds protected the secrets of the trade, and every effort was made to ensure that the German guilds retained a monopoly. The printing process likely would have remained in German hands for much longer than it did had not Adolf of Nassau laid siege to Mainz and captured the city in 1462. German printers fleeing the sword spread throughout Europe, taking with them the secrets of the new technology. Within a decade, Switzerland, Holland, and Italy had major printing houses. Printing was a free enterprise that remained mostly out of the hands of ecclesiastical authorities. It was free from the strictures of prior review and made the transfer of information cheaper and faster than at any time in man's history. Compared to hand-copied manuscripts, a printed book could be purchased at half to a third the price.[7] The bold, dark print was easy to read, although the introduction of the printed book seems to have coincided with the popular use of spectacles. Spectacles had been invented in the twelfth century but only gained popularity during the Renaissance.

Printing's impact on medicine was dramatic. For the first time, medical treatises could be produced relatively cheaply and in large numbers. The press greatly reduced the cost of reproducing medical drawings, a great aid in the revival of anatomical study. Printing books in the vernacular instead of Latin made it possible for medical knowledge to spread relatively easily from one country to another. It also made compendiums of medical information available to those medical practitioners who lacked the means or social status to attend medical schools. Equally important, printing opened up a new avenue for these medical practitioners to communicate with one another and exchange experiences and treatment protocols with little official interference.

One of the more important aspects of medical publishing was the introduction of pocket compendiums of anatomy, complete with medical drawings. The Renaissance saw the rediscovery of empirical anatomy based on dissection and observation, and a number of anatomical texts were printed. Most, however, were expensive and bulky to carry, making them of little use to the military barber-surgeon who was always following the army. (Barber-surgeons were untrained practitioners of folk medicine and surgery whose status as medical practitioners lay in their old practice of cutting the tonsures of monks. They earned a living cutting hair, shaving beards, pulling teeth, dispensing folk remedies, and, later, bleeding and applying poultices to the sick.) The solution was the cheap pocket compendium that could be easily transported and referred to under field conditions. Ambroise Paré's *Anatomie Universelle* probably was published in this format in 1561. In 1601 Joseph Schmidt, a German military surgeon, published his *Mirror of Anatomy* precisely to provide a cheap, portable medical compendium written in the vernacular for the military surgeon's use.[8] These pocket books were the first surgical manuals intended for military use that Europe had seen since the days of the Roman medical service, and military barber-surgeons used them extensively in training and practice.

THE REAPPEARANCE OF THE MILITARY SURGEON

The emergence of the military barber-surgeon as a familiar figure in the armies of the period greatly influenced the military medicine's development in the Renaissance. As in the Middle Ages, the practice of surgery within the traditional medical establishment remained separate from the practice of medicine. Control of the medical profession and its educational establishment remained firmly in the hands of the internist-physicians, while surgeons occupied the lower levels of medical status. Although the medical faculties of the day regarded surgery suspiciously, the formal medical establishment nonetheless recognized educated, medically trained, and licensed surgeons. These "surgeons of the short robe" (physicians usually wore red robes of various lengths) relied upon the distorted works of Galen and Avicenna for their anatomy knowledge, and their surgical techniques had changed little since the Middle Ages.

Quacks, sorcerers, sow gelders, barbers, and other unsavory types mostly practiced the medicine available to common people. This group of practitioners, especially those who attempted surgery, had been outlawed by medical and secular authorities since the Middle Ages. With little financial incentive for the medical establishment to provide medical care to the commoner, these medical mountebanks were the people's only source of medical treatment. Despite their clear legal status as felons, these common practitioners often found their way into military service during wartime. State authorities even impressed them into military service in some instances. These army "cutters" trailed along with the army, tending the wounded for a fee extracted from the soldier himself. Soldiers would often hire these practitioners out of their own pockets to attend the wounded. These quacks probably caused more death and injury, but in an age where medical care was restricted to the officers and others of noble birth, the "cutters" were the only source of any medical attention for the common soldier.

Falling between these extremes were the trained barber-surgeons or military wound surgeons (*wundärtzne* in German), whose profession developed during the frequent wars of the period. These practitioners were almost exclusively of low birth, and many started their careers as common cutters. But they acquired a high level of medical craftsmanship, especially in surgery, through extensive military service. Most often these surgeons had no formal medical education of any sort, although later some of the educated surgeons of the short robe served in the military, a condition that quickly brought their formal training and medical knowledge into collision with the bloody empirical realities of the battlefield. Having no formal medical education, the barber-surgeons were completely unhindered by the distorted medical theories and practices of the period, and they rapidly acquired new knowledge and treatment techniques as a consequence of their raw experience. Barber-surgeons like Paré (1510–1590) became quite famous, served as personal attendants to kings and senior officers, and authored medical books that were printed in the vernacular and thus widely read. These barber-surgeons were responsible for numerous more important advances in the military surgery of the period.

The barber-surgeons' ability to acquire medical reputations and their effective medical techniques gradually made them an important military component of the armies of the day. The more the traditional medical establishment relied upon old doctrines and practices to protect their status and position, the more the empirically accurate and effective medical practices of the barber-surgeons spread in opposition. In this struggle for recognition and status, the printing press played a decisive role in distributing the new medical knowledge as military surgery began to emerge as an important subdiscipline. In the sixteenth century, barber-surgeons published in the vernacular no fewer than forty-five works or parts of works on the subject of military surgery. One work on military pharmacy, one on military hygiene, and eleven on various diseases associated with military service were also published.[9] Where once no such texts had been available, now there were more than two score, all published in a cheap and easily read format that spread the new medical knowledge throughout Europe.

The status of the military surgeons as legitimate medical practitioners gradually became recognized in law, and some of the medical schools admitted them to faculty. In 1506, the Paris Medical Faculty admitted some of these surgeons to the college where they lectured and trained other physicians in surgery.[10] Accompanying this rise in status was the gradual formation of the barber-surgeons into self-governing guilds. As early as 1462, the Guild of Barbers in England became the Company of Barbers under royal charter. In 1492 they obtained a special charter, and in 1540 Henry VIII (1491–1547) united the Guild of Surgeons with the barbers to form the United Barber-Surgeon Company.[11] By the end of the Renaissance, the empirically trained barber-surgeon had become a legitimate member of the medical profession, although he still ranked below the internists and general physicians who continued to control the medical profession for at least three more centuries. Once organized into guilds, the new surgeons established training regimens and licensing requirements for future generations of practitioners. These military surgeons became regular features of the military establishments of the day. Having been absent from the battlefield for more than a thousand years, the true military surgeon, trained in empirical medicine and wound management, had reappeared.

NEW MEDICAL CHALLENGES

The most significant change in military operations of the Renaissance period was the introduction of gunpowder weapons on a large scale. The use of gunpowder in cannon had occurred almost a hundred years earlier, and by the Renaissance cannon had become common military equipment in all armies. While used almost exclusively for siege operations prior to this time, during the Renaissance cannon was commonly used as antipersonnel weapons to disrupt packed infantry formations. This tactic brought into existence canister and grapeshot, or soft metal containers filled with steel balls, rocks, metal shards, nails, and scrap glass. The most lethal gunpowder weapon, however, was the reliable musket and pistol. The musket enhanced the infantry's power against cavalry, but it became vulnerable when cavalry equipped with pistols delivered counterfire. Gunpowder weapons greatly changed the nature of the medical challenges that the military surgeon faced by introducing three new types of battlefield injuries: compound fractures, gunshot wounds, and burns.

The soldiers of ancient armies rarely suffered compound fractures because their muscle-powered weapons could not produce sufficient impact energy to break bones in more than one place. The ancient soldier's edged weapons cut deeply into the flesh but did so relatively cleanly and leveraged the impact of the blow over a narrow area of bone surface. When a bone did break, it usually did so only in one place and along a narrow area, factors that facilitated splinting and setting it if the soldier survived the battlefield. Compound fractures were so rare that Hippocrates considered a compound fracture an almost always fatal wound and one of the few instances when amputation of the shattered limb ought to be attempted.

Gunpowder weapons, however, easily produced the impact energy to shatter a bone in more than one place. More important than the impact energy of a musket ball, however, was the nature of musket shot itself. These early weapons fired a lead ball weighing a half ounce. The projectile's muzzle velocity was relatively slow, and the bullet highly unstable in flight.[12] The lead shot also became deformed as it left the barrel. Solid lead shot, unlike modern copper- or steel-jacketed bullets, did not retain integrity upon entering the body; instead, it spread flat upon impact. This combination of shot weight, deformity, softness, and low speed produced horrible wounds. When the bullet struck a bone, a compound fracture was a common result.[13]

Gunshot-induced compound fractures presented a new medical challenge to the battle surgeon. The common treatment for these fractures was amputation, and it is hardly surprising that the surgical works of the period are filled with references to amputation and contain the first portrayal of this technique for gunshot wounds. The commonality of these gunshot-induced compound fractures stimulated experimentation into effective amputation techniques, which also emerged in the military medical manuals of this period.

The gunshot wound unattended by fracture still produced its own problems. Unjacketed bullets traversing the soldier's clothing at slow speeds often forced bits of cloth and leather into the wounds, increasing the risk of infection. For the first time in history, the battle surgeon confronted the problems of how to remove shattered bullets from the human body and how to determine the circumstances under which the spent projectile could be left within the patient. The common technique of enlarging the wound and then probing for the bullet with fingers or unsterile probes increased infection rates. The old and dangerous doctrine of laudable pus and necessary suppuration led to the common practice of stuffing gunshot wounds with all sorts of foul materials to produce suppuration and promote healing; instead, it resulted in a horrifying rate of wound infection. Likely only a few combatants suffering gunshot wounds healed without infection, if they healed at all.

Confronted with exceptionally high rates of infection for gunshot wounds after traditional treatments, the medical establishment was at a loss. The idea gained currency that gunshot wounds were altogether different kinds of wounds in that they were by their very nature poisonous. The first evidence of this new doctrine appeared in Alsatian Army surgeon Hieronymus Brunschwig's *Book of Surgery* (1497). The doctrine gained wide currency under the influence of Pope Julius II's personal physician, Giovanni da Vigo (1460–1520), who published it in his medical treatise in 1514.[14] Although infection continued to carry off thousands of slightly wounded soldiers, other battlefield surgeons of the period—notably Paré, Hans von Gersdorff (1455–1529), and Philippus Aureolus Paracelsus (1493–1541)—argued from empirical observation that nothing about gunshot wounds was inherently poisonous and that, if left free from the common treatment of cautery and boiling oil, they would heal. The debate continued for almost three centuries with little agreement.

Gunpowder introduced yet another new medical problem, a high proportion of burns. Cannons often exploded as a consequence of defective casting. Soldiers reloading the powder charge after failing to swab the barrel properly suffered flash burns. The production of gunpowder itself was highly dangerous, and flash burns and explosions were common. Unstable powder transported in the baggage trains often exploded. The most common cause of gunpowder burns stemmed from the design of the musket itself. The soldier poured the powder into a flash pan secured to the side of the musket. Under stress, soldiers frequently poured too much powder into the pan, and when the pulled trigger moved the burning punk to ignite the power, it resulted in an explosion. Since sighting over the barrel required the soldier to press the stock to his cheek beneath his eye, these "flashes in the pan" often produced horrifying burns on the soldier's face and blinded him. Paré recalled treating this type of injury.[15] He tried various burn treatments on soldiers' faces, comparing the results while searching for more effective methods. The most commonly used medicines for facial burns were various vegetable and animal ointments that usually produced blistering and scarring. One treatment was to use various inks that contained tannic acid, an effective anti-blistering agent.[16] As recorded in his medical writings, one of Paré's innovations, which he obtained from an old country woman, was a paste of crushed onions and salt that greatly reduced blistering and scarring. American military physicians during World War II noted that Soviet battle physicians used this same treatment in 1945.[17]

The problems that military medical personnel faced in treating gunpowder weapons greatly increased in another way. Because the reliable musket forced infantry formations to spread out to avoid destruction under cannon and rifle fire, armies deployed for battle over larger areas. The combat formations of the past in which densely packed masses of men clashed with one another at close range had made it comparatively easy to locate the wounded once the battle ended. The new dispersed infantry formations left the wounded scattered over a much greater area than ever before, making them much more difficult to locate. Because commanders retained the doctrine forbidding medical aid on the battlefield during engagement, the wounded lingered for hours and sometimes days before any medical treatment could be attempted. Not until the Napoleonic Wars when Dominique-Jean Larrey (1766–1842) invented the "flying ambulances," whose task was to locate and evacuate the wounded, did this situation change even marginally for the better.

The new technology of gunpowder weapons largely shaped the military medical challenges of the Renaissance. That effective medical knowledge concerning infection, amputation, and blood loss had progressed only marginally since the Roman military medical service collapsed more than a thousand years earlier hindered dealing with these challenges. Worse, the entrenched medical establishment regarded surgery and empirical observation as a threat to its position and continued to hamper whatever progress the barber-surgeons made. They upheld the doctrine of necessary suppuration of wounds despite the clinical observations and printed commentaries of the battle surgeons who practiced otherwise. They did the same with cautery and boiling oil in amputation. Although a few bright lights in Renaissance medicine introduced new ideas and treatment protocols, the medicine of the period, even the military medicine, remained largely unchanged from the Middle Ages. Because the new military technology had changed the nature and severity of battle wounds considerably, however, the resulting casualties and the rates of infection not surprisingly increased dramatically.

A few empirically minded surgeons and physicians of the Renaissance, meanwhile, did contribute significantly to the advancement of medicine in that period. Although they differed widely in background and training, they all shared the new empirical clinical perspective and were willing to abandon the scholastic approach to medicine and rely more heavily on their own observation and experience. Some, such as Paracelsus and Andreas Vesalius (1514–1564), were members of the medical establishment and worked to change it. Paracelsus was the major critic of the scholastic approach to medicine and attacked the methodological roots of traditional medical knowledge. He raged against those who opposed the new empiricism and suggested throwing the works of Galen and Avicenna into a bonfire. He is regarded as the essential reformer of Renaissance medicine. Vesalius, meanwhile, had served as a battlefield surgeon in the armies of Charles V. He taught medicine using public dissection, lectured in the vernacular, and accomplished the only physiological experiments in anatomy after Galen and before William Harvey (1578–1657). The publication of his *De humani corporis fabrica* in 1543 obliterated the old Galenic anatomy, which had been based on the anatomy of apes and swine, and was the first comprehensive book on anatomy, complete with medical drawings, produced in almost fifteen hundred years.[18] His work was considered so accurate that others imitated and improved upon it for centuries. Vesalius is correctly admired as the father of modern anatomy.

By far the most important surgical contributions of the period came from the new barber-surgeons, the most important of whom was Paré, the era's most famous surgeon. Born of low station in Bourg Hersent, France, he was a self-taught barber-surgeon. He became the chief military surgeon to four monarchs; wrote important medical treatises, the most important of which was his *Method of Treating Gunshot Wounds* (1545); and served as an army surgeon all his life. Paré invented many surgical instruments, introduced the use of artificial limbs and eyes, wrote of flies as carriers of contagion, attempted implantation of artificial teeth, and tried to organize medical care for the common soldier.[19] All his clinical experience was obtained on the battlefield, and Paré naturally concentrated on diagnosing and treating those medical conditions that arose from warfare.

Paré's most important contribution was his development of successful techniques for performing battlefield amputations. His own experience showed that the traditional practice of amputation accompanied by cautery and boiling oil, a technique that da Vigo had popularized to treat the supposedly poisonous nature of gunshot wounds, more often produced pain and death than recovery. Paré reintroduced the practice of ligature prior to amputation, a procedure lost since Aulus Cornelius Celsus performed it in the second century. This Roman practice greatly reduced bleeding and shock. Paré abandoned the barbarous technique of plunging the amputated stump into boiling elder oil mixed with treacle; instead, he treated the amputated limb with a mixture of egg yolk, oil of roses, and turpentine. The results were dramatic, with infection rates dropping as recovery rates increased. Paré applied similar poultices to regular gunshot wounds, also reducing infection rates. He concluded that nothing about gunshot wounds was poisonous per se and that infection was carried into the wound from external sources. He urged secondary and repeated debridement of wounds to allow healing by secondary intention. Paré used adhesive bandages in closing wounds to facilitate healing and astringent red wine, similar to the Roman acetum, as an antiseptic.[20] Later, Bartolommeo Magi's (1477–1552) experiments with firearms and wounds demonstrated that Paré's assumption that gunshot wounds were not inherently poisonous was correct.[21] Despite Paré's findings, however, traumatic amputation treated by cautery and boiling oil remained a basic application up to the nineteenth century.

Paré's introduction of ligature also allowed him to amputate limbs damaged from other causes, and he appears to have been the first physician since Celsus to successfully amputate live limbs above the wound.[22] Paré's ligature, as important a medical advance as it was, worked primarily upon amputations below the knee that did not require tying off the femoral artery. Like most surgeons of his day, Paré had no experience in amputating above the knee, where his technique of ligature would have been almost useless in any case. In 1718, Jean-Louis Petit (1674–1750) introduced the screw tourniquet, which achieved temporary hemostasis in thigh and leg amputations by effectively compressing the femoral artery in the groin. His advancement helped reintroduce ligature in surgical amputations.[23]

MILITARY MEDICINE IN RENAISSANCE ARMIES

Paré's most significant contribution was his military medical service to several monarchs, and his widely read medical writings raised the status of the battle surgeon and surgery to its highest point in medical history prior to modern times. The needs of kings and nobles for battlefield surgical skills in an age of almost constant warfare greatly aided his achievement; however, increasing medical knowledge and the status of the military surgeon did not greatly improve the medical care available to the common soldier. For the most part, medical care was not significantly different from what it had been in the Middle Ages. Paré and others certainly made attempts to deliver medical care to the common soldiery and regarded it as their duty to do so. But despite advances in medical knowledge, the nature of military medical care remained primitive as armies struggled to find ways to deliver care in a systematic manner. As had been the case for almost a millennium, medical care on the battlefield was still mostly limited to kings and nobles.

Renaissance armies were undergoing a state of transition, moving away from the decentralized and temporary feudal armies of the Middle Ages toward the emerging professional national armies that eventually came to characterize the seventeenth century. Renaissance armies were not yet sufficiently structurally articulated and formed as genuine national armies that could sustain themselves with permanent financial support from their national sovereigns. Consequently, armies of the period contained only the embryonic beginnings of a permanent military medical service to deal with casualties. Also working against the establishment of an effective field medical service was the use of mercenary contingents in the emergent dynastic armies. No national sovereign felt an obligation to tend to the casualties of hired troops. Death and maiming were simply the costs of doing business, and the contract soldier assumed the risk. Although the class structures of the Renaissance states were somewhat looser than those of the Middle Ages, the line between nobles, royals, and commoners were still strictly drawn. Obligations toward one's fellows were limited to equals within the same class. The idea that medical aid should be extended to the common soldier had yet to take root.

In the meantime, the presence of military medical personnel on the battlefield became increasingly common, with the nobles and kings usually being attended by barber-surgeons while at war. The histories of this early period document a number of military surgeons who attended to the armies.[24] The era's first example of a semi-regular use of surgeons on the battlefields can be attributed to the Italian city-states, which seem to have employed surgeons for campaigns as early as the thirteenth century.[25] Even earlier, some Italian states gathered groups of medical practitioners within cities under siege to provide medical support and to enforce hygienic regulations.

The Swiss were the first Europeans of the period to provide regular medical care to the common soldier, perhaps as early as the Battle of Laupen (1339).[26] The Swiss considered themselves a union of free peoples in which the citizens' worth and rights were recognized in law. Because they were a rural people scattered throughout mountainous country, central authority was difficult to maintain, forcing the citizens to rely upon one another. Accordingly, the idea of a citizen's obligation to the state based on general reciprocal commitments was established early. This principle of citizenship fostered the state's obligation to care for those citizen-soldiers who waged war to protect the community.

From 1339 onward, the records of Swiss towns and cantons are filled with accounts of public funds being disbursed to care for the sick, wounded, and damaged of war. Some Swiss public authorities commonly hired barber-surgeons to care for the wounded after battle.[27] By 1405, all Swiss cantons had done so. Later, it became custom to pay the wounded soldier as long as the army remained under arms. In 1476, the archives note that all of the wounded's living expenses should be paid out of the public purse. The Council of Lucerne passed an ordinance that the state should legally guard the property of children orphaned by war. If public officials were deficient in this task, the state was to make restitution to the soldier's heirs. Most enlightened was the decree requiring that the state pay both for the indigent wounded's medical treatment until they were fully recovered and for the family's expenses of the wounded until the damaged soldier could return to work.[28] After the war between Bern and the five Catholic cantons in 1533, sick and wounded war prisoners were allowed to return to their homes without ransom upon payment of the cost of living expenses and medical attention. The Swiss soldier became so accustomed to these military medical benefits that later, when Swiss armies hired themselves out for duty in the service of foreign kings, they routinely included provisions for the pay of medical services and veterans' benefits in their contracts.[29]

In Swiss musters of this period, historians find the first use of the title *feldscher*, or "field-barber," which generally was used to describe the barber-surgeon in the European armies until the present day.[30] Medical personnel in Swiss armies even commonly bore arms and participated as combatants. They treated the wounded only after the battle. Swiss law required that wounded soldiers remain with their units and not seek safety from the fight under penalty of desertion. This injunction made good military medical sense. It prevented the soldiery from scattering all over the battlefield, making it much easier to locate and treat the wounded when the battle was finished.[31] Further, until the middle of the sixteenth century, the victors frequently slaughtered the wounded at will. Wounded men staggering around the battlefield would have been easy prey in an age where the intensity of religious wars severely eroded basic mercy and humanity.

The Swiss military medical service was the first in the Renaissance period; it emerged in a military force recruited from a single nation state bonded by common feelings of national identity. Once other armies of the period began to recruit from their own people instead of hiring bands of mercenaries and thugs, it was to be expected that they would develop the outlines of a military medical service to treat the common soldier as well. Charles VII (1403–1461) of France was the first European monarch to attempt the creation of national forces when he established his *compagnies d'ordonnance* (units of national troops directly under the orders of the king). Henry VII of England (1457–1509) created a similar force in 1485 with his "yeomen of the guard." Maximillian I (1459–1519) of Germany formed a similar national force, the famous Landsknechte (native-born soldiers), drawn from the citizenry. This army was further strengthened and enlarged under Charles V (1500–1556) into a truly national military force.[32] For the first time in a millennium, Europe once again had a formal military medical service.

Leonhard Fronsperger described the organization of the Landsknechte, including its military medical support, in his treatise on *Imperial Courts-Martial* (1555), which Col. Charles L. Heizmann translated.[33] The Landsknechte were aggregated into *hauffen* (units of five thousand to ten thousand men), which were divided into regiments consisting of ten to fourteen *fahnlein* (standard units of four hundred men each). A barber-surgeon was assigned to each of these units of infantry and to each troop of two hundred cavalry.[34] Attached to each hauffen was a field physician in chief, who was responsible to the commander for medical support, and an additional field-barber. The chief marshal of cavalry also had a physician under his command, and a surgeon was assigned to the artillery commander.[35] The regulations clearly make providing medical support a command responsibility, and it ensured that medical supplies, surgical chests, and medical transport were given to the medical complement. The surgeon was required to sleep in the command tent so that he could be easily located should the wounded need attention. Medical personnel received double pay from public funds.[36]

The army also provided wagons to transport the wounded and sick. Each morning, the slightly sick and wounded were transported along with the army, and because no army of this period had yet established a system of military hospitals to tend the wounded, the more seriously ill and wounded were sent to whatever hospitals were in nearby towns. The troops contributed to a common fund out of which they paid a *spital meister*, or "hospital attendant," delegated to look after the sick. When the army moved, couriers were dispatched to locate suitable quarters, including a house where the barber-surgeon could attend patients. In battle, the medical personnel were located with the rear guard, and their orders were to bring the wounded out of the line and find a safe place to treat them. As long as the army remained in the field, the wounded and sick continued to receive their pay.[37]

These regulations governing medical support represent at least the spirit of the new national sovereigns who were attempting to care for the common soldier drawn from the ranks of the citizenry; however, the system was still not very effective in practice. The armies were largely constituted from the dregs of society, and they did not conduct any medical examinations to exclude the mentally or physically unfit. Unlike the Swiss, these armies made no provisions to care for the wounded after military service. A wounded Landsknechte made his way home as best he could and survived upon his own resources, often nursed by one of the many female camp followers who attached themselves to the soldiery as wives and girlfriends.[38] It was common practice to abandon the wounded, who were treated where they lay by bands of roving charlatans and cutters that followed in the wake of the army.[39] The quality of these medical personnel was not likely to give the soldier much comfort. Surgeons and physicians who attended the officers and nobles were probably barber-surgeons with extensive empirical experience but little formal medical training. Those who treated the troops, however, ranged anywhere from the apprentice barber-surgeon who was seriously trying to learn his trade to crude army cutters or sow gelders. The army still impressed common medical practitioners into service, and most of them ended up treating the troops.

The increasing national character of the Renaissance armies stimulated the formation of medical services for the soldier in other armies of the period. In France, the armies of Charles the Bold, Duke of Burgundy, had a surgeon attached to every company of a hundred lancers or eight hundred infantrymen in addition to the personal physicians of the king and nobles. Edward IV of England (1442–1483) had a chief physician, two body physicians, a surgeon, and thirteen assistant surgeons on his staff.[40] At the Battle of St. Quentin in 1557, the English Army had a total of fifty-seven surgeons at its service and established a rudimentary organizational structure of medical care that English authors often cite as the first instance in England's history where a medical service was provided.[41] In Italy, the republics of Florence, Venice, Naples, Ferrara, and Verona had small surgical units attached to their armies, and the galleys of the Genoese Navy had one barber-surgeon and one assistant barber attached to each ship's complement of 210 men.[42] In Spain, each infantry regiment had a physician and surgeon attached to it, and the armada had a hospital ship on which to treat casualties.[43]

These rudimentary medical establishments gradually grew in size and sophistication as the end of the Renaissance approached, and stationary military hospitals were founded and replaced the temporary field hospitals throughout the various European realms. The permanent structures opened the possibility of long-term care for the wounded. The idea of caring for disabled veterans had gained currency as early as 1318, when the Venetians established a home for disabled mariners. A century earlier, Louis IX (1214–1270) had founded an asylum for blind crusaders, and in the thirteenth century a charter was granted to the Chevaliers de l'Étoile (Knights of the Star) to care for the disabled.[44] The earlier medieval hospitals to care for disabled soldiers had their roots in the Carolingian Dynasty (751–987), when the practice was to send the disabled to monasteries, convents, and churches and allow them to earn their keep by performing menial chores as lay brothers.[45] By 1600, this system had been mostly abolished, and in 1605 the French replaced it with the Maison Royale de la Charité Chrétienne, where disabled soldiers were supported by whatever surplus could be extracted from the budgets of various charities.[46] The idea of permanent care for the wounded, first used by the Roman Army, along with pension benefits did not emerge in full form until the modern era.[47]

It can be said that the continuous wars of the Renaissance increased the leadership's concern for their common soldiers' medical care, but this interest was balanced by the fact that the soldiery came from the lowest social orders, and in general the political and military leadership of the day was indifferent to the people's welfare. Rudimentary, unsubstantial efforts at medical care were made, but the effect of the era's advances in medical knowledge on the casualty rate was felt largely among the soldiery drawn from the higher social orders. Since military medical establishments of the time came in and out of existence as the press of war dictated, no corps of military medical professionals developed that could devote its full attention to improving medical care for the soldiery. Further, the degree of organizational articulation of medical support structures remained primitive throughout the period. Military medicine, as distinct from military surgery, for the most part remained dismally behind civilian medicine, which itself was in a less than exalted state.

Military medicine would have been more effective had the leadership given attention to field hygiene. Disease carried off more soldiers than weapons did in every war in history until modern times.[48] Armies lost more combat power to temporary disablement due to illness than to any other cause. Controlling and preventing outbreaks of disease depended on advances in medical knowledge that did not occur until the nineteenth century. Moreover, commanders simply regarded the presence of disease and sickness in the army as a normal cost of war, since it had always been the case as long as anyone could remember.

Disease and illness were such common aspects of civilian life of the period that it is hardly remarkable that no one should have taken much note of it in military life. For centuries, for example, monastic orders had forbidden their members to bathe more than twice a year unless a physician ordered them to do so. Queen Elizabeth I (1533–1603) was horrified at the suggestion of washing herself all over more than once in a year.[49] As noted earlier, the period saw a number of diseases become epidemic to the population, which commonly accepted death and illness as part of the natural order. The medical profession, having forgotten the old Roman notion of preventive medicine, could do little to prevent outbreaks of disease and even less to cure them once they were under way. Little wonder, then, that few commanders gave much attention to preventing disease and illness on military campaigns.

In Heizmann's study of military sanitation and hygiene in the Renaissance, he notes that the proportion of sieges to battles during the period was 2 to 1, probably owing to the introduction of the new heavy artillery. Of the fifty-seven besieged towns studied, twenty-four were eventually reduced by assault, twenty capitulated, and in thirteen cases the siege was abandoned.[50] In almost every case of capitulation or abandonment, one or both armies suffered heavy casualties from disease. In only a single instance, at the siege of Metz in 1552, can one find any attempt by military commanders to prevent disease. So uncommon were such attempts that the siege of Metz is regarded as the period's high-water mark for military sanitation.

The siege provides an example of what happened when one army made attempts at military sanitation and the other did not. Charles V laid siege to the town on October 20 with a force of almost 220,000 men going against the city's force of fewer than 6,000 troops commanded by Francis, Duke of Guise. The besieging army conducted sanitary affairs as usual, and by December 26 it had lost more than 20,000 men to disease. The main killers were typhus, dysentery, and scurvy.[51] Although the losses to disease were not unusually large as a percentage of force for that time, they were great enough to force Charles V to abandon the siege.

Within the walls of Metz, the Duke of Guise proved himself a first-rate medical officer who succeeded in keeping his losses to disease relatively low through applying basic rules of field sanitation. Guise increased expenditures for rations to ensure his troops ate well. Water points were checked for purity and placed under guard. Any soldier who fell ill was immediately isolated from the rest of the garrison in hospitals provided at remote spots within the city. Special units of pioneers cleaned and swept the city streets. Any human waste or animal carrion was thrown over the city walls.[52]

Barber-surgeons were hired to attend the sick within the garrison and in the hospitals, the first time that the physicians of nobles were placed at the regular disposal of the common soldier.[53] Physicians were appointed to oversee the quality and distribution of the food supply. No one was permitted to eat fish, venison, or game birds for fear that they might carry disease.[54] These efforts were so successful that not a single serious outbreak of disease occurred during the sixty-five-day siege.

The siege of Metz is also known for the first instance of the period when a commander showed basic humanity to prisoners. It was common practice to butcher prisoners, especially the sick and wounded, who fell into enemy hands. Guise instead ordered that the enemy sick camps not be burned and that the captured sick prisoners be taken to hospitals within the city and given medical treatment. He communicated with the enemy commander, suggesting safe passage to units designated to police the area for additional wounded and sick, and supplied wagons for this purpose. A number of boats to transport the enemy sick to their home units were supplied, marking the first time since Rome that "hospital ships" were used to evacuate and treat the wounded.[55] Guise's clemency, however, proved a disaster. Once he had transported the enemy sick to the city's hospitals, an epidemic of typhus spread from the prisoners to the larger population, killing hundreds.

Guise's example of humane treatment provoked a remarkable change in the treatment of the wounded that other armies gradually adopted. At the siege of Therouanne in 1553, Spanish troops who had fought at Metz remembered the French example of merciful treatment and did not kill a single prisoner. Again at Thionville in 1558, both sides followed Guise's example. The common practice of massacring those prisoners not reserved for ransom gradually declined. By the seventeenth century, the combatants themselves had established the custom of sparing prisoners, and from it sprung the idea that the wounded and sick should be treated as noncombatants. This idea was codified into international law centuries later in the Geneva Convention.

The Renaissance was more than a "revival of learning" insofar as it saw the discovery and promulgation of new medical knowledge. More important, the period produced a new type of medical practitioner, the military barber-surgeon, who could apply the new empirical medical knowledge on the battlefield. For the first time in a millennium, the soldier had access to some effective empirical medical talent to save his life. At first this talent was reserved for the nobility, but as the feudal armies gradually became national armies drawn from the citizenry, the leadership paid more attention to the medical needs of the common soldier. The first embryonic stirrings of regular medical establishments in the armies of all the major states appeared, and the gradual introduction of humane rules and practices for dealing with the captured, sick, and wounded probably went some distance in reducing casualty rates. The first permanent military hospitals appeared, as did greater concern for caring for the disabled after their return from military service. Yet, it is important to remember that in all these aspects the Renaissance represented only the germination of new military medical ideas and practices. It took another three centuries before any of these ideas were carried to fruition in a manner sufficient enough to make a real difference in the quality of military medical care available to the soldier.

NOTES

1. The dates used here to define the Renaissance period encompass the most important military and medical events of the period. From a literary, cultural, and artistic perspective, however, the Renaissance can be said to have begun much earlier, perhaps as early as the twelfth century.
2. The first outbreak of the Great Plague in Europe occurred in 1348. Outbreaks of lesser intensity occurred in 1361–1363, 1369–1371, 1374–1375, and 1390–1400. Historians have generally come to accept Jean Froissart's estimate that as much as a third of the population of Europe succumbed to the disease.
3. Fielding Garrison, *Notes on the History of Military Medicine* (Washington, DC: Association of Military Surgeons, 1922), 107.
4. The effects of disease and social disorder as they affected socialization mechanisms are found in John Rathbone Oliver, "Medical History of the Renaissance," *International Clinics* 1 (March 1928): 239–62.
5. Among the more important medical humanists are Niccolò Leoniceno (1428–1524), who translated the aphorisms of Hippocrates and corrected the botanical errors in Pliny's *National History*; Thomas Linacre (1460–1524), who translated the major Galenic treatises on hygiene, therapeutics, temperaments, natural faculties, and the pulse; and François Rabelais (1490–1553), who translated the other major works of Hippocrates.
6. It is probable that the first European press was not invented by Johannes Gutenberg but by Laurens Coster of Haarlem in 1440.
7. Fielding Garrison, *Introduction to the History of Medicine* (London: W. B. Saunders, 1967), 193.
8. Le Roy Crummer, "Joseph Schmidt: Barber Surgeon," *American Journal of Surgery* 4 (February 1928): 237.
9. Charles L. Heizmann, "Military Sanitation in the Sixteenth, Seventeenth, and Eighteenth Centuries," *Annals of Medical History* 1 (1917–1918): 283.
10. Garrison, *Introduction to the History*, 239.
11. Ibid.
12. For the dynamics of bullet flight and impact, see D. A. W. Hopkinson and T. K. Marshal, "Firearm Injuries," *British Journal of Surgery* 54, no. 4 (May 1967): 344–53.
13. Firearms experts estimate the muzzle velocity of a black powder smoothbore musket firing

a half-ounce .50-caliber ball at standard charge to be approximately 1,100 to 1,350 feet per second, providing an impact energy of 350 foot-pounds at 50 yards. For comparisons with modern military firearms, see E. Stephen Gurdjian, "The Treatment of Penetrating Wounds of the Brain Sustained in Warfare," *Journal of Neurosurgery* 39 (February 1974): 157–66.

14. See Robert D. Forrest, "Development of Wound Therapy from the Dark Ages to the Present," *Journal of the Royal Society of Medicine* 75 (April 1982): 269. Remarkably, the debate on whether gunshot wounds were poisonous continued until at least the early twentieth century, when in a curious twist it was held that the temperatures generated in firing modern weapons made bullet wounds essentially aseptic! See F. P. Thoresby and H. M. Darlow, "The Mechanism of Primary Infection of Bullet Wounds," *British Journal of Surgery* 54 (1967): 359–69.
15. Henry E. Sigerist, "Ambrose Paré's Onion Treatment of Burns," *Bulletin of the History of Medicine* 15, no. 2 (February 1944): 144.
16. Ibid., 143.
17. Ibid., 148.
18. Garrison, *Notes on the History*, 115.
19. The best short history of Paré's contributions to Renaissance medicine is Owen H. Wangensteen, Sarah D. Wangensteen, and Charles F. Klinger, "Wound Management of Ambroise Paré and Dominique Larrey: Great French Military Surgeons of the 16th and 19th Centuries," *Bulletin of the History of Medicine* 46, no. 3 (May–June 1973): 207–34.
20. Ibid., 214.
21. J. S. Taylor, "A Retrospect of Naval and Military Medicine," *U.S. Naval Medical Bulletin* 15, no. 3 (1921): 575–76. Thomas Gale (1507–1586) of England performed similar experiments with firearms at about the same time.
22. Wangensteen et al., "Wound Management," 213.
23. Ibid., 214.
24. Garrison, *Notes on the History*, 99. Some famous physicians who served in military campaigns were Nicholas Colnet and Thomas Morestede with Henry V at Agincourt, Hans von Gersdorf with the Swiss at Grandson, Gabriel Miron with Charles VII at Naples, Marcello Cumano with the Milanese armies at Novara, and Symphorien Campier with Francis I at Marignano.
25. Heizmann, "Military Sanitation," 284.
26. The only extant work on the subject of Swiss military medicine in the Renaissance was written by Dr. Conrad Brunner, *Die Verwundeten in den Kriegen den alten Eidgenossenschaft* (Tübingen, 1903).
27. Ibid., 57.
28. Ibid., 52–54.
29. Ibid.
30. The Soviet Army used the term "feldscher" as an official title for its combat medics at least until 1990.
31. Modern weaponry's increased killing power necessitated tacticians' spreading out their forces, and the consequential dispersal of the wounded still bedevils modern medical planners. Using medevac helicopters as a solution works only if one controls the air over the battlefield. Otherwise, the helicopters are themselves vulnerable to new long-range weapons, as the Soviets found to their dismay in Afghanistan.
32. The Landsknechte were heavy infantry armed with muskets, halberds, and bows. The state

partially provided their pay, and they were permitted to loot and keep the booty as a supplement to their pay.

33. Heizmann, "Military Sanitation," 284. These early regulations are regarded as the birth of the German military medical service.
34. Ibid., 281–83.
35. Ibid., 284.
36. Ibid.
37. Garrison, *Notes on the History*, 103–4.
38. The thousands of female camp followers who usually attended the armies of the period certainly contributed to the spread of syphilis, which was epidemic.
39. Heizmann, "Military Sanitation," 285.
40. Garrison, *Notes on the History*, 104.
41. Heizmann, "Military Sanitation," 284.
42. Garrison, *Notes on the History*, 105.
43. Ibid.
44. Taylor, "Retrospect of Naval and Military Medicine," 598.
45. Ibid.
46. Ibid.
47. Some idea of how slowly the notion of providing long-term care to veterans developed can be obtained from noting that the disabled veterans of the famous Light Brigade at Balaclava during the Crimean War were not provided any care at all. In desperation, the disabled veterans sent representatives to their commander, Lord Cardigan, and asked him to plead their case with the government. Cardigan sent them away, promising to ask the government to grant a special dispensation so that his troops might be given preference in obtaining beggar's licenses!
48. This remained the case until the Franco-Prussian War of 1870–1871 in which for the first time more men were lost to enemy fire than to disease. The low loss rate to disease resulted in large part from the discoveries of Robert Koch, who developed the theory of the etiology of disease and established regular sanitation officers in German units.
49. Reginald Hargreaves, "The Long Road to Military Hygiene," *The Practitioner* 196 (March 1966): 441.
50. Heizmann, "Military Sanitation," 281.
51. Carey P. McCord, "Scurvy as an Occupational Disease: Scurvy in the World's Armies," *Journal of Occupational Medicine* 13, no. 12 (December 1971): 588.
52. Heizmann, "Military Sanitation," 285.
53. Garrison, *Notes on the History*, 106.
54. Heizmann, "Military Sanitation," 286.
55. Ibid., 287.

3

THE SEVENTEENTH CENTURY
Gunpowder and Slaughter

The new empirical spirit of the Renaissance threatened much more than the storehouse of knowledge inherited from the Middle Ages. The spirit of empirical inquiry was rooted in new notions of individualism, themselves products of the wide-ranging social disruption that the plagues and wars of the period engendered. The same spirit of individual inquiry that made the new knowledge possible also undermined the collectivism that had underpinned the European social order for more than a millennium. It was this "spirit of individual disorder" as much as the plagues, wars, and new technologies of the seventeenth century that weakened the social institutions of the old order.

The old intellectual tradition of inquiry based on scholastic reasoning, first principles, and absolute causes remained strongly in place as the new century dawned. The new empirical knowledge had not yet achieved a level of generalization or acceptance capable of challenging the old approaches to medicine and science on any scale. At the same time, the new knowledge was sufficiently accurate to seriously call into question the ability of scholastic assumptions and methods to explain the physics, science, and medicine of the day. As the intellectuals of the seventeenth century conceived it, the challenge was not to discard the age-old idea of a universal order but to utilize empiricism to demonstrate the validity of that order.

The period was the age of Isaac Newton (1642–1727), himself a devoutly religious man, who wrote his *Principia Mathematica* precisely to demonstrate the empirical reality of a divine order that governed human affairs. The new approach to science was never intended to discredit the conclusions of the old system of reasoning as much as to introduce new methods of demonstrating the validity of those conclusions through empirical observation. The difficulty was that while the new empiricism could collect data that had yet to await eventual theoretical synthesis, the new knowledge created disturbing observable facts that undermined the assumptions upon which the old scholastic approach was based. It resulted in creating as much of a threat to the old intellectual order as if the assumptions of that order had been directly challenged in the first place.

The seventeenth century witnessed the progressive weakening of the old social, political, and epistemological system as the press of epidemics, wars, and social disruption continued to cripple the social institutions that gave expression to the assumptions of the old knowledge in everyday life. The collectivism that had underpinned the old order was also undermined. The old order had been based upon reciprocity of obligations, but the new knowledge was based on rights.

The erosion of the collective spirit brought with it a decline in those social practices that thrived on collectivism, among them organized nursing, charitable care of the sick, well-managed hospitals, and the general power of the church. In its place, the new experimenters could only offer the promise of eventually complete explanations of human events. With the exception of Newton's work, the seventeenth century produced no new tested theories or agreed-upon set of empirical observations. While the period did generate a number of important discoveries in medicine, few of them were integrated into the medical practice of the day.

Among the more important advances in medical knowledge was William Harvey's demonstration of the circulation of the blood in 1616. Harvey proved mathematically that given the volume and speed of blood in the body, there was no alternative to circulation. Harvey's work destroyed the Galenic dictum that blood passed through "pores" in the heart ventricles; instead, Harvey demonstrated that the heart pumps blood to the body and the veins return blood to the heart. Another major invention, the microscope, belongs to this period. While the instrument's origins are obscure, Athanasius Kircher (1602–1680) was probably the first to use the microscope in investigating the causes of disease. Antonj van Leeuwenhoek (1632-1723) made further advances in medical microscopy, wrote more than 250 papers from data assembled from microscopic investigation, and produced the first scientific description of red blood corpuscles. Marcello Malpighi (1628–1694), the father of histology, was the greatest microscopist of the period and introduced a theory of respiration. Franz de le Boë (1614–1672) established the science of physiological chemistry, and Robert Boyle (1627–1691) conducted experiments on gasses that made a cogent theory of respiration possible.[1]

The decline of collectivism was evident in these discoveries. Individuals working in private laboratories with little in the way of institutional affiliation or support achieved most of them. The universities and medical schools of the day continued to cling to Galenic and other theories, and their rigorous enforcement of these perspectives prevented them from attracting the best minds to their faculties. Men associated with universities made few of the era's great discoveries. In an age of individualism, individualism propelled investigation and discovery. Yet, the new knowledge cried out for an integrative theory to oppose the standing scholasticism. The search for a new theoretical structure influenced medicine as well.

The search for an integrative medical theory based on empirical observation manifested itself in the development of two major schools of thought that sought to organize the new medical knowledge into a systematic whole. The pull of universal order, assumed for more than a millennium, influenced medicine as much as it did Newton's laws of physics. The two new schools of medical theory were the Iatromathematical school and the Iatrochemical school.

The Iatromathematical school sought to apply the new principles of mechanics and mathematics to medical investigation. As represented by René Descartes (1576–1650), Giovanni Borelli (1608–1679), and Santorio Sanctorius (1561–1636), the human body was conceived of as a mechanical machine in which all bodily processes—thinking, respiration, digestion, locomotion, and so forth—were regarded as mechanical processes subject to physical and mechanical laws. The Iatrochemical school, represented by Jean-Baptiste van Helmont (1577–1644), Franciscus Sylvius (1614–1672), and Thomas Willis (1621–1675), saw the body as the product of a series of chemical reactions and processes.[2] Both schools ended in sterile failure, as they sought to generalize to operational principles of larger scope without sufficient empirical data upon which the structure of their analysis was built. Both schools were examples of what the new experimentalism was attempting to achieve. Because neither succeeded in enforcing a new theory of medicine upon the discipline, the process of experiment and discovery that characterized the period continued.

A number of important medical advances laid the groundwork for further development in the coming centuries, although few found large-scale application in daily medical practices. The new knowledge of physiological chemistry and of the behavior of liquids and gases was applied to medical experiments. One application was the intravenous injection of drugs, which Christopher Wren (1632–1723) first attempted on dogs. Others experimented with the technique, and Caspar Scotus carried out the first successful intravenous drug injection on a man in 1664. In England, John Graunt (1620–1674) introduced the science of vital statistics by compiling a statistical study of mortality. Stephen Bradwell (1588–1665) published the first handbook on first aid for common injuries in 1663. Daniel LeClerc (1652–1728) wrote the first comprehensive history of medicine, and the newly introduced medical dictionary became commonplace.[3]

The seventeenth century also saw the introduction of copperplate engraving to replace the woodcut, revolutionizing the art of anatomical illustration. Johannes Scultetus (1595–1645) wrote *Armamentarium Chirugicum*, the first complete book of surgical instruments with each instrument drawn to scale and complete with illustrations of their application in surgical settings. It was published posthumously in 1655.[4] Until this time, armorers, blacksmiths, and razor makers had made surgical instruments to individual specification, with little in the way of standardization. Now highly skilled silversmiths, cutlers, and pewterers made these instruments and produced implements of standard design, balance, and quality.[5]

The quality of medical instruction, while still generally poor, was improved somewhat by the gradual introduction of clinical instruction in hospitals. A century earlier the Italians had introduced clinical instruction, and in the seventeenth century it was introduced to the universities in Holland, where it became a model for other medical universities. Dissection as a means of teaching anatomy became more common, especially in Italy, France, and Holland, and the anatomical theater became an established common feature of medical education. While corpses and skeletons were difficult to obtain, dissection increased as a means of instruction and discovery. Raymond Vieussens (1641–1716) is said to have conducted five hundred dissections in the course of his career.[6]

Two other innovations greatly spurred the development and communication of scientific and medical knowledge during this period. The first was the invention of the scientific society. The emphasis on individual efforts of discovery unencumbered by institutional affiliation created the need for a mechanism whereby scholars and scientists could gather, share, and test each other's ideas. The idea for the resulting professional scientific society may have originated during the Renaissance in Italy, where such societies were a well-kept secret lest their members fall afoul of ecclesiastical authority. In 1560, one such secret academic society in Naples was called, appropriately enough, the Secret Academy. In 1603, the Academy of the Lynxes was founded along similar lines in Rome. Thirty-two years later, Cardinal Richelieu

(1585–1642) founded the Académie Française. In 1660, the Oxford Philosophical Society of England opened its first journal book, and two years later Charles II (1630–1685) bestowed its charter as the Royal Society of London. In 1665, Jean-Baptiste Colbert (1619–1683) founded the French Academy of Sciences, and in 1683, the Dublin Philosophical Society came into being. These societies provided invaluable vehicles for transferring scientific knowledge across national borders. The idea survives today in the many societies and professional associations to which scholars, scientists, and other academics routinely belong.

The second stimulus to developing and communicating scientific knowledge was the introduction of periodical literature on a wide scale. First in the form of newspapers, then political tracts, and finally professional journals, these periodicals provided important channels for publishing research results and engendering learned debate. The *French Journal of Medicine* was first published in 1681. The first English medical journal was the *Medicina Curiosa* published in 1684, followed by *Progress in Medicine* in 1695.

The seventeenth century saw the establishment of national medicine in Russia and the United States. In the sixteenth century, Ivan III of Russia (1468–1505) had invited foreign physicians to settle in Moscow, a tradition continued to the end of the Romanov Dynasty in 1917. Both Peter the Great (1672–1725) and Catherine the Great (1729–1796) increased the number of foreign physicians hired. In many ways these foreigners had similar experiences to the Greek physicians in ancient Rome; they were skilled by comparison to Russian folk medicine, but the government and people always regarded them suspiciously for their strange ways. The first native Russian physician was Peter V. Postnikoff, whom Czar Peter sent to study in Padua in 1694.[7]

With regard to Russian military medicine, the first mention of a physician attached to the army appears in 1615. It seems to have been prior common practice for the state to provide money for barber-surgeons to care for the troops during wartime. In the second half of the century, the first regimental dispensaries appeared. Under Peter the Great, the Ministry of Medical Affairs became a chancellery, and the need to provide medical care to his army stimulated Peter's efforts to attract foreign medical talent. By the end of Peter's reign (1725), Russian military medical care was probably on a par with the rest of Europe, and a royal edict assigned each division of the army a physician, a staff barber, and an apothecary. A surgeon was assigned to each regiment and a field barber to each company. As with the armies of the other nations of Europe, the Russian armies also used field hospitals behind the lines. There is no mention in contemporary literature, however, of any provision for the long-term care of the wounded or disabled.[8]

The early settlement of the United States led to the creation of another national medical establishment. Although two doctors, Samuel Fuller and John Winthrop, were among the party on the *Mayflower* in 1620, and the establishment of Harvard College (1636) and the College of William and Mary (1693) gave further impetus to medical training in the early days, Americans traditionally studied abroad at European medical schools. The greatest number of American doctors during the colonial period, however, was trained through apprenticeship programs. Lacking a strong medical establishment made such an innovation possible. Further, the frontier nature of the early American society produced sufficient barriers to education and communication such that on-the-job training and experience were the rule for training physicians. Few of these medical apprentices were encumbered by theoretical knowledge, so similar to the education of the wound surgeons of the Renaissance, observation and experience became the primary emphasis of American medical education. This highly pragmatic emphasis, moreover, distinguishes American medicine to this day. The long-standing conflict between the physician and surgeon that crippled the development of European surgery for more than four centuries never developed in the United States. Meanwhile, in 1663, the first hospital was constructed on Manhattan Island.

Dynastic and religious rivalries caused constant wars that wracked the seventeenth century. The Thirty Years' War and the English civil wars were among the period's major conflicts. The increased number of firearms used by armies and the advent of the mobile field cannon greatly increased mortality rates in these wars, as did epidemic disease. The chief disease killers of the period were bubonic plague, typhoid, typhus, dysentery, and diphtheria. Horrible epidemics were common. In 1665, the Great Plague of London carried off sixty-nine thousand people. In 1679, the plague killed seventy thousand in Vienna. In 1681, more than eighty thousand fell victim to the disease in Prague, and in the Venetian states as many as half a million died.[9] Nathaniel Hodges (1629–1688) was the first physician to conduct a postmortem inspection of a plague patient.[10]

On military campaigns, typhus, typhoid, and dysentery took a heavy toll. Typhus was so common in eastern Europe that it was called the "Hungarian disease," and so many Germany troops died from it that they called Hungary the "Graveyard of the German Army." This area remained a cesspit of infection for centuries, with yet another outbreak of typhus in 1915 decimating the British and Turkish armies there. Smallpox was pandemic in 1614, and a deadly epidemic broke out in England in 1666. Child mortality was high throughout the period, and it is estimated that as many as half of the English children born during the Restoration died from disease.[11] The period's only medical high points were that leprosy seems to have died out almost completely, and the treatment of syphilis by mercurial fumigation and inunction had slowed the rate of the disease's spread.

TRENDS IN MILITARY MEDICINE

The quality of military medicine in the seventeenth century showed no great advance over that of the Renaissance, in large part owing to the rigid divorce of surgery from medicine that had begun under Galen, was maintained by the Muslims, and then standardized into law and custom by the ecclesiastical interdictions of the Middle Ages. As the rivalry among physicians, surgeons, and barbers continued unabated throughout the new century, the battlefield care of the soldier and the common people remained the province of the few qualified wound surgeons and the usual collection of quacks. The number of competent, trained surgeons was very small, or less than a dozen of any note.[12] Tension in the universities between surgeons and physicians produced generally poor surgical instruction even though dissection and the clinical amphitheater had become regular features in medical education. Unifying the barbers and surgeons into common guilds, however, did nothing to reduce the tension or to raise the general status of surgery.

Much of the new anatomical knowledge had yet to be integrated into the medical profession in any practical way, and most physicians still regarded surgery as dangerous. They generally avoided difficult operations on the grounds of legal liability and potential damage to their reputations and positions. Most armies also maintained the rigid separation of physicians and surgeons, with the physician attending general internal complaints while barbers and wound doctors did field surgery.

The generally low quality of military medicine was evident in the sparse publication of new works on the subject. Given the stimuli of the Thirty Years' War and the English Revolution, one might have expected a greater number of original works on military medicine to have been published; however, for the first fifty years of the century, only eight works on surgery—none of them original or very valuable—and only nine on disease were printed. While in the previous century forty-five books had been published on surgery alone, the seventeenth century saw the publication of only thirty-four. While the production of epidemiological works was also sparse, twenty-eight new works on the subject of diseases in the military, two on diseases associated with ship duty, and ten on particular diseases associated with ground force campaigns appeared.[13] A particularly bright light was the book *Medical Observations in Hungarian Camps* (1606) by Tobias Cober, a physician with the army of Bohemia. After seeing seven years' service in the long war between the Hungarians and Turks, Tober provided the first clinical notice of the relationship between pediculosis in military camps and the outbreak of fever, probably typhus.[14] Meanwhile, the era's low level of military medicine was reflected in the rise to prominence of a new breed of field medical practitioners, the executioners! Some executioners acquired medical reputations based on the knowledge they gained while practicing their trade. The idea was that because executioners knew how to break bones, in some manner they also possessed some ability to set them.[15]

The three noteworthy physicians in wound surgery were men who had seen extensive military service in England and Germany. Perhaps the most important was Wilhelm Fabry (also known as Fabriz von Hilden, or Fabricius, 1560–1624) of Germany, who invented a number of new surgical instruments and advocated amputation above the diseased or damaged part of the limb to ensure the stump would be suitable for prosthesis. Fabry also used a primitive tourniquet in which he twisted a strap around a stick. He described the first army field surgical chest, which was based on that first introduced by Maurice of Nassau in 1612. Another important military surgeon was Matthaeus Purmann (1649–1711), a bold German surgeon who sutured intestines and gained extensive experience with gunshot wounds. His *Fifty Strange and Wonderful Cures for Gunshot Wounds* (1693) demonstrates, however, his belief in the magical curative powers of two common but useless methods of treating gunshot wounds—the "weapons salve" and "sympathetic powder," which were applied to the weapon and not to the wound. The greatest English surgeon of his time, Richard Wiseman (1622–1676) was also a soldier. His book *Several Chirugicall Treatises* (1672) reveals a true medical empiricist who performed amputations, treated gunshot wounds, and provided a compendium of empirical military medical knowledge to future generations.

After all is taken to account, however, the seventeenth century did not produce anyone of Paré's stature in military medicine.[16] Even the most empirically oriented surgeons of the period continued to prescribe compounds that ranged from useless to dangerous and to believe in superstitious and magical cures for all kinds of medical conditions. Whatever advances in medical knowledge had been made during the Renaissance were either forgotten or long in coming into vogue in everyday military medical practice.

For the most part, then, the soldier often received indifferent or poor medical care for his wounds. Valid theories for treating the most common military medical conditions were, at best, in their embryonic stages of development. The combination of poorly trained medical personnel, sporadic systems of casualty servicing in the armies of the day, deadly medical practices, increasingly lethal weaponry, poor diet, and a complete lack of understanding of the causes of disease and illness combined to make the lot of the wounded soldier truly pathetic. Throughout the entire century only one voice, that of Polish knight and soldier Janus Abraham Gehema (1647–1715), cried out against these conditions. A combat soldier with extensive battle experience, Gehema wrote numerous short books on caring for the military wounded. Although he himself was not a physician or surgeon, the titles of his works suggest a keen appreciation of the military medical care of his time. His *The Well Experienced Field Physician* (1684), *The Officer's Well-Arranged Medical Chest* (1688), and *The Sick Soldier* (1690) were all attacks on the contemporary military medical practices as being mostly useless, dangerous, and barbaric.[17] In the spirit of the day, however, he was ignored.

WOUND TREATMENT

The seventeenth century saw the continued evolution in weaponry and tactics that had begun during the Renaissance with the introduction of the first practical firearms. The number of firearms to pikes in infantry units increased enormously. Renaissance armies had armed between 25 and 35 percent of infantry with muskets. Gustavus Adolphus's armies almost doubled the rate of firearms to pikes during the Thirty Years' War. On average, 65 percent of his infantry forces carried muskets, and almost all the cavalry were armed with pistols.[18] Swedish armorers redesigned the long heavy musket with a shooting fork to shorten it and made it lighter to allow quicker firing with better accuracy. The introduction of the paper cartridge with its standard powder load reduced the rate of misfires to practically zero, and the introduction of standard-caliber ammunition both increased the weight of the musket ball and eased supply efforts. Standardized ammunition and powder loads propelled the musket ball at a greater velocity than was possible a century earlier and, as noted previously, resulted in bullets becoming more commonly deformed upon impact, creating more ghastly wounds.

Although a number of fundamental medical discoveries had been made in the previous century, the application of this knowledge to military surgery was marginal at best. Wound surgery remained essentially unchanged from the Renaissance. The doctrine of necessary suppuration, long in vogue and buttressed by the still prevalent belief that gunshot wounds were inherently poisonous, led to the practice of attempting to remove the bullets with probes and extractors and increased the chances of infection. Standard surgical practice was not to close the wound but to widen it, allowing the wound to become infected and drain. Surgeons often placed bits of leather and cloth in a minor wound to bring on infection. Draining infected wounds did not become standard practice until Dominique Larrey, the surgeon in chief of the Napoleonic Armies, helped establish it in the nineteenth century.

Military surgeons, faced with an almost 100 percent rate of infection of battle wounds, fell back on miraculous and spurious treatments to combat a clinical condition that rendered them powerless. Physicians of the day placed great faith in a treatment called "the sympathetic powder," which Kenelm Digby (1603–1665), a former privateer and con man, had introduced. Digby saw an opportunity to cash in on the then current propensity of military physicians to try all sorts of pharmaceutical materials. Digby's sympathetic powder was ostensibly made from "moss scraped from a dead man's skull and mixed with powdered mummy's flesh."[19] It is a measure of the low quality of field surgery of the time that this wound treatment gained wide acceptance. No less a figure than Francis Bacon, who advocated the scientific method, included sympathetic powder in his scientific collection of drugs.

Other cures for gunshot included "the transplantation cure" in which a bit of wood was dipped in the blood or pus of the wound and wedged into a tree. If the sliver of wood took root and grew, it was believed the patient would recover. Most amazing was "weapon's salve," an ointment that was applied to the wounded soldier's weapon in the belief that this process created some "influence from afar" that would cause the wound to heal.[20] These attempts to deal with infected wounds suggest how helpless the military surgeons were when confronted with the clinical challenges that the more accurate and highly powered rifles of the period wrought.

The mystical quality of wound treatments during this period is evident from its materia medica, or what is more appropriately called a "filth pharmacopoeia." Part of the problem was the growth of the apothecary guilds that controlled the distribution of medicinal compounds. In 1607, James I (1566–1625) recognized the apothecaries as a special guild distinct from grocers, and throughout Europe the apothecaries soon built a rich and powerful organization. In 1682, the apothecaries won the exclusive right to supply drugs to the army and navy in England. Like any salesmen, the apothecaries needed merchandise to sell.[21] The result was an explosion in spurious mixtures for which all kinds of miraculous claims were made.

The field medical chests that were routinely supplied to the armies provide an interesting glimpse into the pharmacopoeia of the day. A description of a Bavarian field chest that an artillery unit used in the Turkish campaign of 1688 notes that fully loaded the chest weighed 320 pounds and contained thirty surgical instruments. It also held the following medicinal remedies for the wound surgeon's use: powdered sandalwood, rhubarb, palm juice, spermaceti, mummy dust, scorpion oil, rain worm oil, oil of vipers, angle worms, earwigs, zinc oxide, Vigo's plaster of frog spawn, mercury, human and dog fat, aloes, tartar emetic, sugar of lead, alum, sassafras, and opium.[22] Most of these concoctions were not only useless but also often deadly. Almost all provoked infection when applied to an open wound. One marvels at the poor quality of this pharmacopoeia when compared with what Roman field physicians used more than sixteen hundred years earlier. The seventeenth-century pharmacopoeia is a good example of what happens to medical science when practitioners ignore empirical observation and adopt a method of reasoning in which logical elegance and religious superstition is allowed free rein in determining the nature of medical reality.

The musket's increased power made the protective armor of the Renaissance obsolete; it could no longer protect the soldier from the penetrating power of the musket ball. The increasing national identity of the armies of the period led them to wear regulation field dress to distinguish the combatants from one another amid the smoke on the battlefield. They replaced the steel helmet and body armor with standardized uniforms, shakos, and soft hats, and the helmet did not again become a standard item of military issue until the later years of World War I.[23] This change in military costume also introduced a special uniform for the army surgeon that consisted of a tight-waisted long coat reaching to the knees, the usual stockings, and buckled shoes. The civilian physician also copied the military costume as his professional dress and usually wore a red hat.

For the soldier, the disappearance of the protective helmet proved to be a medical disaster, and the rate of head injuries rose considerably. A black powder musket could indeed fire a ball fast enough to penetrate a steel helmet but only at very close range. A musket ball produced approximately 350 foot-pounds of energy upon impact, and the amount of impact energy required to penetrate a steel helmet is approximately 300 foot-pounds. The impact energy of a musket ball, however, dissipates quickly after the first forty yards and then drops off exponentially. At a hundred yards, the impact energy is far less than that required to penetrate a steel helmet.[24] Without the helmet, though, only 90 foot-pounds of energy are required to penetrate the human skull.[25] The impact energy of a musket ball at even two hundred yards is easily enough to penetrate an unprotected skull but insufficient at that range to penetrate a helmeted skull. Thus, the increase in both head wounds and lethality resulted far less from technological improvements to the rifle than from abandoning the helmet and body armor.

It would still have been wise to retain the helmet if only for protection against exploding cannon fragments, grenades, and canister, all of which proved lethal to the soldier not wearing a helmet. These fragments usually did not achieve sufficient velocity to penetrate a helmeted skull, and most struck the soldier when much of their velocity was already considerably spent as a consequence of traversing some distance after the burst. Even in modern times, the helmet is designed more to prevent these kinds of secondary penetrations than to stop a direct hit from a rifle bullet. Abandoning the helmet, therefore, greatly increased the soldier's vulnerability to secondary weapons' effects. Once the idea took hold that the helmet was no longer a valuable protective device, however, the search for effective head and body armor was dropped for three centuries.

The increase in head wounds became a major topic of medical literature of the period. Wiseman, the English battle surgeon, devoted large sections of his writings to head wounds, especially penetrating wounds of the skull. As with the Egyptian physicians more than three millennia earlier, the key distinction for Wiseman was whether the projectile had penetrated the dura of the brain. Wiseman's treatment techniques for non-penetrating head wounds—essentially lifting the depressed bone fragments from the surface of the brain—are remarkably similar to the techniques that the Egyptians invented and that the Greek and Roman military physicians used extensively.[26] The surge in head injuries paralleled the introduction of two new surgical instruments—the crown saw and the circular bit, both of which made skull surgery somewhat easier.[27] Not surprising, this period also saw a great rise in trephining to deal with head wounds.

AMPUTATIONS

Gunshot wounds and the tendency of bullets and shell fragments to shatter limbs resulted in a greater willingness on the part of military surgeons to amputate limbs. The almost inevitable onset of infection in bullet wounds and the inability to combat it in any clinically effective manner convinced surgeons that the best way to treat wounds to the limbs was amputation. The result was an enormous increase in field amputations, no doubt many of them performed unnecessarily. Lopping off limbs under primitive conditions led to thousands of deaths caused by shock and bleeding. Lacking facilities for the soldier's long-term care, the cities and towns of Europe teemed with thousands of crippled and maimed war survivors. The number of crippled soldiers reduced to beggary became such a public problem in France that Louis XIV (1638–1715) issued an edict making begging a crime punishable by death. He had gibbets erected throughout the realm to give credence to the edict.

Although surgeons practiced amputation more frequently in the seventeenth century, they developed little improved technical knowledge or techniques. In most respects, they performed amputations under more difficult medical circumstances than ever. Military surgeries were usually makeshift arrangements with operations performed in barns, tents, or ruined buildings, where elementary concepts of cleanliness were absent. Stench, filth, and decay were common characteristics of these field hospitals. The operating tables became cesspits of infection, and surgeons routinely used the same instruments in several operations after giving them only a slight rinse in a basin of cold water. Leather suture material was also a source of infection. Wounds were left unstitched to allow for early suppuration, and a piece of sponge or lint was inserted into the wound to encourage infection. After amputation surgery, a patient usually ran a high fever while the wound ran with puss. In most cases, the stump was not suitable for prosthesis.[28]

Among the more disastrous and barbaric practices in amputation was the continued use of the cautery, or what Wiseman called the "Royal Styptic." Paré's innovative technique of ligature to control bleeding was not practiced under field conditions. The reason was that amputation required the use of several assistants (whom the physicians commonly called "servants") to aid in the operation. Some held the patient down, others passed instruments to the surgeon, and still others held lamps and candles so the surgeon could see what he was doing. One military surgeon of the day noted that an arm amputation required at least four assistants, including one to offer the patient pain-relieving cordials. Not only were these assistants often in critically short supply, but also there was never enough light in the indoor field hospitals to tie off the crucial blood vessels when attempting ligature.[29] Wiseman, himself a military surgeon in the English Civil Wars, was well acquainted with Paré's ligature technique, but he did not use it because "it required too much light and too many assistants to be ordinarily used in battles on sea and land."[30] Paré's favorite pupil and biographer, Jacques Guillemeau (1550-1613), even gave up the use of ligature in amputations because of the difficulties involved.[31]

Thus overburdened military surgeons greatly relied upon cautery simply because it was more convenient, did not require as many assistants, and did not need much light. The military surgeon Hughes Ravaton (1719–1785) noted that in an average day's work in battle, a surgeon assigned to a twenty-thousand-man force saw two thousand wounded requiring medical attention. This case load was handled by one surgeon, ten surgical aides, and thirty students of surgery to hold lamps and do other chores.[32] As in the Middle Ages, the surgeon administered anesthesia, when used at all, by allowing the patient to breathe a sponge or cloth soaked in a mixture of opium, hyoscyamus, and belladonna.

Most amputations were performed below the knee. The fact that a thigh amputation required fifty-three separate ligatures militated against attempting them.[33] Ligature could only become an acceptable technique for thigh amputations once some method was found to stop the flow of blood in the femoral artery. Some surgeons occasionally attempted thigh amputations, however, with William Clowes (1540–1604) performing one in 1588 and Fabry in 1614. Fabry is generally credited with introducing a primitive form of tourniquet to military surgery when he placed a block of wood under the bandage encircling the limb. Etienne Morel also used a block tourniquet at the siege of Besançon in 1674. As noted in chapter 2, Jean-Louis Petit invented the modern form of the screw tourniquet, but its widespread use was not adopted until the eighteenth century.[34]

FIELD HYGIENE

Military hygiene improved little from the Renaissance period, as a cogent theory of disease transmission continued to elude medical thinkers. While most armies had some primitive hygienic ordinances, few practiced them with any degree of consistency. Disease continued to kill more men than bullets did, a condition that remained unchanged for another three centuries. Disease and sickness were regarded as a normal part of military operations. The English commander of the garrison at

Tangier noted in 1660 that his men had been decimated by disease and that "1200 men will not produce 800 duty men."[35] A sickness rate of 33 percent appeared to be normal.

Few commanders took an interest in camp hygiene. An exception was the Duke of Marlborough (1650–1722), who issued regulations governing the use of water supplies and required camp butchers to bury their offal daily. Animals' and men's quarters were inspected daily, as were the cookhouses and food supplies. Marlborough required that a medical officer accompany the provost marshal on daily inspections. Latrines were filled in and moved every six days, dead animals buried immediately, and anyone found committing "casual disorders" (urinating or defecating) around the camp was liable for severe punishment.[36]

If conditions in a military camp were often primitive and filthy, they were almost always better than conditions found aboard ships. The unhealthy living conditions of sailors had changed little since the days of the Spanish Armada (1588). One commentator described the conditions aboard English ships as "the pox above board, the plague between decks, hell in the forecastle, and the devil at the helm."[37]

MILITARY HOSPITALS

The seventeenth century saw the nationalism of the last two centuries emerge full blown into the national armies of the nation states. Among the most important were France, Sweden, Brandenburg-Prussia, Switzerland, and England. The development of military medical care varied greatly from army to army and conflict to conflict as the century progressed. While the provision of medical care for the soldier had not yet become a recognized and routine function of government, this period saw the beginnings of a movement in this direction. As soldiers were asked to serve in wars on grounds of national identity and loyalty, inevitably governments would come to recognize some responsibility for treating and caring for the sick and wounded as a reciprocal obligation of military service. Staffing armies with surgeons, physicians, and field barbers became a regular practice, but the military establishment had yet to employ professional military surgeons continually. As in earlier times, the shortage of trained medical personnel forced armies to issue orders of impressment to obtain any medical resources at all. In 1628, Charles I (1600–1628) issued such an edict. Apart from the usual collection of barbers and field surgeons, the female camp followers, who routinely accompanied the army, still provided most nursing and long-term care to the soldier.

The period's most advanced system of military medical care available was in the armies of France. The ambulance hospitals that Maximilien, the Duke of Sully (1560–1641), established at the siege of Amiens in 1597 were the starting point for later French monarchs to try and improve the medical care of the soldier. In the first third of the century in France, as elsewhere, no stationary military hospitals were behind the lines of the field armies. Medical care was rendered in mobile field hospitals that moved with the armies. The hundreds of wounded, sick, and crippled men left behind crowded into the civilian hospitals of the towns and cities; consequently, government efforts on improving the soldier's lot focused on the treatment of the disabled.[38]

As noted in chapter 2, Henry IV of France (1553–1610) opened to disabled soldiers the Maison de la Charité Chrétienne, where they received room and board. Shortly thereafter, the privilege was extended to the widows and children of soldiers killed in battle. Louis XIII (1611–1643) allowed this arrangement to atrophy and reestablished the *droit d'oblat* system of the previous century in which disabled soldiers were assigned to monasteries as lay brothers and earned their keep by doing menial chores. Under Louis XIV, the French established a pension system and raised special taxes to care for the sick and disabled soldiery. The soldiers often exhausted their pension money in the first few months and spent the rest of the year begging in the streets. Thus the system was abandoned, and in 1674 the Hôtel National des Invalides was opened to care for the disabled. The facility housed four thousand people, who slept three to a bed. Although basically a warehouse, the soldiers nonetheless received shoes, clothes, food, and a small sum of expense money. Military discipline was maintained, and those who were able were encouraged to work in the workshops. Patients were permitted to take leave and visit their families, and some of the more able were even assigned to military garrison duty at half pay. While care of the military's disabled had been under control of ecclesiastical authorities since the Middle Ages, in France, the system of veterans' hospitals was placed in the hands of an intendant, a government official who reported directly to the minister of war.[39] It was the first clear example of a nation state recognizing its responsibility for the long-term welfare of the soldier.

As social care for the French soldier improved, so did his medical care. In 1627 at the siege of La Rochelle, Cardinal Richelieu assigned Jesuits and cooks to provide bread and soup at the state's expense to the sick and wounded in the field hospitals.

Two years later, Richelieu established the first permanent stationary hospitals in the rear of the field armies.[40] Generally of poor construction, however, these hospitals were little more than spacious halls in which patients slept three to a bed in squalid conditions. These facilities became nests of infection, filth, and death, and contributed greatly to the average soldier's general fear of hospitals. These hospitals' construction and conditions improved over time, and by the end of Louis's reign permanent military hospitals had been built at Arras, Calais, Dunkirk, and Perpignan. From 1666, the famous French fortification engineer Sébastien le Prestre, Marquis de Vauban (1633–1707), routinely provided space and buildings for a military hospital in all the towns for which he planned fortifications.[41]

The French practice of caring for the wounded and disabled was imitated in England. In 1614, Sir Thomas Coningsby (died 1625) founded a relief house for destitute soldiers. During the Protectorate (1653–1659), the English Parliament provided homes and pensions for the disabled who had fought on the Republican side but did not make any provisions for those who fought on the Royalist side. In 1633, a house for disabled seamen was erected at Chelsea, in 1693 a soldiers' home was built in Kilmainham, and a "benevolent institution" was established in Greenwich for destitute sailors in 1695.[42]

The permanent hospital system offered some employment opportunities for medical practitioners with military experience, and in the French armies the provision of combat medical support seemed to improve as the century wore on. While the quality of field medical support remained low, supplying surgeons and barbers to the armies seems to have become routine. In 1674 at the Battle of Seneffe, the French Army's medical chief was able to furnish 230 surgeons assisted by nurses in three field hospitals located in nearby villages. Each of the field stations was adequately equipped with medical supplies as well.[43]

The Swedish Army of Gustavus Adolphus was fairly well equipped with medical personnel thanks largely to the vision of a previous Swedish king, Gustavus Vassa (1496–1560), who first organized the barbers' guild and extracted a pledge from them to tend the troops in time of war. Under Adolphus, the normal medical complement of two surgeons and barbers per regiment was increased to four, and medical support and supply was made a command responsibility. Civilian hospitals were exempt from pillage, and one-tenth of the spoils of war were set aside for the troops in the hospital. Adolphus made it practice to transport the sick and wounded in wagons to the nearest hospital and to leave medical and command detachments behind with the wounded to oversee their care. He began the convention of gathering the enemy wounded to his camp, where they received medical care or were sent to hospitals with his own wounded. At the siege of Dömitz in 1631, the Swedes provided wagons to transport the enemy wounded to hospitals. Upon recovery, they were granted free passes to return to their units. Adolphus's treatment of the men—his own men and that of the enemy—represented a continuation of the Renaissance practice of attending the wounded in a humane manner.[44]

Switzerland, it will be recalled, had the oldest military medical service in Europe. By the Thirty Years' War, Swiss arms had sunk to a low level. The military medical service, however, endured. Muster rolls of various Swiss cantons during the war show that each company of artillery and infantry had a barber-surgeon attached to it at the state's expense. They also had regimental barber-surgeons, and those from the Zurich regiment were the best-trained surgeons in the city. Military physicians received complete medical chests supplied to them at state expense and field manuals on wound management and sanitation. Still, the Swiss military medical system does not appear to have improved much from the previous century when it was the model of European armies.[45] Meanwhile, it had taken the rest of Europe almost a century to catch up.

The field hospitals of the Landsknechte in Germany became the first permanent field hospitals when, in 1620, Maximilian I, Duke of Bavaria (1573–1651), founded field hospitals for the armies of the Catholic League. One of these massive multistoried hospitals served as a clearing station and fed casualties into a larger hospital located in a nearby town. In 1689, Konrad Behrens (1660–1736) drew up a set of regulations for these hospitals, which were situated on high ground near good water supplies and woods from which the staff could obtain firewood for heat and cooking. Patients were segregated by disease into separate wards. The staff consisted of physicians, field barbers, wound surgeons and their attendants, priests, and female camp followers. An officer supervised each entire hospital. In 1685, one of these hospitals handled eight hundred sick and wounded daily. Medical care, as in every army of the period, however, was still rudimentary.[46]

In the armies of Prussia, every regiment had a barber, and every company of infantry and cavalry had a field barber. When in garrison, a physician looked after the troops' sick complaints while a wound surgeon dealt with their injuries. Because of the devastation wrought by the Thirty Years' War, the training of German field surgeons and barbers seems to have been of particularly low quality. Although regulations required military commanders to provide wagons and clean straw to transport the wounded, the Prussian armies had neither field nor permanent hospitals and simply treated the wounded in their barracks.

The English Civil Wars (1642–1651) retarded the development of military medical structures of any sophistication and scope. Oliver Cromwell (1599–1658) did provide his New Model Army with medical officers in 1645, and P. B. Adamson writes that he was the first English commander to assign such officers to the standing army on a permanent basis.[47] By 1700, field medical chests were provided to the military medical service as items of regular issue.[48]

Military medical care during the seventeenth century was not appreciably better than that provided to the soldier during the Renaissance. Although the new nation states took the first tentative steps in recognizing an obligation to care for the wounded and disabled of war, no nation developed a system approaching even rudimentary effectiveness in accomplishing this task. The almost-two-hundred-year-old regulations of the Swiss Army were still more advanced in providing this type of care than anything developed or even contemplated in the seventeenth century. Medical care in the field remained elementary at best and lethal at worst. Separating surgery from the general practice of medicine made it impossible to develop a corps of adequately trained surgeons for the military's use; thus, most of the practitioners who treated the common soldier possessed little medical skills. The soldier was still at as great a risk from his own medical officers as from enemy bullets and perhaps more so.

In some ways medical care actually deteriorated. The increased use of firearms, their greater killing power, their higher rates of fire, and the abandonment of body armor and helmets in favor of standardized field dress exposed the soldier to a much greater risk of death and injury than he had faced a century earlier. A number of advances in medical knowledge and surgical technique, most notably ligature in amputation, were ignored in practice; consequently, the rate of amputations, infections, and resulting death increased. The provision of long-term care in permanent military hospitals did little to aid the wounded's recovery as the hospitals' filthy conditions raised the chances of incurring infection. As it had been for so many centuries, the combat soldier of the seventeenth century remained at great risk to life and limb. That some of the armies provided him with subsistence care if he was disabled did not go far to change this basic fact of military life.

NOTES

1. Garrison, *Introduction to the History*, 245–309. See the chapter on the development of medicine in the seventeenth century.
2. Ibid.
3. Ibid.
4. J. R. Kirkup, "The History and Evolution of Surgical Instruments," *Annals of the Royal College of Surgeons of England* 63 (1981): 283.
5. Ibid.
6. Garrison, *Introduction to the History*, 283.
7. Garrison, *Notes on the History*, 127.
8. Ibid.
9. Ibid., 130.
10. *Encyclopedia Britannica*, 11th ed. (1910), 49.
11. Garrison, *Introduction to the History*, 307.
12. Heizmann, "Military Sanitation," 294.
13. Ibid.
14. Garrison, *Notes on the History*, 130.
15. Jay W. Grissinger, "The Development of Military Medicine," *New York Academy of Medicine* 3, no. 5 (May 1927): 316. A common form of capital punishment at this time was "to be broken on the wheel," where the victim was strapped to a large wheel that was then rotated until his bones were broken.
16. Garrison, *Introduction to the History*, 275–77.
17. Garrison, *Notes on the History*, 133–34.
18. Heizmann, "Military Sanitation," 292.
19. Forrest, "Development of Wound Therapy," 270.
20. Grissinger, "Development of Military Medicine," 316.
21. Roderick E. McGrew, *Encyclopedia of Medical History* (New York: McGraw-Hill, 1985), 253–54.
22. Ibid., 315.
23. Frank Aker, Dawn Schroeder, and Robert Baycar, "Cause and Prevention of Maxillofacial War Wounds: A Historical Review," *Military Medicine* 148, no. 12 (December 1983): 923.
24. I am indebted to Edward Cielecki and Tom Tremonte, experts in the ballistics of black powder weapons, for these figures.
25. Richard A. Gabriel and Karen S. Metz, *From Sumer to Rome: The Military Capabilities of Ancient Armies* (Westport, CT: Greenwood Press, 1991), 63.
26. Charles G. H. West, "A Short History of the Management of Penetrating Missile Injuries to the Head," *Surgical Neurology* 16, no. 2 (August 1981): 146.
27. D. S. Gordon, "Penetrating Head Injuries," *Ulster Medical Journal* 57, no. 1 (April 1988): 3.
28. Allen C. Wooden, "The Wounds and Weapons of the Revolutionary War from 1775 to 1783," *Delaware Medical Journal* 44, no. 3 (March 1972): 61–62.
29. Owen H. Wangensteen, Jacqueline Smith, and Sarah D. Wangensteen, "Some Highlights in the History of Amputation Reflecting Lessons in Wound Healing," *Bulletin of the History of Medicine* 41, no. 2 (March–April 1967): 102.
30. James Young, "A Short History of English Military Surgery and Some Famous Military Surgeons," *Journal of the Royal Army Medical Corps* 21 (1913): 487.
31. Wangensteen et al., "Some Highlights," 103.

32. Ibid.
33. McGrew, *Encyclopedia of Medical History*, 322.
34. Ibid. See also *Encyclopedia Britannica*, 11th ed. (1911), 128; and Robert Lawson, "Amputations through the Ages," *Australian–New Zealand Journal of Surgery* 42, no. 3 (February 1973): 222.
35. Hargreaves, "The Long Road to Military Hygiene," 441.
36. Ibid.
37. Ibid.
38. Garrison, *Notes on the History*, 121–22.
39. Taylor, "Retrospect of Naval and Military Medicine," 589.
40. Grissinger, "Development of Military Medicine," 316.
41. Ibid.
42. Taylor, "Retrospect of Naval and Military Medicine," 317.
43. Heizmann, "Military Sanitation," 291.
44. Ibid., 291–93.
45. Garrison, *Notes on the History*, 124–25.
46. Ibid., 131.
47. P. B. Adamson, "The Military Surgeon: His Place in History," *Journal of the Royal Army Medical Corps* 128 (1982): 47.
48. Weston P. Chamberlain, "History of Military Medicine and Its Contributions to Science," *Boston Medical and Surgical Journal* (April 1917): 237.

4

THE EIGHTEENTH CENTURY

The First Effective Military Medical Systems

Medicine in the eighteenth century centered around the effort to develop complete theoretical systems to explain disease and other medical phenomena. This approach was the logical consequence of the nascent empiricism that had emerged two centuries earlier during the Renaissance and had been given strong scientific impetus by the success of Newtonian inductionist approaches to understanding and explaining reality characteristic of the previous century. Medical investigators attempted to systematize medical knowledge along the lines of a single major force or cause that could be demonstrated to rest at the base of all medical phenomena. Medical investigation was attempting to do for medicine what Newton had done for physics and what Thomas Hobbes (1588–1679) had claimed to do for politics.

Searching for underlying unifying principles of medical knowledge, a kind of grand theory of synthesis, helped inform Herman Boerhaave (1668–1738). This great Dutch physician and teacher explained all pathological conditions in terms of chemical and physical qualities, such as acidity and alkalinity or tension and relaxation.[1] William Cullen (1710–1790), a Scottish physician whose thinking had a major impact on American medicine at the time, believed that disease could be explained by either an excess or an insufficiency of nervous tension in the nerve pathways of the body and brain.[2] Others argued for varying degrees of animism or excitation in the body's organs. Few of these approaches produced anything of lasting medical value, for the complexity of medical phenomena repeatedly confronted these theoretical schemas with observations that could not be explained by their premises. Nonetheless, the search for the grand medical synthesis continued throughout the century.

The search for theoretical explanations did not hinder the development of an empirical approach to medical research. Indeed, it was precisely the establishment of the empirical method that forced medical theoreticians to continually reexamine their premises as observations time and again produced discoveries that could not be reconciled with theoretical approaches. The empiricism of the Renaissance combined with the rigorous thinking of Newtonian inductionism to produce a method of medical investigation that was soundly grounded in empirical observation. Unlike the scholastic approach to medicine that had characterized the search for knowledge during the Middle Ages, an approach that for centuries permitted empirical data to be rejected on the grounds that it did not satisfy the elegance of logic, the new method did not end in the mind. The willingness of eighteenth-century physicians to attempt to integrate new medical data into mental schemata prevented the development of a complete single-cause theory of medicine from gaining acceptance precisely because such theories did not square with empirical observation. The tyranny of scholastic logic finally came to an end and in its place arose the new methods of empirical observation and experiment. In this sense, the eighteenth century can be said to have laid the methodological groundwork for the progress in medical knowledge and clinical technique that was to follow in the next two centuries.

An individualistic approach to medical investigation had marked the previous century. Much of this trend continued in the eighteenth century and produced a number of important discoveries and surgical advances. The end of the religious and dynastic wars provided some breathing space within which the medical establishment continued its work. The period of peace, interrupted nonetheless by four major wars and three revolutions, also permitted some stability to permeate the social order of the day.[3] As a result, the medical profession became institutionalized and medicine became a respected profession with practices passed from father to son. University education for physicians became commonplace. Dissection became a common method of medical study, as did clinical observation in teaching hospitals. Famous professors established a number of private medical schools and gathered students to their practices as a means of providing medical education. The most noteworthy of these students was Scottish-born John Hunter (1728–1793) in England and three generations of Monros in Scotland. Eventually, both schools became associated with universities, bestowing greater prestige on the study of medical pragmatics than ever before. For the first time in history, medicine was separated from superstition and ecclesiastical control, and the foundations of medicine as a science came into being.

In an equally important development, surgery finally became a legitimate discipline, respected even by the physician internists, and slowly began to develop its own teaching institutions. In 1731, the Académie Royale de Chirurgie (Royal Academy of Surgery) was established in Paris with Jean-Louis Petit as its first director. Later, the École Pratique de Chirurgie was established with François Chopart (1743–1795) and Pierre-Joseph Desault (1738–1795) as its first professors. The press of war placed a premium on training surgeons for the army, and for the first time military medical schools were established in Prussia, Russia, Austria, and France to meet the armies' needs for surgical personnel. Greatly aiding these developments were significant improvements in surgical medicine as a consequence of the renewed empirical emphasis on anatomy and pathology. The greatest of the anatomist-pathologists was Giovanni Morgagni (1682–1771), who pioneered the science of postmortem investigation in an effort to link diseases to their specific anatomical effects. Morgagni was the first writer of a systematic treatise on morbid anatomy. The brilliant surgeons of the day, Hunter and Alexander Monro I (1697–1767), had begun their careers as anatomists, which helped them develop effective surgical techniques that gained wide acceptance. From this point forward, medical education began with studies of human anatomy, and for the first time in history, anatomical knowledge was generally accurate.

Surgery ceased to be merely a technical craft practiced by physicians of low status. Of course, the usual collection of barbers and quacks continued to exist, mostly in the armies, but gradually even their quality began to improve. The military's need for surgical personnel led to regular examinations for candidates for surgeon's mates and orderlies, and some countries provided medical training in special schools to even the lowest ranks of military surgical personnel. The millennia-old distinction between physician and surgeon, a distinction that had hindered medical progress for a thousand years, was gradually disappearing, with overall beneficial results for the civilian and the soldier alike.

Medical publishing was established on a large scale, and books and periodicals were readily available to the professional order as vehicles for expanding and spreading medical knowledge. Anatomical illustration reached great heights. The old copperplate method gave way to the steel plate and made producing anatomical illustrations in color possible for the first time.[4] The advances in surgery also were evident in the proliferation of new surgical instruments designed for specific purposes. Pierre Dionis (1643–1718) published the *Cours d'opérations de chirurgie* in 1708 and presented complete sets of surgical instruments specific to particular operations. In

1782, Giovanni Alessandro Brambilla (1728–1800) assembled a folio of virtually all surgical equipment in his *Instrumentarium Chirurgicum militare Austriacum.*[5] Near the end of the century, the numbers and types of surgical instruments had become so complex that the first catalogs for surgical instruments were published.

The eighteenth century can be characterized as the time when medicine first became a science complete with a new empirical approach that emphasized hard data. There emerged a new intellectual habit, first evident in the Renaissance, and a willingness to reject theoretical premises when they were shown to run contrary to clinical observation. The emphasis on anatomy gave physicians and surgeons more accurate medical knowledge, and the erosion of the social barriers between physician and surgeon finally permitted the latter to represent a legitimate branch of the medical discipline. Formalizing medical education permitted the transmission of accurate anatomy and new techniques to fresh generations of students in a more systematic and complete manner than ever before. Moreover, the stimulus of war forced the contemporary military establishments to pay greater attention to the soldier's medical needs. More than in any century that preceded it, the eighteenth century witnessed the beginnings of truly modern medicine in both its civilian and military aspects.

TRENDS IN MILITARY MEDICINE

In the eighteenth century, the state government recognized its function of providing medical care for its soldiers and provided and paid for it as a matter of course. At the beginning of the century, the pattern of military medical care remained essentially as it had been in the previous century. By mid-century, however, all major armies of the period had moved considerably toward establishing institutionalized systems of military medical care.

This achievement was part of the nation states' larger effort to improve the general quality and organization of their armies as the age of nationalism came to fruition. Armies encouraged voluntary enlistments, adopted limited periods of military service to replace the old practice of lifelong service, implemented regular medical examinations for recruits, issued standard uniforms, provided daily food rations that were paid for by the state treasury, and housed their soldiers in barracks instead of the usual inns, private houses, and barns. Military organizations generally became more structurally articulated as the century wore on, and permanent ranks, pay systems, and combat formations appeared. Armies were almost exclusively armed with firearms, and field artillery became more mobile. The first military medical schools were established, as were the first journals and periodicals devoted exclusively to military medical matters with articles written almost entirely by military physicians, surgeons, and medical officers. Advances in hospital administration were made, and some attempts were also made to prevent disease and generally improve and maintain the soldier's health.

Armies became structurally organized into companies, battalions, and regiments with an increasingly professional corps of officers and noncommissioned officers to lead them. In their organizational realignment to increase control of the armies, the leadership put the troops in barracks and gave them regular rations. The old practice of billeting the troops with the citizenry or in rented inns had become increasingly unpopular, and the new system made controlling desertion easier.[6] The British Army established its first barracks in Ireland in 1713. Barracks were introduced in Scotland two years later, and George I (1660–1727) constructed the first military barracks in England at Berwick-on-Tweed in 1723.[7]

The introduction of voluntary enlistments proved attractive mostly to the urban poor and surplus landless population that had manned armies for centuries. No longer driven by the cudgel or impressment, these social elements were attracted by the prospect of regular food and pay. The health of these recruits, however, proved to be as generally poor as it had historically been. In times of social disruption or difficult economic times, recruits flooded the recruitment stations, and large numbers of marginally healthy adults with poor sanitary habits entered military service. The huge losses to disease in the wars of the period led military officials to launch regular physical examinations for recruits. For the first quarter century, however, the unit or regimental commander conducted only cursory examinations of recruits. Beginning in 1726, the French Army instituted regular medical examinations. After 1763, each recruit regiment had a surgeon whose duty was to examine recruits for physical fitness and weed out those whose health failed during the training process. In France, an inspector general of recruiting was appointed in 1778 and charged with the task of overseeing the selection and health of new troops. Mandatory medical examinations were not instituted in the British Army until 1790. Prussia, meanwhile, had required regimental and battalion medical officers to conduct regular physical examinations of all soldiers since 1788.[8]

France was the first country to institute uniform clothing as early as the 1670s.[9] English regulation military dress was mandated in 1751, following similar regulations by Frederick Wilhelm of Prussia (1688–1740) a few years earlier.[10] As noted in chapter 3, the purpose of uniform clothing was to facilitate identifying friendly units on the smoky battlefield, but the leadership gave little thought to the effects of this clothing on the health and endurance of the soldier. Uniforms were most often made of cheap cotton that provided little warmth in cold climates and no protection from the rain. Tight stockings often restricted circulation and had no padding for the leather buckle shoes, which offered little defense against frostbite or trench foot. Adorning the uniform with tight buttons and belts often restricted the soldier's breathing, and with high crowns, the heavy shakos and hats added to the soldiers' load but did not prevent head wounds from enemy shell fragments and bullets. It would be at least another two centuries before anyone seriously considered designing a uniform for battlefield use while taking the health, comfort, and protective needs of the soldier into consideration.[11]

The standard military ration, meanwhile, did much to improve the soldier's general health, and most soldiers ate better and more regularly in military messes than they had in civilian life.[12] Rations were provided by a central commissary and at government expense as a matter of right.[13] In France, the soldier's daily allowance was twenty-four ounces of wheat bread, one pound of meat, and one pint of wine or two pints of beer. Frederick the Great provided his soldiers with two pounds of bread daily and two pounds of meat a week.[14] Unfortunately, the promise of regular, good-quality food was more often broken than honored. All European armies relied on a supply system in which commissary officers contracted with provisioners, sutlers, and transporters for supplies. This arrangement led to common abuses of fraud and theft, and the pressure to keep expenditures down often reduced food for the troops to less than sufficient quantities or quality.

Before examining the improvements in military surgery, it is worth exploring the casualty burdens that the medical establishments of armies under fire encountered. By the eighteenth century, the armies were universally equipped with more accurate and deadly firearms, and the introduction of truly mobile artillery of increased ranges had the inevitable effect of greatly increasing casualties. Even in the early part of the century, these innovations had an enormous impact on casualty rates. For example, during the War of the Spanish Succession (1701–1714), the allied armies at the Battle of Blenheim in 1704 suffered 5,000 dead and 8,900 wounded. British forces alone endured 670 dead and 1,500 wounded, while the Bavarian armies suffered 12,000 dead and 14,000 wounded. Two years later at Ramillies, the French lost 2,000 dead and 5,000 wounded. It was not unusual during this period for armies to suffer similar casualty rates, with the usual effect of overwhelming the primitive field medical establishments of the day.

In this era, military medical surgery improved markedly and introduced a number of new techniques. Some of the old wound treatments—such as sympathetic powder and wound salve, mainstays of the previous century—disappeared, giving rise to the more extensive use of styptics to stop minor bleeding. Pressure sponges, alcohol, and turpentine came into widespread use for minor wounds. Military surgeons still cauterized arteries, but less frequently, as they widely began to use the new locked forceps as ligatures. They increasingly applied Petit's screw tourniquet, which made thigh amputations possible and greatly reduced the risk associated with amputations above the knee. Military surgeons placed greater emphasis on preparing limbs for prosthesis, and flap and lateral incision amputations became common.

Although more surgeons questioned the need for the inevitable suppuration of wounds, many still provoked infection by inserting charpie and other foreign matter into wounds. While they continued to use the old oils and salve dressings for wounds, the new technique of applying dry bandages moistened only with water held much practical promise. That many of the old chemical and salve treatments endured is not surprising, since doctors often prepared and sold these potions themselves at considerable profit. The practice of enlarging and probing battle wounds continued unabated, but the new debridement treatment was gaining acceptance as an alternative procedure. Despite a literature that established clinical circumstances and guidelines for carrying out the procedure, the improvements in amputation surgery inevitably provoked a spate of unnecessary operations that continued for many years. Yet, without doubt, military surgery was improving at a rapid pace as military surgeons learned new and improved techniques of wound treatment.

John Hunter is generally credited with the first real improvements in understanding the nature of wound treatment. He began his career as an anatomist, only later becoming a surgeon. His training in linking anatomy to clinical signs of pathology served him well. He accepted a commission in the middle of the Seven Years' War (1756–1763) with France and gained valuable surgical experience at the Battle of Belle Île (1761). Afterward he argued against the normal practice of enlarging gunshot wounds and against bloodletting, pushing instead for a conservative approach to treating gunshot wounds. In 1794, he published his *Treatise of the Blood, Inflammation, and Gunshot Wounds*, which is regarded as a major milestone in the surgical treatment of battle wounds.

Pierre-Joseph Desault coined the term "débridement" and recommended not enlarging wounds as common practice. His new technique recommended cutting away only the necrotic tissue within the wound to remove a source of infection. Desault was the first to use the technique for traumatic wounds.[15]

For decades bullet wounds to the head had produced great risk of infection. Because doctors believed that blood that accumulated in the extradural or subdural spaces would eventually become pus, they allowed it to remain as a seat of infection. The military surgeon Percival Pott (1713–1788) was the first to argue against this practice, suggesting that this residual blood could be extracted by cranial draining. His contribution is often cited as a major advance in cranial surgery.[16] For decades surgeons commonly operated on all head wounds with experimental trephination. Many of these operations were unnecessary and exposed the patient to great risk of infection. Near the end of the century, Sylvester O'Halloran (1728–1807), an Irish surgeon, demonstrated that experimental trephination was usually not needed. Within a decade, the practice generally came to an end. O'Halloran was also the first to improve the treatment of penetrating head wounds by regularly utilizing debridement.[17]

Habits of personal, medical, and surgical cleanliness were still dismal during this period, and the soldier faced a greater risk to his health while in the hospital than on the battlefield. It has been estimated that in the American Revolutionary War (1775–1783), the Continental soldier had ninety-eight chances out of a hundred of escaping death on the battlefield, but once he was hospitalized, his chances of survival after medical treatment and exposure to disease and infection fell to 75 percent.[18] Some surgeons, however, did perceive a relationship between cleanliness and surgical infection. Claude Pouteau (1724–1775) a French surgeon, made cleanliness a requirement in his operating area and achieved the remarkable result of losing only 3 of the 120 lithotomies performed in his surgery to infection. John Pringle (1707–1782), the famous English physician and surgeon, first coined the term "antiseptic" in 1750 and in 1753 published the results of forty-three experiments performed over a three-year period that confirmed the antiseptic value of mineral acids.[19] In 1737 Alexander Monro I claimed to have performed fourteen amputations at his Edinburgh surgery with no hospital mortality. By 1752, he had performed more than a hundred major amputations with a hospital mortality rate of only 8 percent. This achievement was all the more remarkable given that for the next century the mortality rate for hospital surgery was generally between 45 and 65 percent.[20] Monro also had a fetish for cleanliness. Despite overwhelming evidence of the relation between cleanliness and infection, however, the work of surgeons Pringle, Monro, and Edward Alanson (1747–1823) was largely ignored until the next century when Joseph Lister (1827–1912) introduced general antisepsis. One can only guess how many soldiers would have survived their wounds had they not been exposed to infection while recovering in the hospital.

While the eighteenth century saw numerous improvements in the establishment and organization of military hospitals, especially in the introduction of the mobile field hospitals that accompanied the armies on the march, they still offered the unsanitary and dismal-quality care as they had in the previous century. Hospital buildings were often little more than rapidly constructed huts in the field.[21] While every army had a hospital medical organization to provide treatment and administration, they were rarely fully staffed. Moreover, there was a notorious lack of coordination between regimental, field, and general rear area hospitals, especially in the provision of medical supplies. Few armies had any organized and dedicated transport to move the wounded from the front to rear area hospitals, and it was not uncommon for a third of the patients to die en route. No army developed a satisfactory solution for extracting the wounded from the battle line, and troops usually made their way to the medical facilities as best they could. As in the previous century, some armies, notably Prussia's, actually forbade attempts to treat the wounded until the battle had ended. No one seems to have thought of copying the Romans' stationing of combat medics within the battle units themselves.

Disease continued to be the major threat to military manpower despite military physicians' many attempts at preventive medicine. Among Continental soldiers in the American Revolution, disease caused 90 percent of all deaths; among British regulars, the figure was 84 percent.[22] Hughes Ravaton, the French physician, noted in 1768 that one of every hundred soldiers in the French Army would be unfit for duty because of illness at the beginning of a field campaign. Halfway through the campaign, another five or six would drop out of combat because of disease. By the campaign's end, ten to twelve more soldiers would be too ill to fight. By comparison, the death and injury rate from combat fire was approximately one per ten men.[23]

The range of diseases that afflicted the troops had changed little from the previous century. Respiratory illnesses were most often seen in cold weather and dysentery-like conditions in hot climates. Disease diagnosis had not yet become a science, and descriptions of disease from this period cannot be entirely trusted. The common "intermittent" and "remittent" fevers of the day were most probably malaria, a disease widespread in Europe and the colonial dominions. Those conditions called "putrid," "jail," or "hospital fever" were probably typhus or typhoid. Dysentery and other stomach disorders were rampant, often as a consequence of poor field hygiene conditions. Venereal disease was almost epidemic. Pneumonia and pleurisy also presented a common threat. The records of the period also show that scabies was endemic. This infestation caused scratching, which produced serious infections requiring medical treatment. Although not fatal, scabies brought more patients to British Army hospitals during the Seven Years' War than did any other medical condition.[24] Scabies continued to plague armies into modern times. In World War I, scabies or the pyrodermas produced by constant scratching caused 90 percent of the illness for which Allied troops sought hospitalization or field treatment.[25]

Smallpox was among the most debilitating and dangerous diseases that afflicted field armies, with numerous examples of entire campaigns being halted as a consequence of outbreaks. In 1775, Gen. Horatio Gates (1727–1806) had to break off the American Northern Army Command's campaign for five weeks because an outbreak of smallpox sent 5,500 of his 10,000 troops to the hospital.[26] The disease afflicted the civilian population without mercy in multiple epidemics that marked the period.

The prevalence of smallpox in the civilian and military populations drove one of the more important medical advances of the century, inoculation. Credit for introducing smallpox inoculation is generally given to Edward Jenner (1749–1823), but in fact, inoculation against smallpox was already an established practice long before Jenner formalized the method. The practice of using cowpox inoculation to prevent smallpox disease was common in the Ottoman Empire before it was introduced into Europe. Lady Mary Wortley Montague, the wife of the British ambassador to Constantinople, knew of the practice as early as 1718 and had herself and her two children inoculated against the disease.[27] In 1721, a smallpox epidemic broke out in Boston, and Dr. Zabdiel Boylston (1679–1766) used inoculation to prevent its further spread. He inoculated 247 persons with a loss rate of only 2 percent, compared to the usual 15 percent death rate.[28] Jenner's contribution to inoculation seems to have been that he was the first person to conceive of inoculating whole populations against the disease, and he developed the popular support to carry out his idea. Jenner did not perform his first smallpox inoculation until 1796.

The first army to try wholesale inoculation on its soldiers was the American Army. In 1775, noting General Gates's debacle while confronting smallpox, Gen. George Washington (1732–1799) obtained the approval of the Continental Congress to inoculate recruits upon their entering into military service.[29] The program was less than successful, however, and we do not know how many soldiers actually received inoculations. The British Army did not allow inoculation against smallpox until 1798, when the Sick and Wounded Board authorized the procedure at military hospitals for those who wanted it. As the century ended, there was still no mandatory inoculation for British troops.[30] The successful immunization of military forces had to await the next century, when inoculation became more generally accepted. Holland and Prussia were the first countries to require inoculations of all their troops, while the French and English continued to lag behind. In the Franco-Prussian War of 1870–1871, unvaccinated French prisoners suffered 14,178 cases of smallpox, of which 1,963 died. The vaccinated German troops suffered only 4,835 cases of the disease, of which only 178 died, or a mortality rate of less than 4 percent.[31]

Recognizing the importance of military medical care in maintaining the fighting ability of their armies, some states established mechanisms for ensuring an adequate supply of surgeons and other field medical personnel. In the first quarter of the century, the French established schools for training surgeons and mates at a number of army and navy hospitals. The most important medico-military institution of the century was established when the French opened the Académie Royale de Chirurgie in Paris in 1731. That five of its seven directors and half of the forty members nominated by the king were prominent military surgeons who had served in battle attests to the academy's dedication to military medical matters. Further, army and naval surgeons wrote more than a third of the period's four volumes of medical papers.[32] Saxony followed the French example and established an army medical school in 1748. Additional military medical schools were established in Austria in 1784 and in Berlin in 1795. In 1766, Richard de Hautesierck (1712–1789), inspector of hospitals, published the world's first medical journal devoted exclusively to military medicine.[33]

Gradually armies established regular field medical facilities. In 1745 at the Battle of Fontenoy, the British military medical service treated the wounded on the first line and collected them at ambulance stations. Surgeons performed capital operations at medical stations behind the lines and then transferred the more seriously wounded to hospitals prepared for them in nearby cities and towns. When these hospitals became overcrowded, the army made arrangements to ship the wounded farther to the rear. Although this model was becoming commonplace in all armies of the period, military medical facilities did not operate so efficiently as a matter of course. More commonly medical facilities were understaffed, were poorly supplied and had little transport, and generally were overwhelmed by large numbers of casualties. Nonetheless, the structural articulation that the armies of the day were demonstrating in other areas was also evident in their attempts to provide better medical care for the soldier. It would take yet another century, but eventually the seeds of a full-time professional military medical service sown in the eighteenth century would come to fruition.

Before examining the development of the national military medical services, it is worth noting another development that did much to foster medical care in the armies of the period. Exempting the wounded from slaughter or imprisonment had begun in the seventeenth century, and the idea gained added support during the eighteenth century. In July 1743 at the completion of the Dettingen campaign, both sides signed an agreement that declared medical personnel serving in the armies would be considered noncombatants and not taken as prisoners of war. In addition, medical personnel would be given safe passage back to their own armies as soon as practical. Most important, both sides agreed to care for the enemy wounded and sick prisoners as they would their own and provide for their return upon recovery.[34] While the Dettingen agreement was important for its humanity in dictating the treatment of the sick and wounded, it was also a significant spur to the further development of military medical facilities. While the old system of slaughtering the wounded reduced the casualty load for the medical facilities, the Dettingen agreement forced armies to increase their medical staffs to deal with the enemy wounded as well.

While military medical care had improved greatly over that of the previous century, by any objective standard it was still poor. This situation was not so much a consequence of poor medical knowledge but developed because no army succeeded in organizing a permanent medical care system that was adequately staffed with trained personnel, provided for the prompt removal of the wounded, ensured adequate medical supplies, and established hygienic hospitals. As in the previous century, command of the armies remained in the hands of temporary commanders of the nobility, and the extent to which any planned medical facilities actually were constructed and operated depended greatly upon the degree to which the respective field army's commander was prepared to provide the necessary resources. Thus, whatever military medical facilities were available during the last war or campaign had to be totally reconstructed from scratch for the next war. The old lessons had to be relearned, with the inevitable result that the medical care provided to the soldier suffered accordingly.

NAVAL MEDICINE

The first literary evidence of medical support provided aboard ship is found in the *Iliad*, where Homer recounted his shipboard surgeon, Machaon, treating his soldiers' wounds. In the *Odyssey* (700 BCE), Homer writes of Ulysses ordering the bodies of the slain to be covered with sulfur and burned, the first account of sulfur fumigation in history. In Roman times, naval surgeons were common fixtures in the medical service. The first evidence of a naval surgeon is taken from the tombstone of N. Londinius, who was the physician on the *Cupid*, a quinquereme of the Roman Navy. During the reign of Hadrian (76–138 CE), each Roman naval ship carried a medical officer, and the fleet strength of the naval medical service was approximately one physician for every two hundred men. This figure compares favorably to the ratio of six and a half naval physicians for every thousand U.S. naval personnel in World War II. Because the Roman Navy enjoyed the lowest prestige of all the empire's military forces, the Romans sometimes had difficulty recruiting naval physicians. Next to the names of some naval physicians is the term *duplicarius,* indicating that they received double pay.[35] The Romans used hospital ships for the transport and care of their sick and wounded. The evidence is inferential and based on the Greek and Roman practice of naming their ships to reflect the purpose for which they were used. There are records of a Roman vessel named *Aesculapius* (the god of medicine), which may have served as a hospital ship.[36]

During the Middle Ages it was common practice to have a physician aboard ship. The navies of this period with the most complete records available are the maritime republics of Genoa and Venice, and both had naval physicians aboard ship as a matter of course. During the Crusades (1095–1291), as ships ranged farther away from home port, navies established shore-based medical facilities to treat the sick and wounded. The medical officers of Genoa and Venice issued the first health certificates to naval crews and originated the practice of quarantining ships to protect against the spread of disease.[37]

Although physicians had served aboard ships since ancient times, naval medicine did not become an important branch of military medicine until the age of Christopher Columbus (1451–1506). Previously, most voyages were along the coast and of short duration, making it possible to provide adequate water and provisions to ensure the crew's health. The proximity of port facilities, including land-based hospitals, made treating the sick and wounded a less pressing matter than it became when ships began venturing upon the open sea for months at a time. Only then did maintaining the health of the crew and treating battle wounds become a real necessity.

In the colonial era (1500–1750), the ship of the line became a new and important instrument in the equation of national power. States wishing to compete in the expanded geographic arena of international politics developed large naval forces to press their interests far from their national home bases. The navy became the main method of projecting power internationally. Accordingly, the navies of France, Spain, Italy, and England expanded greatly during this century, giving rise to a new branch of military medicine.

Medical conditions in the armies of the day were poor, and they were even worse in the navies of the world. The ships of this period were 150–220 feet long and 40 feet wide and displaced two hundred to seven hundred tons. The vessels required a large amount of muscle power to operate, and crew strength ranged from 800 to 950 men. Eight men manned each of the forty to seventy-five guns aboard a frigate. By comparison, a modern frigate is between 500 and 800 feet long with a beam of 70–100 feet and is manned with between 500 and 800 men. The overcrowded ships of the eighteenth century were nests of disease and infection.

Service aboard ship was dangerous business. Crews were jammed into three and four decks, where the air was fetid and ventilation nonexistent, causing even minor outbreaks of disease to spread to the entire crew. In 1753, Stephen Hales (1677–1761) devised a system of small hand-driven pumps to pump fresh air belowdecks. The British Navy was slow to adopt this idea, even though naval commanders recognized its positive effects on improving the sailors' health. Lord Halifax noted, for example, that for every twelve men dying from disease on an unventilated ship only one died on the new ventilated ships.[38]

The method of ship construction also contributed greatly to the ill health of the sailor. Ships were built of green timber in the mistaken belief that unseasoned wood better resisted the sea rot caused by salt water. Shipbuilders soaked the wood in brine and pickling solutions to harden it against the corrosive effects of salt water and worms. These green timbers were a constant source of dampness below decks, and the habit of washing the decks daily with salt water added to the dampness. Naval ships were always dank, damp, dark, and cold, and these conditions produced high rates of rheumatism and consumption among naval crews.

Discipline in national navies was harsh. Flogging was a routine punishment for even minor offenses and produced open cuts on the sailor's back that became seats for infection. Sailors in the British Navy were not provided with regulation uniforms until 1857.[39] Until that time they provided their own clothing, which was often little more than a collection of rags that the men never washed or even changed during the entire voyage. These poor habits produced frequent outbreaks of disease and infection. The practice of impressment also added to the health risks at sea. Press gangs "shanghaied" all manner of urban poor from the city streets for forced military service.[40] The health of these marginal elements of the population was almost universally poor and often broke completely under the rigors of sea duty. Changing crews at sea brought newly impressed sailors into contact with healthier crews. With the navy failing to require either medical examinations or quarantine periods for the impressed sailors, disease and infection were constantly being reintroduced to the fleet at sea.

The nature of naval combat often produced even more horrible wounds than those suffered by the ground soldier. Heavy iron cannon balls fired from ships shredded the wooden deckhouses, decks, railings, and masts, producing showers of wooden splinters moving at high speed. When they struck a sailor, they produced horrible wounds. Explosions from poorly cast cannons produced further injury. The necessity of storing powder on deck near the guns posed the threat of explosions and flash burns, presenting yet another hazard to the sailor.

Poor diet—usually little more than hard biscuits, salted meat, and pumpkins—and crowded conditions made scurvy the most common disease of the sailor. It was a great killer of naval forces. It was not uncommon for a ship to lose between a third and a quarter of its whole crew to the disease on a long voyage. James Lind (1716–1794), the famous Scottish naval physician, recorded that in a single voyage of three months' duration, the Channel Fleet reported twenty-four hundred cases of scurvy.[41] Lind noted in his work in 1754 that regularly issuing lime juice could greatly prevent scurvy, but not until 1796 did the British Navy finally include lime juice a part of the sailor's rations.

Medical care aboard ship was almost universally poor. Because of its low social status, poor living conditions, and long voyages at sea, the navy attracted the lowest-quality surgeons, assistants, and physicians, and most had little training. Surgeons were required to purchase their own instruments, and many who could not afford them borrowed saws, knives, and sewing instruments from the ship's sailmakers and carpenters to perform surgery. Shipboard surgery and medical treatment were performed in a small room deep below deck called "the cockpit" that was poorly ventilated and lit, and the ceiling was too low for a man to stand fully erect. No system existed for evacuating the wounded from their battle stations and transporting them to the surgery. Most often a sailor dragged himself or a friend helped him to the cockpit. This practice was dangerous, however, since a sailor helping a wounded friend could be flogged for deserting his battle station. The small complement of medical personnel had no system of triage and enforced no priority of treatment. The wounded simply lined up for medical attention. It was not uncommon for a slightly wounded sailor to be treated while the more severely wounded succumbed to shock and bleeding while waiting their turn.[42]

The French and Spanish navies made an effort to return their dead to home port. Not so the British. Indeed, a wounded man aboard ship who was unable to make his way to surgery was likely to be thrown overboard while still alive. Usually an officer or petty officer—not the medical officer who, in any case, was far below deck attending to the wounded—led this "selection process."[43] When Lord Horatio Nelson was fatally wounded at the Battle of Trafalgar (1805), he begged the ship's captain not to have him thrown overboard. Capt. Thomas Hardy agreed, and when Nelson succumbed to his wounds, his body was sealed in a cask of brandy for transport back to Nelson's father's parsonage for burial. To this day the daily brandy ration issued to British sailors is called "Nelson's blood."

Surgery aboard ship often involved amputation. British naval surgeons heated their knives in scalding water in the belief that a hot knife caused less pain than a cold one. American medical officers imitated this practice, which had the unintended effect of providing some degree of antisepsis. The patient was given liquor or opium, if available, and a piece of leather to chew on while the cutting was accomplished. Because of the low degree of surgical training, the poor operating facilities, and the heat of battle, naval surgeons seemed not to have given much consideration to preparing the stump for prosthesis. The mortality rate was, of course, horrendous.

The care of the shipboard sick was equally primitive. Ships were not usually equipped with sick bays as such. The more customary arrangement was to leave the sick person to recover in his own hammock. Sometimes a small area belowdecks separated from the rest of the crew by canvas partitions was provided, but these primitive sick bays were located out of the way in the darkest, least-used, and unventilated areas of the ship. Also, although vaccination was now becoming commonplace in armies and other navies, the British Navy did not require vaccination against smallpox until 1858.[44] Under these conditions, smallpox epidemics were commonplace aboard naval vessels.

Shipping large ground forces to colonial areas for military operations increased overcrowding; consequently, losses to disease aboard ship were often even higher than normal. To deal with this problem, the navy provided "hospital ships" to accommodate the sick. These vessels usually had no medical personnel aboard, and the ships' physicians were forbidden to leave their own vessels to treat the sick. These hospital ships became little more than disease-ridden floating warehouses where the ill remained until they either recovered or died. A physician accompanying Lord Cathcart's campaign in the West Indies in 1739 describes the conditions aboard one of these hospital ships anchored in Cartagena Harbor: "The men were pent up between the decks in small vessels where they had not room to sit upright; they wallowed in filth; myriads of maggots were hatched in the putrefaction of their sores, which had no other dressings than that of being washed in their own allowance of brandy."[45] The sailors threw the dead overboard, where they floated on the surface while sharks and birds of prey fed upon them in full view of the surviving patients.

These conditions did not escape the attention of physicians, and some undertook efforts to correct them. Among the more important naval medical reformers of the period were Lind, Thomas Trotter (1760–1832), and Gilbert Blane (1749–1834). Lind published three major naval medical treatises: *A Treatise of the Scurvy* (1754), *An Essay on the Most Effectual Means of Preserving the Health of Seamen in the Royal Navy* (1757), and *An Essay on Diseases Incidental to Europeans in Hot Climates* (1768). As noted earlier, Lind recommended lime juice be added to naval rations to prevent scurvy. He also argued for special tenders on which impressed recruits could be examined and quarantined before being allowed aboard ships of the line, and the navy adopted this reform in 1781. Further, Lind advocated for an improved diet, better uniforms and in sufficient number to permit regular changes, the use of quinine for malaria, and the regular issue of soap for bathing. Trotter became a strong advocate of vaccinating naval crews and recommended it be made compulsory. He also suggested ventilating the lower decks and using chemical disinfectants to clean the ships' compartments. In his *Medicina Nautica: An Essay on the Diseases of Seamen* (1797), he recommended creating a naval health board to compel ships' captains to implement basic sanitary measures, including more beds, more fresh air, and the liberal use of soap.

The navy implemented few of Lind's and Trotter's suggestions with any degree of regularity; however, Gilbert Blane, a scholar, used his political influence, reputation, and writings to provoke the navy to use many of their ideas. In 1785, Blane published his *Observations on the Diseases of Seamen*, which finally moved the naval authorities to exercise reforms. Blane succeeded in having the medical supplies of ships improved, soap issued on a regular basis, and the assignment of a regular space for use as sick bays. As a result, the British seaman's health improved dramatically. In 1782, before these reforms, of the 100,000 sailors and marines in the British Navy, the proportion of sick sailors transferred to hospital to fit sailors was 1 to 3.3. Thirty-one years later, after many of Lind's, Trotter's, and Blane's reforms were effectuated, of the 140,000 sailors and marines in the navy, the ratio of sick to fit personnel was only 1 to 10.75.[46]

The prevailing conditions, however, remained common until well into the nineteenth century when the permanently standing national naval medical services applied the national armies' lessons pertaining to health and surgery to naval medicine. The introduction of the iron ship near the end of the century also altered the nature of the medical challenges aboard ship. Large enough to carry sufficient provisions and to distill its own drinking water, the modern naval ship's conditions drastically reduced the health threats that sailors faced. But the nature of the ship's construction created new problems for medical treatment while under battle stations. Replacing the old problem of flying wooden splinters was a new threat of airborne metal, fire, explosions, crushing injuries, and steam burns. Naval personnel closed their new ships' watertight compartments when under fire, effectively making it impossible for the medical staff to reach the wounded and increasing the likelihood of wounds becoming infected. As in times past, the sailor had to depend on his mates sealed with him in his compartment to provide sufficient medical treatment to keep him alive until he could be transported to a naval surgeon. If a lull occurred in the battle, the men could remove some casualties to clearing points. Usually, however, the wounded sailor on the iron ships had to await the end of the battle before receiving treatment from medical personnel. Sometimes, as in the Battle of Tsushima Straight in 1904, the casualties had to wait until the ships disengaged and were safely out of harm's way before they could be treated. Many of the Russian wounded lingered eight days before being attended to by the remaining members of the ship's medical staff.

ENGLAND

The total medical staff of the British Army in 1718 was 173 medical officers, staff, regimental surgeons, garrison physicians, and surgeons' mates for a field army of eighteen thousand men on campaign.[47] In peacetime, few physicians or surgeons were regularly assigned to military postings. The few evident career medical personnel were some staff members and a few surgeons' mates. In garrisons, officers and medical personnel were commonly granted extended leaves. In colonial garrisons, medical officers could be away for months, leaving these garrisons without any medical support. In 1751, English surgeons were permitted to wear the uniform of the troops to which they were attached. A law was passed in 1783 prohibiting the sale of surgeon positions in the army; however, the abuse continued for almost another century.[48]

Mention has already been made of John Hunter's contributions to British military medicine and treatment of gunshot wounds. John Pringle, also made a number of significant contributions. In 1752, Pringle published what was perhaps the best work of the century on military hygiene, *Observations on the Diseases of the Army*, and set forth the principles of military hygiene with a special emphasis on the need to ventilate military hospitals. Pringle had noticed that soldiers treated in crude, drafty regimental hospitals often had far lower rates of wound infection than those treated in the large rear area hospitals. In addition, he suggested constructing barracks hospitals, identified hospital and jail fevers and proposed treatments for them, anticipated the practice of antisepsis, and used the term "influenza" for the disease that later came to be named such. Other major contributors to military hygiene were Richard Brocklesby (1722–1797), who wrote *Economical and Medical Observations on Military Hospitals and Camp Diseases* in 1764; Hughes Ravaton, a French surgeon, published *Chirurgie d'armée* in 1768; and Jean Colombier (1736–1789) published the *Code de médecine militaire* in 1772. All these works suggested great improvements to prevent and treat disease in the armies of the day. Unfortunately, the armies adopted few of the comprehensive approaches to military medical care on any scale until the next century.

An important advance of this period is attributed to the British Navy. Although notorious for the terrible medical conditions aboard its ships, the British Admiralty in 1798 authorized the discharge of patients from military service on the recommendation of military surgeons and physicians. For the first time, illness and disease in the military became a question of medical importance and not one of morale and discipline.[49] More important, now a surgeon as well as a physician could authorize a medical discharge, clearly demonstrating that the old barrier between the two disciplines had finally eroded to the point where, at least in the military, the surgeon was achieving equal status and influence with the physician.

The organization of the British military medical service was quite good, at least theoretically. During the Seven Years' War, each regiment was assigned a surgeon and a mate; some regiments had two mates. In cantonment, the army usually requisitioned a building or house and converted it into a regimental hospital. In the large towns to the rear, general hospitals were constructed to treat the more serious cases. The surgeons and mates attended the wounded on the field and sent them to houses or tents located in nearby towns and villages. The marching or "flying" hospital with its own tents, transport, medical, and nursing personnel followed behind the army. These mobile hospitals could handle approximately two hundred casualties at a time. When the army moved on, these hospitals retained responsibility for the care of the sick and wounded until they could be sent to the general hospitals located along the lines of communication twelve to forty miles to the rear.[50]

This organizational structure remained the basic model for British military medical care until mid-century, when the flying hospitals were discontinued. Changes in the general hospital allowed the army to abandon the mobile field hospital. In the past, the general hospital had been a permanent fixed-base structure, but by mid-century "the hospital" had really become only a hospital staff.[51] The medical staff marched along with the army, setting up medical facilities wherever they were needed. The army's goal was to place a cadre of trained medical personnel at the regimental hospital's disposal and deliver better-quality care closer to the front. The plan's shortcoming was that because the new hospitals no longer had the tents, transport, and supplies that had accompanied the flying hospital, they had to rely exclusively upon the field commanders for these items.[52] An emphasis on mobility underpinned this change in the British military medical system, because the British forces were expected to deploy and fight far from their homeland. Continental armies, meanwhile, usually fought on their own territory, so they retained the idea of military hospitals as fixed and permanent buildings.

The British closed their general hospitals at the end of the campaign season and reopened them when the war resumed. When a hospital closed, the sick and wounded were transferred farther to the rear at great cost in pain, suffering, and epidemic. While moving, the men suffered harsh conditions, and since most regimental surgeons and mates were required to remain with their units to tend the troops in regimental hospitals, few medical personnel accompanied the patients on the trip. Often a third of the casualties died from exposure, disease, or injury. In 1743, the British shuttered its hospitals in Germany after the campaign season and shipped their sick and wounded to a general hospital at Ghent. Of the three thousand sick and wounded who began the trip, half died on the way.[53]

In winter quarters, the regimental surgeons and mates provided medical treatment. While the quality of these personnel was generally lower than that found in the rear hospitals, in fact soldiers retained in regimental hospitals often had a better chance of survival than if they had been evacuated. First, they were spared the hardships of the evacuation. Second, the regimental hospitals were usually makeshift buildings with better ventilation than the general hospitals had. Third, the patient load was considerably lower, reducing crowding and the risk of epidemic and infection. The last point is important, for hospital mortality from disease was a major killer of military casualties. Between 1715 and 1748, the mortality rate from disease in British military hospitals was 20 percent.[54]

Medical care in rear hospitals was not good. The chief matron described the largest British military hospital at Albany in the American colonies from 1756 to 1760, for example, as "little better than a shed."[55] These hospitals were invariably too small to handle a significant flow of casualties, and the practice of placing two patients to a bed did little to prevent infection. The hospital staff included a director, who was often not a medical man; a physician and surgeon; a purveyor responsible for purchasing supplies; an apothecary for mixing drugs; a chief female matron to oversee the nursing staff; and a large number of cooks, orderlies, laborers, and chaplains. With the exception of the senior physician and surgeon, few of the other personnel were well qualified. The low salaries and poor living conditions worked to dissuade many competent physicians and surgeons from serving in the military. Turnover in the nursing staff, which soldiers' wives often filled, was high. The purveyor's responsibility to keep costs low often led to supply shortages and corruption, to the great detriment of the quality of medical care.

Although women had accompanied armies since ancient times and often been pressed into service as nurses, the British were the first to establish some regularity to the practice. By 1750, almost all nurses in the British Army were females, although some males served in that capacity as well. Most nurses were wives and widows of soldiers, but the British made efforts to plan for regular staffs of nurses in their hospitals. The position of chief matron was a regular and respected medical post and appeared in the table of organization for the medical service. A number of women made military nursing a career, and the leadership commonly assembled nursing staffs in England prior to a campaign and deployed them with the army in the field.[56] The army generally planned for a nurses-to-patients ratio of 1 to 10.[57]

Regimental medical services also left much to be desired. The quality of regimental surgeons and mates was the lowest in the army, and when a regiment occupied more than one cantonment, total responsibility for the men's medical treatment fell upon the untrained surgeons' mate. Few of the mates had any medical training prior to enlistment, and many joined the army to obtain that very training, hoping for some sort of medical career afterward. The surgeons' mate was not a full-time position, so warrant officers of the line doubled as mates. When the army was engaged in battle, however, these warrant officers took their positions in the line, leaving the regimental medical staff without any help at all to treat casualties. Regimental surgeons commonly purchased their positions, and it was not unusual for a mate to secure his appointment by favoritism or by purchasing his surgeoncy and later be elevated to a staff position in the general hospital, all without any training whatsoever.

A regiment's usual casualty load ranged from five hundred to seven hundred men who needed some sort of medical treatment in the regimental hospitals. At the Battle of Albuera (1811), one surgeon described a situation in which he had three thousand wounded but only four wagons to transport them to the nearest general hospital seven miles away. Sir James Henry Craig (1748–1812), general of the British Army in Flanders in 1794, provided an apt description of the conditions that the soldier at the regimental level endured. Craig wrote, "Some kind of medical staff was improvised out of drunken apothecaries, broken down practitioners, and roughs of every description who were provided under some cheap contract . . . the charges of respectable members of the profession being deemed exorbitant. . . . The dreadful mismanagement of the hospital is beyond description."[58]

Military medical care also suffered as a consequence of the organizational relationship between the regimental and general hospitals. Senior medical personnel were quite aware of the poor quality of medical care found in regimental hospitals, and sometimes they pressured the field commander to forbid regimental surgeons from treating all but the most minor wounds. In particular, surgery was often prohibited. Regimental surgeons were encouraged to pass the more serious cases or those requiring surgery to the general hospitals in the rear. Given the nature of emergency medical treatment on the line and the uncertainty of medical transport, these well-intentioned regulations usually resulted in an increased casualty mortality rate. Moreover, the general hospitals' staffs, themselves of uncertain quality most of the time, were not adequate to handle high casualty loads, especially when a high proportion of them required surgery. Thus, for example, in 1742 in Flanders the general hospital had only one physician, one surgeon, one apothecary, and six surgeons' mates to handle the entire casualty flow.

The practice of closing hospitals at the end of each campaign season or disbanding them at the end of each war meant that almost the entire military medical system had to be reconstructed with new personnel whenever it was needed. Whatever expertise that had been acquired during the last war was inevitably lost. As a result, hospital staffs often performed dismally at the beginning of a campaign. As the war went on, however, these staffs improved as they gained experience. Mortality statistics from the War of the Austrian Succession (1740–1748) demonstrate this improvement. From the first large-scale landings of troops on the continent in 1742 until October 1743, 6,104 casualties were admitted to the general hospital, and 1,241 died, or a mortality rate of 20.3 percent. From 1744 until the end of the war in 1748, 24,612 casualties entered hospital, and 2,411 died, or a mortality rate of 9.8 percent.[59] Upon the conclusion of the war, however, the experienced medical staffs of the military hospitals were released from service, taking their valued experience with them.

FRANCE

In terms of the *structure* of military medical care, the French system was the envy of other European armies. No monarch of the period did more to make military medical care of the soldier a formal state function than did Louis XIV. In 1708, the king issued an order that required physicians, surgeons, and hospitals to attend to the sick and wounded on the march. The order established a formal complement of two hundred physicians and surgeons for an army in the field. Moreover, special boards had to examine these medical personnel and ensure their competence. Louis also appointed 4 medical inspectors general to oversee the entire system, 50 advisory physicians to ensure quality medical practice in the military hospitals, 4 surgeons major to inspect military forts and camps, and 138 surgeons major to provide care for the armies in the field.[60] At the same time, eighty-five military hospitals were ordered constructed or improved in the major fortified towns and cities of France.[61]

A major reform was accomplished with the establishment of mobile field hospitals that followed the armies and augmented the care provided by the general hospitals. For the first time in any army of the period, these flying hospitals were not only staffed with adequate numbers of surgeons but also provided with their own independent source of supplies and transport, reducing the old problem of forcing medical units to beg the field commanders for them.[62] While the French field hospital had been available for at least fifty years in one form or another, its lack of transport and supplies had always hindered its practical ability to aid the wounded. Without tents or wagons of their own, these early field hospitals often failed to reach the battlefield in time to do much good. It was not unusual for the soldier to lie on the field for a day or two, awaiting the medical units' arrival.[63]

The mobile hospital system, while a great improvement in the formal structure of military medical care, did not usually work very well in practice. Dedicated transport and supplies surely helped, but these units still had to rely on the combat units' manpower for evacuating the wounded. It was not until the Napoleonic Wars that the army regularly provided to field hospitals the manpower assets to act as litter bearers and surgeons' helpers.[64] The resources and management of the field hospitals fell not under military command but to civilian contractors, a practice that often led to fraud, abuse, and lack of provisions. The same contract system was used to provide resources to the general hospitals, frequently with the same results.

The Enlightenment in France led to an emphasis on scientific and statistical approaches to medical management in general. The emergent concern with the health of the general citizenry and the state's provision of health and medical care encouraged a similar movement in military medicine.[65] In 1718, the first formal hospital regulations were issued for the military medical service in a document of sixty-two paragraphs. These regulations were so comprehensive that they served as the basis for all future French military medical regulations for the next century. They included detailed instructions for hospital personnel, the medical treatment of patients, hygiene regulations for medical attendants, administrative practices for controlling hospital supplies, and military hygiene regulations aimed at preventing disease among the soldiery. The monthly pay of surgeons and physicians was moderately increased, and annual courses in anatomy were prescribed for all military surgeons. Most innovative was the regulation that the cost of the military medical service was to be paid entirely from the king's purse, without taking deductions from the soldier's pay as reimbursement.

In 1775, a royal order authorized the opening of lecture rooms for instruction in military medicine at the hospitals in Metz, Lille, and Strasbourg. This decree marked France's first attempt to create an army medical school. In 1782, the *Journal de médecine militaire,* the first French periodical devoted exclusively to military medicine, was established in Paris. The French experience in the wars of this period revealed that the general military hospitals often failed to provide adequate medical care because of their distance from the fighting and the rampant corruption and mismanagement that characterized their operation. To improve the medical care for the troops closer to the battlefield, the French military abolished general hospitals and created new regimental hospitals. In 1788, new regulations were issued assigning control of all military hospitals to a new military medical directorate composed of military physicians. A new sanitary council was established to oversee disease prevention and hygiene in the armies. The tide of the French Revolution (1789–1799), however, swept away these untested organizational improvements.

The French medical system was similar to the British system in that the wounded were evacuated to hospital clearing stations located near the battle lines. Here the regimental surgeon attended the soldier. Major surgery was sometimes performed in these regimental hospitals, but for the most part they treated only the lightly wounded and prepared the more serious cases for shipment to the rear hospitals. If the patient survived the twenty- to forty-mile trip to the general hospital, he would undergo surgery there.[66]

The French had no systematic method for evacuating the wounded from the front lines. Either a fellow soldier brought his wounded comrade to the medical tent or the wounded soldier made his way to the rear as best he could. The most seriously wounded moved from the regimental hospitals along the roads leading to the base of communications in the rear. Transport was sometimes provided for the medical units, but usually they used the empty food carts and supply wagons that had previously delivered supplies to the front. The wagon drivers were not military personnel but hired contractors who often treated the wounded cruelly, charged them a fee, robbed them, and even abandoned them on the side of the road if the highway became too crowded. Usually medical personnel did not attend the wounded in transit. When medical personnel were available, their numbers were invariably small. The horrors associated with moving the wounded provided an additional stimulus to reform the medical treatment system and to give the field medical detachments their own wagons and the necessary personnel to oversee the transportation of the wounded.

Even with reform, the system remained fragile in times of high casualties. Military medical texts of the period note that it was not unusual for an army to suffer eight thousand wounded in a single day.[67] Under these conditions, it was neither practical nor possible to assign field medical units the necessary personnel or transport to move sufficient numbers of wounded on any regular basis. Much as in modern wars, the medical services of the eighteenth century frequently became overloaded and broke down, with much attendant human suffering.

For all its problems, however, the French military medical service on the eve of the Revolution was seen as the model for other countries, and Austria, Prussia, Denmark, and Sweden all reorganized their military hospital systems on the French model.[68] The social disruption of the French Revolution, however, dashed the old system. In 1792, the new French Republic declared war on Austria. Motivated by the Revolution's sense of national patriotism, fourteen hundred physicians and surgeons applied for service with the new French national army.[69] In August 1793, the National Convention placed all physicians, surgeons, and apothecaries at the service of the Ministry of War. By the end of the year, 2,570 medical officers of various types attended to the needs of the revolutionary armies.[70] Within a few months, their number grew to more than 4,000, and by the end of the war in 1794, 8,000 medical personnel of various types had seen service with the armies.[71]

The war and social revolution had near catastrophic effects on the educational and organizational structure of the French medical establishment. In 1792, the National Assembly voted to abolish the eighteen medical faculties and fifteen medical schools in France, including the older schools in Paris, Strasbourg, and Montpelier and the Académie Royale de Chirurgie and the Société Royale de Médicine. In 1794, the state ordered the creation of medical schools for the express purpose of providing sufficient medical personnel to the armies. These schools trained only military medical personnel. After the disruption of the medical establishment, however, the quality of training in these schools fell drastically. Worse, the practice of medicine was thrown open to anyone of any status and education who could afford to pay for a license. Although the number of military medical assets available to the armies increased, the quality declined drastically. The French persisted with this system of military medical training until Napoleon ended it in 1804 and completely reorganized the military medical establishment.

The French military medical system was still the most structurally advanced of all the armies of the period. Moreover, the revolutionary emphasis on equality provided a further impetus to provide good medical care for the soldier. The French armies were the first genuine citizen armies of the modern period, and while the sacrifice of the citizen's life to the cause of the state was generally accepted as a cost of military service, the state recognized its obligation to provide for the citizen soldier's medical treatment. As the eighteenth century came to an end and the specter of Napoleon loomed over Europe, the armies of the continent realized their military forces were no match for the French unless they resorted to national conscription and patriotic appeals to raise large armies. As part of their new bargain with formally excluded social elements, the continental armies began to explore ways to improve the medical care for their soldiers. In this sense, the spirit of the French Revolution spurred most of Europe's armies to begin providing what would eventually become the modern system of military medical care.

PRUSSIA

The centralization of governmental power that marked most of the previous century in England and France occurred much later in Prussia, with the result that its centralized control of governmental functions lagged behind even that of the other continental powers. In the area of military medicine, this delay worked against establishing a government-sponsored military medical service in Prussia until late in the century. Even then the degree of its organizational sophistication remained low. For most of the eighteenth century, the Prussian military medical service and the degree of care and resources it provided to field medical units depended, as it had in the seventeenth-century England and France, primarily upon the army commander's willingness to arrange it for a given campaign.

The first military hospital in Prussia, a "medical house" near the Spandau Gate in Berlin, was constructed in 1710, but it was only officially established as a regular military hospital fifteen years later.[72] Meanwhile, in 1705, Prussia had a standing army of thirty-five regiments; however, only six of them had a normal complement of regimental surgeons and mates.[73] In 1712, for the first time in the Prussian Army, supervision of company surgeons was transferred from officers of the line to the medical officers in the regiment. The status of Prussian barber-surgeons was so low that they ranked below the chaplains and only slightly above the drummers. Regimental surgeons still had to shave company officers, and senior officers could subject them to public whipping for the slightest offense.[74] The barber-surgeons were forbidden to treat the wounded except under supervision of the regimental surgeons, who themselves usually had poor skills. Company surgeons were allowed to visit the sick and wounded and to report their condition to the regimental surgeons. Long after the distinction between surgeon and physician had begun to diminish in the other armies of the day, in Prussia the rigid separation lasted well into the nineteenth century, thereby preserving the regimental surgeons' low status and training. The Prussian Army did not even have an officially commissioned surgeon general until 1716.

Frederick Wilhelm I appointed the first chief physician of the army in 1724. This officer was charged with presiding over all physicians and surgeons in the army and standardizing regulations governing medical competence. For the first time, both physicians and surgeons received the same training in the army.[75] The army commonly withheld part of the company barber-surgeons' pay to offset the cost of the regiment's medical supplies. Jews were not admitted to military medical practice, and in Austria at the beginning of the Seven Years' War, Protestant surgeons had to convert to Catholicism or leave the army.[76] Some German states authorized surgeons to wear regular uniforms, and others forbade them to do so. The staffing of regimental hospitals with apothecaries was poor at best, and unlike in England at this time, nursing was not organized.

Frederick Wilhelm issued regulations requiring all military surgeons to be examined before the medical college as a test of competency, a regulation probably only rudimentarily enforced. Frederick made use of at least twelve French surgeons in his army, but little effort seems to have been made to have them train Prussian medical personnel. This lack of serious concern over military medical matters was evident in the infantry regulations of 1726 that still forbade medical attention to the wounded until the battle was over, a practice that other continental armies had long abandoned. The regulation read: "When the battle is over each regiment shall seek out its wounded and bring them to a definite place where they can be bandaged and cared for; no wounded may be recovered during the battle."[77] The same regulation noted that a military hospital was to be established in the nearest village or town to which the warring party's sick and wounded could be sent. Each battalion was assigned a barber-surgeon and two attendants to provide medical care. The barber-surgeons were only supposed to attend the lightly wounded and to send others to the rear. Although general hospital personnel in the town hospital were presumably better trained, this was seldom the case. If the army moved on, a noncommissioned officer without medical training was assigned to remain with the sick and wounded. He was allotted a sum of money to help care for the patients and to purchase whatever medical help and supplies were available in the area. Although the field apothecary was also designated to remain behind and provide drugs, no one remained behind to tend the wounded. All other trained medical personnel moved forward with the army. When the sick and wounded required transport, the army used whatever wagons were available for it had no systematic provision for transport. In all these respects, the Prussian medical system in the first half of the century fell far short of the quality of medical care that soldiers in other armies received.

The army of Frederick the Great made a number of improvements to this system. Still, the system itself was more the responsibility of the field commanders than of the national government. Frederick had a personal interest in medical matters, and his concern for his troops grew as much out of his genuine concern for their welfare as from the fact that the population of Prussia was small and every fighting man was a precious national resource. As a field commander, Frederick often personally selected locations for unit dressing stations when determining the battle plan. He ordered that these stations be appropriately fortified and protected from enemy fire and cannon shot.[78] He introduced the old Roman practice of guarding safe water points and mixing a small amount of vinegar with water to make it more potable. He was personally solicitous of the medical care of his troops and ordered incompetent surgeons flogged. While the care of his own wounded had priority, Frederick issued orders that the enemy wounded should be cared for as time and supplies permitted.

As time went on, Frederick's battle losses in his frequent wars forced him to take military medical care more seriously. Although he attempted several remedies to improve care, as the century ended Prussian military medicine remained considerably behind that of other armies. Frederick ordered the creation of permanent, fixed-site military hospitals at Breslau, Glogau, Stettin, Dresden, Torgau, and Wittenberg and introduced the use of forward field hospitals. Each regiment was provided with a barber-surgeon and four company barbers to provide first aid. While no dedicated personnel or transport were used to evacuate the wounded, Frederick dictated that regular detachments be assigned from the regiment's manpower to accomplish this task. Efforts were made to draw these transport detachments from the regiments that had suffered the fewest losses in the day's battle.

Prussia did not open its first military medical school, the Pépinière (later known as the Frederick Wilhelm Institute), until 1795. Austria had established the Josephinum, an academy for imperial army surgeons, ten years earlier.

RUSSIA

Russia's long years of isolation from the European mainstream caused by its geography, religion, and foreign occupation left it far behind the continental powers in almost all aspects relating to military affairs, including military medicine. The condition of general medicine was also quite backward, and the number of trained medical personnel of any sort, in the army and society, were extremely few. Peter the Great, whose interest in medical affairs stemmed largely from his own suffering from various medical conditions, attempted to remedy this situation with numerous reforms.

The lack of native-trained physicians and surgeons forced Peter to rely on foreign doctors for his military forces. Although some were successfully recruited for short periods, the difficult living conditions, harsh terms of service, low pay, and the general suspicion that most Russians had for all foreigners made the program largely unsuccessful. In 1700 during the Great Northern War, Russia had fewer than sixty military surgical personnel in the army, and few of them had any formal medical schooling or training.[79] In 1706, Peter reorganized the primitive military medical service, and each soldier was required to contribute a small sum from his pay to offset the cost of medical treatment. Regimental surgeons, usually ill-trained barber-surgeons, were appointed. The surgeon had to select a soldier from each company, at double pay, to shave the men and apply plasters. These soldiers also served in the line and were not full-time medical assistants.[80] Peter's "improvements" were actually old practices that the European armies had instituted a century earlier. Even the Russian surgeons' mates, positions that hardly attracted the epitome of medical talent and training in the West, were far less skilled than those found in Western armies.

Forced to deal with a constant shortage of trained medical personnel for his armies, Peter founded the Gospitali with the express purpose of training military surgeons. The institution was placed under the direction of Nicolass Bidloo (1674–1735), the famous Dutch physician and surgeon, who arranged the curriculum along the lines of clinical empirical medicine characteristic of Dutch medical schools. From the outset, the institution had difficulty attracting the talented sons of the middle and upper classes, and for most of its history it drew its students from the lower classes. The school was under constant pressure to provide mates and surgeons for the armies; indeed, the director had to allow students to enter military service who had received only marginal training. In 1708, Peter ordered the college to provide twenty medical students for the army. Even by the low standards of Russian military medicine, the director agreed to send only six.[81] The constant drain of half-trained medical students to serve as surgeons and mates almost forced the school to close. The school produced only ten graduates a year, and from 1712 to 1727 every member of every graduating class was sent into military service.

These difficulties aside, the number of trained medical personnel available to the army increased, albeit slowly. In 1713, the Apothecary Bureau reported that 262 medics of all types were assigned to military service. In 1720, the Baltic Fleet employed 102 medics, and seven years later, the number had increased to 165. The Russian Army's medical branch was formally established in 1716, and medics were assigned to each regiment, apothecaries provided in the field, and field hospitals organized for the first time. In 1720, the navy was ordered to construct a similar medical system.[82]

The success of the Gospitali in providing military surgeons lent impetus to the construction of other medical facilities. The military itself began to construct military hospitals to care for its wounded and at the same time to serve as training facilities for medics. In 1715 the Petersburg Admiralty Hospital was founded. To provide military surgeons for the army, Russia built other hospitals at Reval (1717), Kronstadt (1717), Tavrov (1724), Astrakhan (1725), and Archangel (1733).[83] Regardless of the effort, however, Russia continued to remain far behind the military medical facilities provided in other armies. It took more than a century, until the Russo-Japanese War of 1904–1905, before military medical care in czarist armies was on par with those found in armies of the West.

THE AMERICAN COLONIES

The close relationship between England and the American colonies for more than a hundred years before the American Revolution exerted a considerable influence upon the development of military medicine during the American War of Independence. Most of the doctors with a formal medical education had been educated in England or Scotland, although some had received their medical training at Leyden in Holland. Only two medical schools existed in the colonies during the colonial period.[84] Meanwhile, the garrisoning of English troops in the American colonies, the direction of state militias by British officers, and the numerous skirmishes that the Indians and the French fought with British and American forces for almost fifty years had the effect of introducing the American military forces to British military medical practices.

As early as 1676, the Massachusetts Bay Colony provided medical support for its militia when it appointed a surgeon at public expense to attend a force of five hundred troops. In addition, a special house was constructed to care for the sick and wounded.[85] In 1762, a military hospital was built at state expense in Albany to care for the casualties of the French and Indian War (1754–1763). In imitation of the British practice of the time, a surgeon and one surgeon's mate routinely attended militia companies. As in British units, American regimental colonels appointed their surgeons, who, in turn, selected the mates. Not surprising, many of the problems of competency and training associated with these British Army practices were also present in the colonial militia armies.

Massachusetts was the first colony to create the position of medical commissioner, whose charge was to purchase, store, and issue medical supplies to the armies. In May 1775, the colony rented buildings in Boston to billet and care for the troops, established separate hospitals to deal with smallpox cases among the soldiery, and made provisions for caring for the "insane of war."[86] In early June, a medical committee was appointed to devise means for providing the troops with medicine and supplies, and another committee was created to prepare plans and regulations for hospitals. These steps were taken before the outbreak of open hostilities. When war broke out with England, the Committees of Safety purchased medical chests and surgical instruments at public expense for the state regiments' use and a complete set of medical instruments for each corps. At the Battle of Bunker Hill on June 17, 1775, however, the American casualties were so heavy that the planned medical system collapsed under the load.

It became evident early on that the quality of medical personnel available to the army posed a serious problem. Massachusetts took the lead in establishing a board of medical examiners to examine all candidates who applied for the positions of surgeon and surgeon's mate. Although the regimental commander could submit the name of candidates, the board certified the military surgeons. For the most part, its examinations were thorough and difficult, although somewhat spotty in other states. Throughout the war, each colony remained responsible for providing medical personnel and supplies for its home regiments.

In July 1775, Congress authorized the establishment of a "hospital for the army," a term for the medical department for a force of twenty thousand men. Following the British pattern, the hospital was really a medical staff whose task was to follow the army and set up ad hoc medical support behind the lines. The British pattern was followed in all important details, with the hospital comprising a director, one chief physician, four surgeons, one apothecary, twenty surgeon's mates, one clerk, two storekeepers, one nurse for each ten sick, and one nurse matron.[87] A total of three hospitals were created for the Northern, Middle, and Southern Departments (theaters of operation) of the armies. It developed two separate medical systems—one responsible to national authority and the other responsible to state authority—resulting in inevitable confusion, lack of supply, and poor coordination that hindered the provision of medical care to the field armies.

If the states did not provide sufficient medical supplies—and most often they either did not or could not—the regimental surgeon was largely on his own since there were no provisions to supply him regularly through national authorities. Medical tents were usually unobtainable, and when the army was garrisoned in a city, the regimental barracksmaster was responsible for finding a building suitable for use as a hospital. In winter encampments such as Valley Forge, makeshift log huts served as hospitals and housing. Beds and bedding were rarely provided to the hospitals, which were forced to rely on the regimental supply officer for these items. Each company was required to carry extra bed sacks to be filled with straw when the sick needed them, and the soldier provided his own blanket in the hospital. Without a dedicated supply train for the medical units, even these items were reserved for the wounded, but no provisions were made for the sick.

As in the English Army, there were no transport vehicles organic to the colonial medical service. It did not use any special ambulance vehicles, and what wagons were from time to time available were drawn from the regular army stores. The arrangements for evacuating the wounded were so poor that surgeons were instructed to find handbarrows to move the wounded to the hospitals. Any manpower that was made available for this task came from the largesse of the field commander. The manning levels for the medical service were low, with a single surgeon and five mates for every five thousand men. Further, the English blockade made it difficult to import medical supplies from abroad, the usual source for colonial physicians. An inventory of medical supplies on hand in February 1776 for an army of 16,877 men revealed only nine sets of amputating instruments, twenty pocket cases, two cases of lancets, twelve cases of crooked suture needles, two cases of surgical knives, twenty-four tourniquets, 859 bandages, and twelve pounds of surgical lint.[88] Surgeons were instructed to use razors to perform operations in lieu of adequate surgical instruments. Six months later conditions had not improved. Four days before the Battle of Long Island (August 1776), the army's total medical supplies on hand consisted of only five hundred bandages, twelve fracture boxes, and two scalpels.[89]

In the early days of the war, patriotic fervor prompted large numbers of citizens to enlist in the army. With no medical screening examinations for recruits, the American Army soon became a walking health disaster. Military medical officers attempted to establish field hygiene practices and encourage daily shaving and regular bathing to reduce the spread of disease. The American force was composed mostly of country boys and the urban poor, neither known for their cleanliness habits. Disease became the army's constant companion throughout the war, and the overall death rate from disease was ten times higher than from enemy bullets.[90] Disease was so common that it became increasingly difficult to recruit sufficient manpower as men now avoided military service out of fear of epidemic.

The frequent incidence of disease in the revolutionary army is easily discernible from the following figures. In February 1776 the army of 16,877 men had 3,765 men, or 22.3 percent of total its strength, listed as unfit for duty due to illness.[91] At Crown Point, New York, that December the nation's largest military hospital listed 3,000 patients in that single hospital. In the first year of the war, more than 5,000 men, or 25 percent of the total force, were lost to death, illness, or desertion.[92] In December 1777, 2,898 men of the 11,000-man force at Valley Forge were unfit for duty because of illness. By February 1778, 4,000 men were unfit because of illness and injuries from cold.[93] The American Army was the first army to attempt widespread vaccination of its troops against smallpox, but the use of smallpox inoculation at Valley Forge sent 3,000 men to the hospital with reactionary cases of the disease. "Jail fever" (typhus), for example, was an ever-present danger in close quarters. In a three-month period, four hundred of the seven hundred prisoners died of jail fever and were buried in a common grave.[94] The Valley Forge encampment of Washington's army was a medical catastrophe. The encampment lasted from December 17, 1777, to June 19, 1778, or a period of six months. Some ten thousand soldiers had entered the encampment. By June, twenty-five hundred to three thousand had died of disease, exposure, or malnutrition.[95]

The field hospitals in the Valley Forge cantonment were primitive, constructed largely of log huts. These "flying hospital huts" were twenty-five feet long and fifteen feet wide by nine feet high and covered with boards or shingles for roofs. Windows were placed on each side and a fireplace and chimney at one end. Two hospital huts were authorized for each brigade, but the space was never sufficient to handle the number of casualties and the sick from a single brigade. Hospitals were established in rear area villages and towns, but the local populace always raised considerable opposition to placing a hospital in their midst. The fear of epidemics, the requisitioning of buildings for military use, and the widespread fraud in purchasing supplies led the locals to treat the military suspiciously. Sometimes the number of casualties brought to a small town or village exceeded the number of residents.

Of the thirty-five hundred colonial physicians and surgeons in America in 1775, only four hundred of them had medical degrees or formal medical education.[96] In Virginia, only one in nine practicing physicians had received any formal medical training.[97] These figures, however, do not provide an accurate portrait of the quality of medical personnel available to the military.[98] Unlike in Europe, where strong guilds perpetuated the strict separation between surgeons and physicians, that practice never developed in America. American medicine was in the hands of the general practitioner who healed, operated, and mixed and prescribed his own medicines. His medical training was largely achieved less through formal education than through an apprentice system. General Washington realized that the states provided many physicians whose technical competence left much to be desired, and he pressed Congress to require surgeons and mates to take examinations before being assigned to military units. Congress yielded to pressure from the states, though, and didn't take any action.[99] Gradually the states enacted examination and licensing procedures, but Congress did not establish a screening board for military surgeons until 1782. Because of the apprentice system of medical training, however, the quality of military medical personnel was as good as, and in a number of ways even superior to, that available in European armies.[100]

The pragmatic bent of American medical practice unhindered by the social distinctions between surgeon and physician was evident in the appointment of John Jones (1729–1791) as the first full professor of surgery at the Medical School at King's College, New York.[101] Jones wrote *Plain, Concise Practical Remarks on the Treatment of Wounds and Fractures*, the first surgical text published by an American in the United States in 1775. The book appeared in time for the war and became a basic training and field text for military surgeons.[102]

The Revolutionary War provided a strong stimulus to developing military and general medicine in the colonies. The early problems of the military doctors' competency forced states to adopt stringent examinations and licensing requirements that persisted after the war, generally raising the quality of medical practice. The war also gave physicians who heretofore were isolated in small rural communities an opportunity to interact with other physicians and to exchange ideas, treatments, techniques, and drug formulas. American doctors also came into contact with the medical staffs of their French allies and acquired skills on hospital administration for which the French were noted. Although expressly forbidden by both civil and military law, undoubtedly battlefield surgeons experimented on the bodies of the dead to improve their anatomical knowledge.[103] Furthermore, because the severance of commercial ties with Britain removed the main source of medical equipment and drugs, the Americans were forced to develop their own substitutes.

The quality of American medical thought and innovation during this period was evident in the publication of a number of American medical books. Jones's book, already noted, became the definitive text in the field. *Recommendations of Inoculation According to Baron Dimsdale's Methods* (1776) by John Morgan (1735–1789) influenced the American Army to adopt inoculation as a preventive for smallpox. Morgan became the first director general of the American military medical service. William Brown (1754–1808), an army doctor, wrote a *Pharmacopoeia for Use of Army Hospitals* (1778), the first book of its kind in the colonies.[104] Benjamin Rush's (1745–1813) *Directions for Preserving the Health of the Soldier* (1778) became the handbook for field hygiene, as did his other work, *Regulations for the Order and Discipline of Troops of the US*. Hospital administration and health care were the focus of James Tilton (1745–1822). He wrote about his experiences as a physician and surgeon in the war in *Economical Observations on Military Hospitals and the Prevention of Disease Incident to an Army* (1813). Ebenezer Beardsley (1746–1791) wrote an account of the cause, spread, and treatment of dysentery in colonial regiments. All of these works made significant contributions to the theory and practice of military medicine and reflected the pragmatism that continues to characterize American medicine to the present time.

The care of veterans had long been a tradition in the American colonies. As early as 1636 the Plymouth colony passed a law providing for the support of the crippled soldier, and in 1644 the Virginia Assembly created a system of relief for the soldier maimed in battle. Immediately after the start of the Revolutionary War, Congress ordained that soldiers incapacitated by war should receive half pay, similar to the British practice of caring for their wounded veterans. In 1792, Congress passed a pension law for veterans.

Congress always viewed its raising of a national army to fight the War of Independence as a temporary measure forced by difficult times, and when the war was over, the national army was demobilized. By 1783, the entire national armed force of the United States, renamed "The Legion," consisted of fewer than a thousand men. With the army's demobilization also came the dismantlement of the military medical service. Regimental surgeons and mates stationed with the troops in camp hospitals had provided the soldier's medical care. The U.S. military continued to operate without a systematic military medical service until the War of 1812, when military necessity again forced the country to devise ways to provide medical care for its soldiers.

To recap, in the eighteenth century the centralized power of the nation state reached a level of organizational control that it had sought for three centuries. This centralization enabled the aggressive monarchs of the period to consolidate their power within their domestic realms and to expand it beyond their borders. Inevitably, the price of this expansion was war. With the improvements in military technology came a greater demand for large numbers of soldiers, a demand that could only be filled through voluntary enlistments. To encourage recruitment, the armies of the day had to improve the soldier's living conditions. This effort also required developing better military medical care and establishing veterans' programs. Consequently, the provision of organized military medical care became a recognized and regular function of government.

Improvements in the general quality of medical education and training in civilian society enabled armies to enlist trained medical personnel to treat the soldiers. The advances in medical knowledge and technology inevitably, if slowly, found their way into the military medical organizations. Only the navies of the world, where medical care was as dismal as it had been during the Middle Ages, remained the exception to this general trend. The final liberation of surgery from the social and political tyranny of the physician establishment also elevated the quality of medical care for the soldier.

As the nineteenth century dawned, armies had gained considerable experience in providing medical care to their troops in the field. In times of peace the medical service structures took the opportunity to improve their quality and, most important, to plan for providing medical care before the next actual fight. The stability of the organizational structure permitted the introduction of medical advances accomplished in the civilian sector much more quickly than before. Finally, the graduates of the first national medical schools of military medicine were reaching the peaks of their careers in the military bureaucracies, providing the armies with generally well-trained and experienced medical officers to manage the problem of medical care in wartime. The armies of the eighteenth century were poised on the edge of developing a modern military medical service in its degree of organizational articulation. Once the structure was in place, incorporating the medical innovations of the next century into the armies was relatively easy, thereby raising the quality of medical care available to the soldier to heretofore unachievable heights.

NOTES

1. Mary C. Gillett, *The Army Medical Department, 1775–1818* (Washington, DC: Center of Military History, U.S. Army, 1981): 1.
2. Ibid.
3. Garrison, *Introduction to the History*, 397.

4. Ibid., 335.
5. Kirkup, "History and Evolution," 284.
6. H. A. L. Howell, "The Story of the Army Surgeon and the British Care of the Sick and Wounded in the British Army, from 1715 to 1748," *Journal of the Royal Army Medical* Corps 22 (1914): 324.
7. Ibid., 323.
8. Heizmann, "Military Sanitation," 295.
9. Ibid., 296.
10. Ibid.
11. The first attempts to adopt clothing for purely military use were intended to afford the soldier greater concealment on the battlefield. The British Army abandoned the traditional red coat during the Second Afghan War and adopted khaki uniforms to better blend in with the light and sandy background of the country's terrain. After the Franco-Prussian War, the Germans rid themselves of their brightly colored regimental uniforms and adopted the famous *feldgrau*, or "field gray"–colored, uniforms that are worn to this day.
12. Starvation and poor economic conditions have driven military recruitment since time immemorial. The large contingents of Irish serving in the British armies since the Great Famine is an obvious example. A great number of soldiers in Gen. George Custer's command were Irish immigrants. Much of the American frontier army was comprised of immigrants, free blacks, and other minorities (Mexicans and native Indians) as a consequence of the lack of opportunity for these groups in the larger society.
13. Officers, however, continued to pay for their rations and still do in most modern military establishments.
14. Heizmann, "Military Sanitation," 296.
15. John Thorne Crissey and Lawrence Charles Parish, "Wound Healing: Development of the Basic Concepts," *Clinics in Dermatology* 2, no. 3 (July–September 1984): 554.
16. West, "A Short History," 147.
17. Gordon, "Penetrating Head Injuries," 5–6.
18. Howard Lewis Applegate, "The Need for Further Study in the Medical History of the American Revolutionary Army," *Military Medicine* (August 1961): 617.
19. Wangensteen et al., "Some Highlights," 105.
20. Ibid., 106.
21. However, the disease and infection rates among soldiers in these primitively constructed hospitals were often much lower than in the larger hospitals. The poor construction left these makeshift hospitals subject to drafts, which provided ventilation and renewed the stale air within the wards. See Young, "Short History," 488; and Howard Lewis Applegate, "Effect of the American Revolution on American Medicine," *Military Medicine* (July 1961): 552–53.
22. Gillett, *Army Medical Department*, 3.
23. Ibid., 8.
24. Ibid., 6.
25. Grissinger, "Development of Military Medicine," 317.
26. Abram S. Benenson, "Immunization and Military Medicine," *Clinical Infectious Diseases* 6, no. 1 (January–February 1984): 2.
27. McGrew, *Encyclopedia of Medical History*, 155.
28. Benenson, "Immunization and Military Medicine," 1.
29. Ibid.

30. Taylor, "Retrospect of Naval and Military Medicine," 594.
31. Garrison, *Notes on the History*, 374.
32. Heizmann, "Military Sanitation," 297.
33. Ibid.
34. Howell, "Story of the Army Surgeon," 333.
35. For more on the military medicine of the Roman Navy, see Richard A. Gabriel, "The Roman Navy: Masters of the Mediterranean," *Military History*, December 2007, 37–43.
36. Ibid.
37. The term "quarantine" comes from the Latin *quarantine*, which means forty. Tradition has it that the original period of quarantine for crews on commercial vessels was forty days, the same length of time that Christ was said to have spent being tempted in the desert.
38. Taylor, "Retrospect of Naval and Military Medicine," 596.
39. Uniform clothing was not issued to the sailor as a health measure. The officers recognized that uniforms made sailors more easily identifiable on shore, an advantage in curtailing desertion.
40. The term "to shanghai," meaning to impress a person forcefully into naval service, refers to the port of Shanghai, China. The idea is that once caught by the press gangs, the sailor's next stop was Shanghai.
41. Taylor, "Retrospect of Naval and Military Medicine," 596.
42. Lawson, "Amputations through the Ages," 223.
43. Taylor, "Retrospect of Naval and Military Medicine," 600.
44. Ibid., 601.
45. Howell, "Story of the Army Surgeon," 327.
46. Taylor, "Retrospect of Naval and Military Medicine," 603.
47. Howell, "Story of the Army Surgeon," 321.
48. Chamberlain, "History of Military Medicine," 240.
49. Nonetheless, armies persist in defining medical conditions as discipline and morale problems. Soviet frostbite casualties were so high during World War II that Joseph Stalin issued an order that any soldier careless enough to get frostbite would be shot. In Vietnam, American soldiers who contracted venereal disease were subject to punishment. Psychiatric conditions of the "silent" type often are still treated as discipline problems.
50. Howell, "Story of the Army Surgeon," 332.
51. Paul E. Kopperman, "Medical Services in the British Army, 1742–1783," *Journal of the History of Medicine and Allied Sciences* 34, no. 4 (October 1979): 428–29.
52. Howell, "Story of the Army Surgeon," 332.
53. Ibid., 331.
54. Ibid.
55. Kopperman, "Medical Services," 430.
56. Ibid., 437.
57. Ibid., 438, citing Robert Jackson, *A System of Arrangement and Discipline for the Medical Department of the Armies* (London: J. Murray, 1805), for these figures.
58. Taylor, "Retrospect of Naval and Military Medicine," 596.
59. Kopperman, "Medical Services," 454.
60. Garrison, *Notes on the History*, 138.
61. Edgar Erskine Hume, "The Days Gone By: Military Medicine in the Eighteenth Century," *Military Surgeon*, October 1929, 563.
62. Ibid.

63. Chamberlain, "History of Military Medicine," 240.
64. Ibid.
65. Louis S. Greenbaum, "Science, Medicine, and Religion: Three Views of Health Care in France on the Eve of the French Revolution," *Studies in Eighteenth-Century Culture* 10 (1981): 373–91.
66. Heizmann, "Military Sanitation," 299.
67. Hume, "Days Gone By," 564.
68. Heizmann, "Military Sanitation," 298.
69. Garrison, *Notes on the History*, 139.
70. Ibid.
71. Ibid.
72. Ibid., 141.
73. Taylor, "Retrospect of Naval and Military Medicine," 606.
74. Ibid.
75. It should not be assumed, however, that the physician and surgeon came to military service with the same educational background. The most that can be implied is that both received the same military medical training after entering military service.
76. Taylor, "Retrospect of Naval and Military Medicine," 607.
77. Garrison, *Notes on the History*, 142.
78. Taylor, "Retrospect of Naval and Military Medicine," 566.
79. The best English work on military medicine in Russia during this period is John T. Alexander's "Medical Developments in Petrine Russia," *Canadian-American Slavic Studies* 8, no. 2 (Summer 1974): 207.
80. Ibid.
81. Ibid.
82. Ibid., 210.
83. Ibid.
84. L. G. Eichner, "The Military Practice of Medicine during the Revolutionary War," lecture presented at the Tredyffrin Easttown History Society, Pennsylvania, October 2003, 25.
85. Edwin P. Wolfe, "The Genesis of the Medical Department of the United States Army," *Bulletin of the New York Academy of Medicine* 5 (September 1929): 823.
86. See Ibid., 613; and Taylor, "Retrospect of Naval and Military Medicine," 627.
87. Wolfe, "Genesis of the Medical Department," 613.
88. M. A. Reasoner, "The Development of the Medical Supply Service," *Military Surgeon* 63, no. 1 (July 1928): 7.
89. Taylor, "Retrospect of Naval and Military Medicine," 613.
90. David B. Davis, "Medicine in the Canadian Campaign of the Revolutionary War," *Bulletin of the History of Medicine* 44, no. 5 (September–October 1970): 461.
91. Reasoner, "Medical Supply Service," 7.
92. Ibid., 9.
93. William Shainline Middleton, "Medicine at Valley Forge," *Annals of Medical History* 3, no. 6 (November 1941): 465.
94. Ibid.
95. Eichner, "Military Practice of Medicine," 27, for a list of the specific medical conditions that caused death.
96. Howard Lewis Applegate, "Preventive Medicine in the American Revolutionary Army," *Military Medicine* 126 (May 1961): 380.

97. Blair O. Rogers, "Surgery in the Revolutionary War: Contributions of John Jones, M.D. (1729–1791)," *Plastic and Reconstructive Surgery* 49 (January 1972): 3.
98. Davis, "Medicine in the Canadian Campaign," 461.
99. Eichner, "Military Practice of Medicine," 26.
100. Rogers, "Surgery in the Revolutionary War," 9.
101. The name was changed from King's College to Columbia University during the Revolutionary War.
102. Jones had been a military surgeon in the French and Indian War, an experience that prompted him to write his manual for wound treatment. The practical value of his manual, appearing as it did at the outbreak of the war, is obvious from the table of contents. Jones's book contains chapters on inflammation, superficial wounds, general wounds, penetrating wounds, simple fractures, compound fractures, amputations, head injuries, concussions, skull fractures, gunshot wounds, and how to set up and manage a military field hospital.
103. Applegate, "Preventive Medicine," 551.
104. Allen C. Wooden, "Dr. Jean François Coste and the French Army in the American Revolution," *Delaware Medical Journal* 48, no. 7 (July 1976): 398. While Brown's work was the first of its type written by an American in the colonies, Coste had authored a small military pharmacopoeia for the French troops' use that had gained wide readership among American physicians.

5

THE NINETEENTH CENTURY
The Age of Amputation

The nineteenth century was the period in which the principle of empirical observation finally triumphed in medical matters over the influence of cosmological theorizing. As the century progressed, medical clinicians and researchers gradually worked out the methodological problems associated with discovery, innovation, and verification; abandoned old theories of disease; and established criteria of proof for new medical information. While the century was replete with new approaches and discoveries, the evolution and systematic application of new methodologies marked the century as the true beginning of modern scientific medicine. Table 7 presents a list of the most important medical advances and innovations relative to the wars that occurred in the nineteenth century.

The century was also marked by significant contributions that military physicians made to medical advances and the development of military medicine along modern lines. Military physicians applied to the battlefield various medical discoveries and techniques that the civilian medical establishment developed and greatly improved the organizational structures required to deliver effective medical care to the soldier in the field. Few armies began the period with anything approaching a systematic military medical service, but by the century's end, all major combatants had set up independent military medical departments capable of dealing with mass casualties. The stimulus for these developments was, of course, the frequency of wars.

The wars of the nineteenth century were fought with increasing ferocity and lethality as a consequence of the technological advances in the killing power of weaponry. The French Revolution had created a new kind of army, an army of citizens, who, in exchange for the burden of conscription, expected better military medical

Table 7. Major Medical Advances of the Nineteenth Century and the First Half of the Twentieth Century

Year	Medical Discovery	British War
1815		Waterloo (1815)
		↑
		40 years
1846	Ether (John Snow)	
1847	Chloroform (J. Y. Simpson)	
1852	Plaster of Paris (Mahijson)	↓
		Crimea (1854–56)
		↑
1867	Pasteur (Bacteria)	
1868	Lister (Carbolic)	
1878	Thomas Splint (Dormant till 1914)	40 years
1885	B. Tetanus isolated (Nicolaier)	
1890	A.T.S. (Behring)	
1895	Konrad Roentgen	
1898	R.A.M.C.	↓
1899	T.A.B. (AlmrothWright)	Boer War (1899–1902)
		↑
1901	Landsteiner (Blood groups)	14 years
	(1914–18 Experimental)	↓
	(1939 Organized B.T.S.)	World War I (1914–18)
		↑
1931	T. Toxoid (Ramon)	20 years
1935	Sulphonamides (Domagk)	
1939	Blood Transfusion	
1940	E.M.S. Hospitals	
1943	Penicillin	↓
1943	D.D.T.	World War II (1939–45)

Table by author.

care. The extremely high casualty rates caused by more lethal weapons forced political and military authorities to improve medical care as a way of conserving expensive manpower. Although few armies at the start of the period had learned these lessons, all major combatants had institutionalized their practices to establish adequate military medical services by the end of the century.

Few periods can compare with the nineteenth century in terms of the sheer frequency and destructiveness of warfare. The century began with the decade-long wars of the French Revolution only to witness, after a short respite, their continuation in the guise of the Napoleonic Wars. Across the Atlantic, the Americans fought the War of 1812 and the Mexican War of 1846–1848, both significant conflicts for the emerging United States. The Crimean War, which pitted the Russian Empire against a European alliance, caused so many casualties from weapons and disease that the public outcries of the combatants' civilian populations forced significant military and medical reforms. The American Civil War, the world's first truly modern war, shocked not only the United States but also caused European leaders to search for ways to increase the combat power and manpower assets of their own armies in anticipation of having to fight such wars themselves. France's wars with Italy and Germany were bloodbaths, revealing the West's complete inability to avoid horrific slaughter in its own backyard. In the end, the strategists and tacticians abandoned the search for solutions and resigned themselves to the fact that slaughter could not be avoided. Unwilling to abandon the structures and tactical principles, along with the accompanying privileges and social status, that had marked the military establishments of Europe for a century, the military thinkers of the late nineteenth century seem to have comforted themselves with more traditional doctrines of war fighting. When once again the major powers of Europe stumbled into conflict in the early twentieth century, these illusions evaporated overnight and left in their wake the most horrible slaughter ever wrought between contesting armies.

If war provided the stimulus for improved military medical care, the technological innovations of the Industrial Revolution provided the opportunity. The wars of the French Revolution and the Napoleonic era that followed interfered with the transfer of medical knowledge across national borders. The location of these wars and their long duration effectively forced medical research and discovery back within respective national borders. After 1815, wars of the period were fought on the periphery of Europe (Crimea) and outside Europe (the Mexican War, the Civil War) and were of short duration (France-Italy, Franco-Prussian War). The period following the

Napoleonic Wars also saw great improvements in travel and communication. Medical discoveries and new treatment techniques were shared through printed books, newspapers, and medical and scientific journals, often transmitted telegraphically or through regular mail service that spanned the oceans in a few weeks. For the first time since the Roman Empire, the development of medicine could be viewed as a coherent whole rather than applying only to separate countries. A general commonality of medical knowledge and practice began that connected the efforts of researchers and practitioners across national boundaries. Only Russia—because of its geographic and, to some degree, cultural isolation—and Germany, because of its political fragmentation, remained apart from the stream of medical discovery and practice.

Neither medical nor military men could have anticipated the changes that occurred in warfare and military medicine during the nineteenth century. When the century began, the long-established tensions among the physician, surgeon, and barber-surgeon that had retarded the application of practical medicine to the soldier continued to strangle the medical profession. By the end of the century, except in Russia, the military barber-surgeon had disappeared, and surgery had finally established itself as an equal partner in the medical profession. A similar status was finally conferred upon military medical officers for the first time.

When the nineteenth century dawned, medical practitioners believed that the suppuration of wounds was a natural, inevitable, and beneficial part of the healing process, and they accepted the deaths of thousands of soldiers to wound infection as an unavoidable cost of war. By century's end, however, discoveries in bacteriology made antiseptic and, later, aseptic surgery a common practice, and the death rate to wound infection dropped dramatically. Also at the beginning of the century, pain was the expected price of surgical application. Within fifty years, the introduction of anesthesia banished pain from the operating room and gave birth to the new science of anesthesiology. With pain alleviated, the necessity for surgical speed was reduced, opening up the possibility of more complex surgical procedures. Most military surgeons at the turn of the eighteenth century had not yet mastered ligature or the tourniquet; thus, amputation, the most common surgical procedure performed on the wounded, remained a traumatic and risky business. By the end of the nineteenth century, however, both ligature and tourniquet applications were normal practice, as was the use of the hemostat and surgical clip. Cautery was finally banished from the surgeon's kit.

The greatest killer of soldiers at the beginning of the century was still disease, and it routinely carried off eight soldiers for each one felled by an enemy bullet. The advances of bacteriology, nutrition, and military and public sanitation, along with antiseptic surgery, finally made it possible for an army to kill more of the enemy with hostile fire than were killed by deadly infectious microbes. The Franco-Prussian War was the first war of any magnitude in which the number of soldiers lost to hostile fire was greater than to disease.

At the start of the nineteenth century, no army had established an independent military medical service under the control of medical officers for treating the sick and wounded. No nation could provide a trained medical staff, supply structure, transport, and medical personnel adequate to handle the usual casualty loads. By the end of the century, every major army had an independent, professionally trained, and sufficiently manned military medical service complete with an ambulance corps for reaching and evacuating the huge numbers of casualties that had never before been seen on the battlefield. If war finally reached modern proportions in all its respects in the nineteenth century, it is also fair to say that military medicine achieved a similar stature.

ANESTHESIA

Effective and safe anesthesia was introduced to military medicine in the nineteenth century. The term "anesthesia" is generally credited to Oliver Wendell Holmes Sr. (1809–1894), to describe the effects of ether.[1] Prior to the discovery of ether and chloroform as anesthetics, the most commonly used agent against pain was opium administered in liquid or powdered form. Other methods of rendering a patient unconscious or semiconscious for surgery were to reduce the blood supply to the brain either by compressing the carotid artery until the patient passed out or by bleeding the patient to a state of near total unconsciousness. Immediately prior to the introduction of ether anesthesia, some surgeons, including the famous English surgeon Sir Robert Liston (1794–1847), used hypnotic suggestion to induce sleep.[2] All of these methods produced semiconscious states of only short duration, requiring the surgeon to complete the surgical procedure quickly.

The first gas recognized as having anesthetic properties was nitrous oxide, which Joseph Priestley (1733–1804) identified in 1772 as part of his experiments with oxygen. For several years the gas was thought to be deadly. In 1795, the chemist Humphry Davy (1778–1829) inhaled nitrous oxide and, noting its pleasant effects, named the mixture "laughing gas." In 1800, Davy published a monograph in which he described the use of nitrous oxide to relieve the pain of an inflamed gum. More important, he suggested its use as a surgical anesthetic. Eighteen years later, Davy's student, Michael Faraday, noticed the anesthetic effects of sulfuric ether and compared them to the effects of nitrous oxide. In 1842, Henry Hill Hickman, a member of the Royal College of Surgeons of London, performed the first operation with an anesthetic on animals.

None of these experiments evoked any serious interest. Although nitrous oxide and ether were well known by mid-century, the medical community still showed no systematic interest in using it for surgery, perhaps because of the widespread belief that pain was natural to illness. Medical students were aware of the anesthetic properties of both nitrous oxide and sulfuric ether, and they commonly used them at university parties to induce silly behavior. In January 1842, William E. Clarke, a student of chemistry, convinced Elijah Pope to extract a tooth from a patient anesthetized by ether. Two months later a Georgia dentist, Crawford Long, removed a tumor from the neck of a patient who was anesthetized by ether. After William T. G. Morton, a Boston dentist, extracted a tooth from a patient to whom he had administered ether in 1846, he published the results of his work in the *Boston Journal*. Morton was heretofore regarded as the discoverer of ether as a surgical anesthetic. In October 1846, Morton administered anesthesia while Dr. John Collins Warren removed a tumor from a patient's jaw. The use of ether as a surgical anesthetic quickly spread to Paris and to London, where, in December 1846, Sir Liston performed a thigh amputation on an etherized patient and publicly proclaimed the new anesthetic a major medical innovation.

The U.S. Army was the first to formally issue ether for anesthetic purposes, having allotted supplies to the physicians and battle surgeons who accompanied Maj. Gen. Winfield Scott's men in the 1847 landing at Veracruz during the Mexican War. That March or early April, Edward H. Barton, surgeon of the Third Dragoons, Cavalry Brigade, Twiggs's Division, anesthetized a teamster of the U.S. Army's logistics train to amputate his leg, which had been shattered by an accidental musket blast. The operation marks a military field surgeon's first use of the ether anesthetic.[3]

Samuel Guthrie in the United States, Eugène Soubeiran in France, and Justus von Liebig in Germany almost simultaneously discovered chloroform in 1831.[4] Chloroform was not used as an anesthetic, however, until 1847.[5] Chloroform had a number of advantages over ether for military applications. The simple "rag and bottle method" of administering chloroform was easier to use since it did not require an inhaler. Smaller quantities were required to induce anesthesia, and chloroform could be more easily stored and transported in the battle surgeon's pocket while in the field. Most important, unlike ether, chloroform was not explosive, an important consideration in a time when most operations were performed by candle or lantern light in close quarters. Given these advantages, it is difficult to explain why chloroform was so slow to catch on, especially among English military surgeons. From 1847 to the early days of the Crimean War in 1853, there was not a single documented instance of a British military surgeon using chloroform for anesthesia.[6] John Snow (1813–1858) was the first physician to calculate specific doses for ether and chloroform as surgical anesthetics. He personally administered chloroform to Queen Victoria (1819–1901) during the births of the last two of her nine children, leading to the widespread acceptance of the use of anesthetics among English physicians. Although the French military had used it as early as the Paris revolt of 1848 and the Prussians likely used it in the Danish-Prussian War of 1848–1851, British military medical doctors did not begin to use chloroform until the first few months of the Crimean War. A British naval surgeon aboard the HMS *Arethusa* was the first to administer chloroform at sea in 1854.[7]

AMPUTATION

Anesthesia revolutionized military surgery, especially in the area of battlefield amputation. Without anesthesia, speed was the surgeon's primary qualification. Sir Liston, the famous English surgeon, reportedly could amputate a leg in twenty-eight seconds. Even less skilled military surgeons could accomplish the task in less than a minute. Moreover, the doctrine of primary amputation advanced early in the century by Dominique-Jean Larrey, Baron Pierre-François Percy (1754–1825), and George James Guthrie (1785–1856) was gradually accepted as the century wore on, and under the influence of Sir Thomas Longmore (1816–1895) and George H. B. MacLeod in the Crimean War, it became established practice for military surgeons. Anesthesia made it possible to operate more slowly, to take the time to effect more complete hemostasis (stopping blood flow), and to prepare the stump for prosthesis. Although early in the century surgeons maintained that the pain associated with surgery was actually beneficial in that it kept the body's systems fighting to survive, in fact the use of anesthesia greatly reduced the incidence of death by surgical shock.

The problem of hemostasis remained a serious obstacle to battlefield surgery, however. A common method of hemostasis during amputation was to put pressure on the femoral artery. Liston preferred this technique to the tourniquet. Ligature gained more acceptance as surgeons trained in battlefield surgery gradually learned how to accomplish it. At the beginning of the century, surgeons found that a ligatured artery formed a clot within the ligature. Military surgeons often left the ligatures long so that the suture could act as a drain outside the wound. A common practice until after the Civil War, this technique allowed the exposed suture to act as a wick along which infection could be transferred deep within the wound, provoking a secondary hemorrhage that was often fatal. Since the ligature material was not sterile, even a short ligature left in the wound provoked infection and secondary hemorrhage. Philip Physick (1768–1837), a Philadelphia surgeon, made some progress in this area. He experimented with ligatures made of buckskin and parchment to make them absorbable. Horatio Jameson (1778–1855) of Baltimore continued the work and, in 1824, introduced absorbable ligatures made of kid and chamois.[8] The medical community, however, was slow to accept both advances. Until after the Civil War, most ligatures were still made of harnessmaker's silk, horsehair, and catgut. Dr. Joseph Lister experimented with treating catgut with carbolic and tannic acid to make it sterile, but using these materials produced high rates of tetanus, anthrax, and gas gangrene in amputated limbs.[9] Meanwhile, some advances in hemostasis were achieved. In 1829, Karl Ferdinand van Gräfe developed a lock to hold the hemostat closed, and more technical advances were made along the way until William Steward Halsted invented the modern hemostat in 1879.[10] Spencer Wells contributed greatly to the introduction of bloodless surgery in 1872 when he used small arterial clips to close off blood flow temporarily during surgical procedures. In 1873, the German military surgeon Friedrich von Esmarch invented the Esmarch elastic bandage, which served as a battlefield tourniquet and promised the possibility, although unrealized, of bloodless surgery.

The large numbers of experienced surgeons on the battlefield over the course of the century generally improved the overall competence of surgical procedures and stimulated solutions to problems that they had commonly encountered. Thus, the French surgeon Charles Pravaz, searching for a way to administer drugs more efficiently, developed the hypodermic syringe in 1853. René Laennec, another military surgeon, carried out experiments with the stethoscope (published in 1819) and introduced this vital piece of diagnostic equipment for use on the battlefield.[11] Wilhelm Röntgen's discovery of the X-ray in 1895 became a revolutionary way of determining the position of projectiles buried deeply inside the body.[12] Unknown military staff physicians in the Seminole War (1841) discovered that regular doses of quinine were a safe and effective preventive for malarial fever.[13] In 1900, the U.S. Army Yellow Fever Commission, consisting of Walter Reed, James Carroll, and contract surgeons Jesse Lasaer and Aristide Agramonte, proved experimentally that yellow fever was transmitted by the bite of a mosquito. In 1898 American Army physician William Gorgas was assigned to eradicate Cuba of yellow fever, and his efforts later made the building of the Panama Canal possible.[14] As important as these advances were, though, little progress in the field of military surgery and hygiene would have been possible without the discoveries in the field of bacteriology, which, for the first time, made it possible to prevent infection, the primary killer of wounded soldiers.

BACTERIOLOGY AND THE MICROSCOPE

By 1830, improvements in the microscope began to open up the microbial world to medical investigation. Even so, by mid-century no one had made a systematic investigation into microbes as agents responsible for disease, although medical thought had already started to move in the direction of specificity of disease analysis. The most commonly held theory of disease causation at the time was that all sorts of foul matter, or miasmas, transmitted by air and water caused diseases. While medicine at least had abandoned the idea that evil spirits produced illness, conceptions of disease agents had not moved much beyond those of the Roman engineer Marcus Terentius Varro (177 BCE–27 BCE), who speculated that little animals too small to see invaded the body by respiration and breaks in the skin to cause diseases. It was the specific nature of these "little animals" that continued to elude scientific investigation.

Disease and infection continued to kill thousands of soldiers, especially those who succumbed to postoperative infection. In the early 1860s, Joseph Lister found that infection carried off 80 percent of the patients who underwent amputation of the femur and 50 percent who underwent amputation of the tibia in the Male Accident Ward at London Hospital.[15] During the Crimean War, infection produced a mortality rate for thigh amputations of 62 percent, a scant improvement on the 70 percent mortality rate for similar operations during the Battle of Waterloo (1815).[16] Until bacteriology was able to determine the specific cause of infection and disease, no serious attempt at preventing surgical infection was likely to succeed.

Between 1857 and 1863, French chemist Louis Pasteur (1822–1895) conducted a series of experiments on fermentation and putrefaction, successfully demonstrating that different microbe agents caused fermentation in different substances. Pasteur also proved that these agents were not spontaneously generated, a view that enjoyed wide currency at the time, but entered the substance from outside. Pasteur became the most forthright proponent of the germ theory of infection and, in 1878, presented a paper asserting that microorganisms were responsible for disease and infection. Because Pasteur's results were hardly convincing, his new theory was not readily accepted.

After the Franco-Prussian War, Edwin Klebs (1834–1913) furnished convincing proof of the role of microorganisms in surgical sepsis. The most important evidence came with the publication of Robert Koch's *Investigations into the Etiology of Traumatic Infective Diseases* (1879). Not only did Koch (1843–1910) establish through studies of the anthrax bacillus that microorganisms caused specific diseases, but equally important for future investigation, he established the methodology for testing the causative nature of disease-specific agents, one still in use today.[17]

The discovery that microorganisms were responsible for infectious diseases made the advent of antiseptic surgery and the prevention of postoperative infection possible. The idea of antisepsis had been around a long time, but medical practitioners focused on the use of disinfectants in hospital wards. Carl Wilhelm von Scheele had discovered the antiseptic properties of chlorine in 1774, and Bernard Courtois discovered iodine in 1811. Since 1820, chlorine and iodine solutions had been used as "deodorants" along with creosote and turpentine to clean hospital wards and equipment. At the time, a number of published articles suggested using chlorine and iodine solutions as hand rinses for surgeons, but the practice never attracted much attention.[18] Carbolic acid, discovered in 1834, had been used to treat sewage in waste plants for some time, and it is likely that Joseph Lister's experience with carbolic acid at the treatment plant in Carlisle, England, led him to use it in his experiments in antisepsis in the 1860s.

Lister was the son of an amateur microscopist and received early training in the use of the microscope. After completing his medical training, Lister was placed in charge of the Male Accident Ward at London Hospital as a professor of surgery. His own experience with amputation showed that the mortality rate in amputation cases ran between 45 and 50 percent from postoperative infection. Lister's interest in microscopy led him to pay attention to Pasteur's work long before its validity had been demonstrated. Believing Pasteur was correct in his assumptions, Lister began the search for a substance that would kill bacteria. In August 1865, Lister used bandages soaked in carbolic acid for dressing a compound fracture of the tibia. In May, he repeated the procedure on another compound fracture of the leg. Both patients recovered. Lister then developed a systematic procedure for keeping operative wounds wrapped in dressings soaked in carbolic acid. He had hit upon two major medical innovations—*antisepsis*, which involved destroying infective agents that had entered the wound, and *asepsis*, which prevented an infective agent from entering the wound. In March 1867, Lister published his results in the *Lancet.*

Although by 1869 the surgical mortality rate from infection had dropped from 45 percent to less than 1.5 percent in his accident ward, the reaction to Lister's innovation remained mixed. To accept Lister's method, one also had to accept Pasteur's theories, and the latter were hardly demonstrated facts at this time. Resistance to Lister's practices remained strong in France, England, and the United States, where, in 1882, the American Surgical Association officially rejected Lister's doctrines and practice. Only in Germany was Lister regarded as a hero, and the German Army was the first to implement his antiseptic surgical procedures on a wide scale. This practice paid off handsomely during the Franco-Prussian War, when German military surgeons saved thousands of lives by using Lister's technique.

The German medical establishment's acceptance of Lister's work provoked further investigations into bacteriology and antisepsis, such as the work of both Edwin Klebs and Robert Koch, who were also Germans. The Germans pioneered the use of steam sterilization of instruments, sterile operating gowns and masks, and rubber gloves.[19] They were the first to abandon the crowded surgical amphitheaters for smaller disinfected operating rooms. While other countries gradually adopted these procedures, in no other country were they so widely, systematically, and rapidly adopted as in Germany.

These innovations only slowly seeped into the military medical services of other countries.[20] For instance, the American Army made antiseptic surgery part of its official military medical practice in 1877.[21] In 1899, the U.S. Army medical officers officially began using rubber gloves and then widely practiced antiseptic surgery in the Spanish-American War. By 1909, 60 percent of all operations in the American military featured rubber gloves, and by World War I, antiseptic surgery with rubber gloves and sterile surgical drapes was standard doctrine.[22]

The great strides in medical care that were made in the nineteenth century turned upon three major discoveries: anesthesia, bacteriology, and antiseptic surgery. These discoveries revolutionized medical care and opened the door for further research that produced remarkable advances in disease prevention and surgical procedures in the next century. Military medical men were among the first and most enthusiastic practitioners in adopting the new techniques to their task of caring for the sick and wounded, and most of the innovations of this period found their first large-scale use in the military medical environment. The task of treating the suffering and human wreckage of war has always forced the military medical mind into a more practical than theoretical bent and toward a propensity for utilizing what seems to work regardless of the larger theoretical issues involved. The increased degree of institutional development evident in the military medical institutions of the time positioned them perfectly to recognize and adopt new techniques much faster than the civilian medical establishments could. The nineteenth century, after all, was the period in which, by mid-century, every major army had developed a professional military medical service of some institutional stability and competence.

THE FRENCH REVOLUTION AND THE NAPOLEONIC WARS

The armies of revolutionary France were huge for their time and presented a serious problem for their opponents' well-disciplined linear armies. The use of "horde tactics" and frontal assaults produced horrendous casualties. After a poor start, the revolutionary armies succeeded in placing thousands of medical officers in the field. All civilian surgeons and physicians were placed under military conscription and control in August 1793, and in an attempt to abolish privilege, all medical schools were closed and medical practice was opened to anyone who could afford a license. Although the numbers of medical officers were sufficient, the quality of medical care provided to the soldier was often dismal. Inspector General Hercule Sieur of the French medical service called this period "the darkest period of French medicine."[23]

When the Revolution suddenly swerved to the right with the fall of Maximilien Robespierre in 1794, the concern for all social welfare services, including military medicine, declined. Although the medical service had lost six hundred officers in the wars between 1794 and 1795, it remained the object of political scorn and interference. By 1795, the French military medical service had been placed under the political control of various ministries, which changed its organizational structure at whim. It no longer had a clear hierarchy of officers, a system of litter bearers, or a medical supply service, and medical personnel were subordinated to political administrators.[24]

To comprehend the opposition to an established, independent military medical service, it is important to remember that despite the slogans of the Revolution, within the military itself the spirit of privilege and caste was very much alive. The artillery arm had only recently attained equal status with the infantry and cavalry, and it strongly opposed extending similar status to the engineers and medical corps. By 1796, political authorities assumed control of the military hospitals, removed the mobilization and disposition of the ambulances from the authority of the chief surgeons, and appointed political officers from Paris to whom all medical officers in the field were subordinated. Medical service chiefs in hospitals were forbidden to interact with the administration of the hospitals themselves.[25]

The one positive effect of these "reforms" was to drive the best physicians and surgeons from the hospitals into the field to treat the wounded, thereby providing an excellent opportunity to develop a corps of experienced battle surgeons. Nonetheless, between 1800 and 1802 the number of military doctors attached to the armies fell by half, and the number of serving surgeons did not reach the original number again until 1809. By that time, however, the armies had doubled in size. In 1800, 210 physicians and 629 surgeons were in the army. By 1802, the number of physicians had fallen to 62 and the number of surgeons to 500.[26] Napoleon compounded the disaster in 1803 by reducing the number of military hospitals in France to only thirty while simultaneously closing the military teaching hospitals that had been established during the Revolution.[27] Napoleon also refused to make the commissions of military doctors permanent, and despite pleas from Larrey and Percy, he would not establish an independent military medical service.[28]

The results of these misguided policies made themselves felt in the enormous levels of French battle casualties suffered in the Napoleonic Wars. Of the 4.5 million soldiers who served in the revolutionary and Napoleonic armies, 2.5 million died in hospitals from wounds and disease.[29] Another 150,000 were killed in action. During the Egyptian campaign (1798–1800), a force of 30,000 men suffered 4,758 dead in action and 4,157 to disease and infection. The army suffered almost 30,000 cases of ophthalmia, and the death rate from all diseases was 109 men per 1,000.[30] When the sick and wounded were transported home, the mortality rate in transit reached 41 percent.[31] The Russian campaign (1812) began with 533,000 men in Napoleon's invasion force. By the time the army reached Moscow, disease had shrunk the force to 95,000, even though it had fought only two battles along the way. The retreat from Moscow was even more devastating, with thousands of men abandoned to die of disease and cold.[32] Of the total force that began the invasion, only 40,000 lived to reach France. Of these men, fewer than 1,000 were able to return to duty.[33] The death rate among military medical officers was equally appalling. At the start of the campaign,

876 medical officers of the Service de Santé (Health Service) attended the army. By the end, only 276 had survived, representing a loss of 551 officers, or 63 percent, to battle, cold, disease, or capture.[34] To make matters worse, the quality of military surgeons had fallen so low in the Napoleonic armies that Baron Percy, the chief surgeon of the army, called them *chirurgiens de pacotille,* or "slop-shop surgeons."[35]

There were exceptions to this general trend of poor quality, and Larrey, Napoleon's medical director and chief surgeon, was first among them. Larrey took part in twenty-six campaigns, sixty battles, and four hundred engagements and was wounded three times. After Waterloo, the Prussians captured Larrey, but a Prussian surgeon recognized the famous military surgeon and saved him from execution. Marshal Gebhard von Blücher, whose son Larrey had treated before the war, ordered him released. Larrey's memoirs, *Memoires de Chirurgie Militaire et Campagnes* (1812–1817), are the definitive source of information concerning military medicine in this period and make truly adventurous reading. At the Battle of Eylau (1807), Larrey operated for twenty-four hours without rest in weather so cold that his assistants could not hold the instruments. At Borodino (1812), by his own account, he performed no fewer than two hundred amputations in a twenty-four-hour period. His own experience with amputation led him to become an early advocate of the doctrine of primary amputation in contradiction to the then accepted advice of John Hunter. Larrey is recognized as the first military surgeon in Europe to advocate primary amputation. As a student of Desault's, Larrey espoused and practiced debridement of necrotic tissue, and he realized the danger of closing traumatic wounds prematurely. Larrey stipulated basic clinical rules for determining when amputation was required, and these guidelines and the doctrine of primary amputation remained standard military medical practice until after the Russo-Turkish War, when a Russian military surgeon, K. K. Reyer, demonstrated that the majority of gunshot-induced fractures could be salvaged with the aid of antisepsis and early debridement.[36] Larrey was also among the first surgeons to recognize the value of immobilization in healing, and he used the starch splint to reduce the pain that casualties suffered during transport.

Larrey had begun his military medical career in the armies of revolutionary France, where he was quick to recognize the poor quality of medical training and knowledge available to the hastily recruited medics of his day. To correct this problem, Larrey established ad hoc training classes in anatomy and surgery at each of his postings no matter the duration. In Egypt, he became aware of the dangers of disease contagion through his experience with infectious ophthalmia. His list of hygiene instructions to his surgeons was remarkable for its prescience. Larrey prescribed special surgical garments for doctors and nurses made of oiled cloth or rubberized taffeta. If these items were not available, he ordered that gowns should be made of tightly woven linen dipped regularly in vinegar water. He designed special wooden shoes coated with turpentine for use in medical wards. He directed that faces and hands were to be washed regularly in vinegar water, and when undertaking surgery, doctors had to wear linen surgical masks dipped in vinegar water. Larrey's surgeons were required to change the patients' dressings regularly and to minimize physical contact with the patient's wound. Old bandages and bedding were to be burned immediately and instruments washed frequently and kept in an airy place. Before leaving the hospital, surgeons and physicians were required to change their outer clothing and underwear and wash their bodies with vinegar water.[37] As contradictory as it seems, however, Larrey remained a believer in the necessary suppuration of wounds and recommended using charpie as a suppurative.[38]

Larrey may also have been the first to introduce a formal policy of combat triage among his battle surgeons. He ordered that the old practice of treating the officers and rankers first regardless of their degree of injury be replaced with preference for treatment going to the most severely wounded. His instructions to send the slightly wounded back to the second line were especially directed at officers "because officers have horses."[39]

The Flying Ambulance

France's most enduring contribution to the military medicine of the period was the innovation of an effective ambulance corps for evacuating casualties. This development was also a product of Larrey's ingenuity. Under Louis XVI (1754–1793), the French were the first to introduce hospital wagons, and these wagons were still in service at the time of the revolutionary wars. They were very large, carried great amounts of equipment, and were staffed by 134 medical personnel, including thirty-one surgeons and thirty-one trained male nurses. The wagons' colossal size required forty-nine horses to tow each one.[40] Because of their size and slow speed, army regulations required that the wagons remain three miles behind the battle line. Even in the armies of revolutionary France medical personnel were forbidden to treat casualties until the battle had ended, but with the roads around the battlefield clogged, these hospital units normally reached the wounded twenty-four to thirty-six hours later. The huge wagons were often abandoned in retreat, leaving the wounded to their uncertain fate.[41]

The wagons were designed to bring medical treatment to the soldier, but the French Army had no means of evacuating casualties to aid stations or rear area hospitals. The problem of casualty evacuation led Percy, chief surgeon to Gen. Jean-Victor Moreau's Army of the North, to introduce a lighter medical ambulance. Called by the German troops "Percy's Wurst"—after the sausage—these new wagons packed sufficient medical supplies and instruments to treat twelve hundred casualties. The wagons had a complement of eight surgeons who sat atop the vehicle and eight surgical attendants who sat on the medical chests on the floor. Stretchers were stowed under the driver's seat. Towed by six horses, these wagons were only slightly more mobile than the earlier collossi and were not integrated into an overall system of casualty evacuation.[42] Moreover, while sitting atop the wagon, the medical personnel made easy targets for enemy riflemen. Percy's most important innovation was the creation of a corps of litter bearers who could reach the wounded on the battlefield and move them to the medical wagons. These bearers (*brancardiers*) were first employed in the Spanish campaign (1808). Larrey then integrated the stretcher bearers into a modern system of evacuating and transporting casualties to clearing stations.

Larrey was a field surgeon with the Army of the Rhine in 1792 when he introduced his ambulance system. The idea was born from watching the newly mobile horse artillery—the *artillerie volante*, or "flying artillery"—moving horse-drawn guns, crews, and ammunition in independent mobile carts. Larrey designed and had built the prototypes of a new style of mobile field ambulance constructed on special springs to ease the wounded's transport. Each wagon was covered and equipped with ventilation holes and mattresses that swung out on wheeled pallets to make loading and unloading easier. These ambulances came in both a light two-wheeled, two-horse variety and a heavier four-wheeled, four-horse design. The ambulances were to drive as close as forty feet to the battle line and deploy litter bearers to reach the wounded still under fire and transport them to the ambulance. Once aboard, the ambulances would move the casualties to nearby dressing stations. When the ambulances returned to the line for more casualties, they also would bring fresh medical supplies. Larrey was the first since Roman times to propose evacuating casualties from engaged battle formations in a military medical ambulance corps. His major innovation was to man these wagons with a corps of trained personnel assigned specifically to drive the ambulances, to carry the litters, and to remove these medical resources from the quartermaster's control.

Larrey was also the first military medical officer to fully appreciate the value of concerted action between line and staff assets for the benefit of the wounded. To place the medical organization on a par with the military organization he had to redesign the division's entire medical support system. The essence of his plan was to have a medical unit available for each military unit based around the division, and in 1793 he reorganized the medical units of the Army of the Rhine along genuinely modern lines. Larrey divided the medical responsibilities of the division into two sections. The first section comprised a commissary and other subordinate units in which twelve surgeons and twenty-five attendants were designated to provide medical and surgical services to the wounded. In another interesting innovation, probably adopted from the mounted artillery, he provided the surgeons and some attendants with mounts so they could move from behind the lines to where the casualties were heaviest. The second division was an ambulance corps of twelve light carriages and four heavier wagons doubling as medical supply transports. Each wagon had a man in charge, a driver, a horseshoer, and a bugler who also served as medical assets exclusively, and unit commanders could not commandeer them. One hundred and thirteen medical personnel staffed the division section. Subordinate units could be created ad hoc, each with a directing surgeon and fifteen assistant surgeons. Medical personnel staffed the aid stations close to the lines. After the ambulance corps brought casualties to these collecting points, those wounded requiring further treatment were sent along predesignated routes to the general hospitals farther to the rear. Everything in the modern casualty evacuation systems was included in Larrey's organization, and he may be genuinely credited with creating the first modern casualty handling system in the West.

Larrey's medical organization was tested at the Battle of Metz (1793) and was so successful that he was ordered to assemble the new ambulances and equip all fourteen armies of the Republic.[43] Quartermaster general Jacques-Pierre Orillard de Villemanzy ordered a few prototypes to be built. Unfortunately, the idea came to the attention of the political authorities, who ordered a national contest to determine the best design. This committee's interference delayed the ambulances' introduction for more than two years.[44] By the time a design was settled upon, political instability and the lack of a centralized medical organization resulted in the ambulances never being produced in sufficient quantity. It was not until Larrey served as chief surgeon under Napoleon that the new medical organization was finally tested.

Napoleon's attitude toward providing military medical care for his men was curiously ambivalent. On the one hand, he was personally solicitous of any wounded soldier, at times forcing his officers to walk while their horses carried the wounded.

In Egypt, he gave up his own mount to the medical service and walked with the troops. On the other hand, Napoleon seems to have shared the traditional view of the officer corps and nobility of the ancien régime that soldiers drawn from the lower social orders simply did not count for much. After the Battle of Eylau, for instance, Napoleon walked the battlefield, noting that his casualties amounted to only "small change." At the same time he was personally fond of Larrey because he had proven himself a true soldier by being wounded, so Napoleon gave him free rein to design a medical service for the Imperial Guard. But again, Napoleon's attitude was contradictory. Throughout the wars, both Percy and Larrey pressed him to establish an independent medical service and make the commissions of physicians and surgeons permanent. Napoleon refused. And while the medical support for the Imperial Guard was the best in Europe, Napoleon never saw fit to extend this support to the rest of his army. Thus, during the Austrian campaign of 1809, while the casualties of the Imperial Guard were treated and evacuated immediately, the other French wounded were still left on the battlefield without medical attention three days after the battle ended.[45]

The medical service for the Imperial Guard consisted of a *division d'ambulance* for each corps, with one surgeon first class, two surgeons second class, and twelve surgeons third class supported by twelve hospital attendants (*infirmiers*). All of these people were mounted for increased mobility. Forty-four additional hospital attendants were available on foot and supported by selected officers and noncommissioned officers seconded from the line for medical duty. The transport train consisted of twelve ambulances, eight two-wheelers, four four-wheelers, and four heavy wagons of the Percy design outfitted as mobile casualty clearing stations. For the first time a primitive first aid kit of bandaging material was provided to designated officers and enlisted men in the medical units. The system apparently worked very well. At Aboukir (1799), none of the French wounded were on the ground for more than forty-five minutes. Later, at Austerlitz (1805), Napoleon's bloodiest battle, the medical service reached and treated all casualties of the Imperial Guard and evacuated them to hospitals in less than twenty-four hours.[46]

The weak point of the Napoleonic military medical care system was the general hospitals. Napoleon reduced the number of military hospitals in France to fewer than thirty. Because the Grand Armée fought mostly on foreign soil and was always on the move, the available hospitals were mostly makeshift affairs in churches, houses, factories, and other accessible buildings. Because the best doctors served in the field to avoid the political interference and difficulty attendant from Paris, the general hospitals were either understaffed or staffed by incompetents. These makeshift hospitals became pesthouses, and "military hygiene in the modern sense was almost non-existent, and the sanitary status of the hospitals was almost the lowest in recorded history."[47] So many men died of illness and disease in these charnel houses that they became known throughout Europe as the "tombs of the Grand Armée."[48]

British Medicine

Although French military medicine was poor, with the exception of that provided to the Imperial Guard, the ranks of the British-led alliance that opposed the Napoleonic armies during the Peninsular Campaign (1808–1814) received more terrible care. The British military medical system had not changed in a century. The Army Medical Board, consisting of a physician, a surgeon, and an inspector general, was charged with overseeing the few peacetime hospitals and providing for a surgeon and a surgeon's mate in each regiment. The medical resources of the army on campaign remained under the control of the regimental officers of the line. The system for supplying doctors, medical materials, hospitals, transport, and nurses had to be re-created each time the army took the field. There were no intermediary hospitals between regiment and the general hospitals, and because the medical service had no organic resources, transport, or supply services, it still had to rely on the largesse of the field commander in any given campaign for these provisions. The commanders' need to keep the army mobile and ready to move necessitated sending the wounded to the rear. Since the regimental surgeons were expected to move with the army, they had to abandon the wounded. From time to time, members of the regimental band were pressed into service as litter bearers.

The typical military surgeon in the British Army had little or no formal training; was inferior in status to the military physician, who had a university education; and thus occupied one of the lowest ranks in the military hierarchy. The high casualties that resulted from the engagements with the French in 1790–1791 increased the demands for greater numbers of military surgeons. While the French solved their manpower problem through impressment, the British simply lowered their already low standards to attract any young man with even the most rudimentary medical or pharmaceutical training to military service. George James Guthrie, the most famous British military surgeon of the day, noted that "surgeons were appointed without having served a single day in a regiment."[49] British regimental medical units often lacked a specified set of instruments, and still without an official sanitary code, the problem of field hygiene was left to the unit commander.

The medical experience of the British units at Walcheren, Holland, in 1809 was so horrible that it prompted reform of the medical system. In April, 39,214 men were shipped in 245 transports to the island of Walcheren to mount an attack against Napoleon's naval base at Antwerp. Deployed in a disease-ridden swamp, 3,000 men were down with fever by August. By September, 14,800 were sick. A month later, only 4,000 men of the original force were fit for duty. When the army finally withdrew in February 1810, of the original force, 4,000 had died of disease, 11,000 were still in hospitals, 106 men had been killed by enemy action, and another 100 had died of wounds.[50] The disaster resulted in the replacement of the Army Medical Board, whose members were replaced with experienced military surgeons and physicians. A new medical director, James McGrigor (1771–1858), was assigned to the staff of Maj. Gen. Arthur Wellesley, Duke of Wellington (1769–1852), in the Peninsular War.

Until the breakthroughs in bacteriology in the last quarter of the nineteenth century, disease often devastated armies and presented medical officers with insurmountable problems. Since the armies were large and remained in the field for long periods, the death rates from disease were higher in this era than ever before in history. The following data provide some insight into the problem. During Napoleon's attempt to conquer Santo Domingo in 1802, a 20,000-man army under Gen. Charles-Victor-Emmanuel Leclerc lost 15,000 men to yellow fever.[51] During the Peninsular campaign, the average British sick rate was 210 per 1,000 men annually,[52] while the annual death rate from disease was 118 per 1,000 men.[53] Of 61,511 men, the British lost 24,930 from disease and 8,889 to enemy fire.[54] During the Mexican War, 100,000 American soldiers saw field service. Only 1,550 were killed or died of wounds, 10,900 were lost to disease, and another 12,280 were discharged from service for illness. At any given time, the sick rate for the army ran between 17 and 27 percent.[55] Overall losses in the Crimean War were equally horrible. Although four thousand men died from wounds in the British Army, sixteen thousand perished from disease. On average, three of every ten men perished from disease each year of the war.[56]

When Wellington's new chief medical officer arrived on the Peninsula in January 1812, McGrigor found that the common practice was to dump the wounded at makeshift collection points behind the lines where there were few hospitals to treat them. The army had made no provisions for medical supplies, and the hospital system was widely scattered, unregulated, and disorganized. Further, the large general hospitals, created ad hoc, could handle only three hundred casualties. McGrigor immediately overhauled the medical supply system and standardized the flow of medical supplies to the front. He also instituted regular procedures at the hospitals, appointing inspection teams to enforce hygiene measures to reduce disease. He introduced weekly medical inspections for the rank and file and a sanitary code for the regiments.

McGrigor knew that Wellington's army was always short of manpower. He observed that once a wounded or sick soldier was sent to the rear hospitals, they had no provision for systematically returning him to his unit. McGrigor attacked the problem by requiring that standard medical report forms be submitted on a weekly basis. He moved the convalescing soldiers out of the hospitals to temporary collecting centers, where they were housed in prefabricated huts shipped from England. McGrigor was then able to establish a regularized system for returning recovered soldiers to their units.[57] Prior to the Battle of Vitoria in 1813, McGrigor was able to return almost a full division of men to combat duty.[58]

Wellington's tactics continually worked against McGrigor's efforts to establish an efficient medical treatment system, however. Outnumbered, Wellington pursued a strategy of mobility, conducting deep, quick strikes into the enemy lines and retreating rapidly to prearranged defensive assembly areas. Wellington's priority was to keep his army on the move. He continually rejected McGrigor's attempts to requisition wagons and create an ambulance service, fearing it would clog his lines of communication and disrupt his artillery and logistics train. McGrigor adapted his medical system to these realities and created fully equipped mobile regimental hospitals to move with the army. Instead of evacuating the wounded to the rear, McGrigor attempted to bring the surgeons closer to the wounded at the battle line.[59] By the end of the war, the system was working relatively well. At Toulouse in April 1814, 13 percent of the English force became casualties. Two deputy medical inspectors, ten staff surgeons, six apothecaries, and fifty-one assistant surgeons administered medical treatment to 1,359 wounded soldiers and 117 officers on the line.[60]

Unfortunately, the system of medical treatment developed during the Peninsular War was solely a product of the personal trust and working relationship that McGrigor and Wellington developed, and it represented no permanent change from the traditional pattern of establishing ad hoc military medical services. The army did not adopt any of McGrigor's innovations on an institutional basis, and when the war was over, the army and McGrigor's medical service were both demobilized. The trained corps of medical personnel was pensioned off at half pay. When the British met the French at Waterloo a year later, the British medical service already had fallen back into the old disorganized pattern that had characterized it for more than a century before the Peninsular War.

Waterloo

The Battle of Waterloo was fought on June 15, 1815. It lasted nine hours and ranged over five square miles of ground. Napoleon's army numbered 70,000 men and the allied armies under Wellington, 60,000. When the battle was over, Napoleon's force suffered 25,000 dead and 8,000 taken prisoner. The British and Hanoverian elements of Wellington's army had lost 10,700 men killed and another 7,000 wounded.[61] The Prussians lost 7,000 soldiers killed and another 7,000 wounded.[62] Within an area slightly larger than New York's Central Park, 56,700 casualties lay strewn across the blood-soaked ground.[63] The French casualties continued to lie unattended for days, their medical service having been destroyed or disorganized in the battle. The British system was almost nonexistent, and as late as eleven days after the battle, British and French casualties were still awaiting treatment. The failure of the allied armies to prepare adequate general hospitals in Brussels and to provide transportation for the wounded meant that even when the wounded reached the rear hospitals, little medical treatment was available. Waterloo was a military medical disaster of enormous proportions.

Having dismantled their medical service a year earlier, the British were caught without any meaningful medical support at all. In theory, each battalion of six hundred men was authorized only one surgeon and two assistants. In reality, of the forty British battalions at Waterloo, only twenty-two had their full complement of medical personnel. One unit, the Twenty-Eighth Foot, suffered 50 percent casualties and had only one assistant surgeon to treat them.[64] Few of these newly appointed surgical assistants, however, had any medical training. Without a corps of litter bearers, it was not uncommon for several men to help a wounded comrade to the medical tent and then refrain from returning to the battle. Wellington noted that 1,875 men were unaccounted for after the battle. They were later found to have helped their comrades to the medical tents and remained there until the battle ended.[65] No provisions were made for wagons to serve as ambulances. Wellington had moved so fast to Waterloo that much of his wagon train, including the few medical assets available, were still miles away when the battle began. What few carts and wagons that the medical service could scavenge were useless as the roads to Brussels were choked with the soldiers and wagons of Wellington's army as it withdrew. The general hospitals deep in the rear had only fifty-two surgeons and physicians to staff them. Under these conditions, the hospitals at Ostend, Brussels, Anvers, Ghent, and Bruges were useless.[66] With its regimental hospitals designed to handle merely sixty casualties, the British medical service was quickly overwhelmed and collapsed. Only 273 medical officers were at Waterloo to serve the entire army, and at least a third of them had neither medical training nor combat experience.[67]

Thus the quality of medical care, especially surgery, left much to be desired. Amputations were frequent, with a mortality rate approaching 40 percent. The surgeon usually operated in the open, often on the ground, and without assistance. Even the general hospitals did not have operating rooms, and surgery was performed on makeshift tables. Unlike Larrey's system, the British had no triage system, and the wounded often waited their turn in line regardless of the severity of their injuries. The largely untrained personnel of the medical service had little experience with ligature and the other means of hemostasis, and their delay in reaching the wounded proved fatal in thousands of cases. Bleeding the patient was still a common practice, and one can only guess how many wounded soldiers lost their otherwise salvageable lives because of it.

The one bright spot was English surgeon George James Guthrie, who accompanied Wellington on all his campaigns and was called "the English Larrey." Guthrie's experience with military surgery convinced him that Larrey was correct in his advocacy of primary amputation. In 1827, Guthrie published his *Treatise on Gunshot Wounds: Inflammation, Erysipelas, and Mortification, on Injuries of Nerves*, which established the doctrine of primary amputation in England and became the basic manual of British and U.S. military surgery until the Crimean War.[68]

McGrigor, who had been appointed director general of the Medical Department prior to Waterloo, held the post until the Crimean War. The medical disaster at Waterloo led him to attempt reform, but once again the government demobilized the army and drastically reduced funds for support its medical services. Curiously, Wellington did little to reverse this state of affairs. McGrigor tried to raise entrance standards for the medical service, purchased textbooks, began a medical library, and finally established an army medical school at Fort Pitt, England. Together with army doctor Henry Marshall (1775–1851), McGrigor attempted to institutionalize the practice of regular medical reports on the health status of the army, but this reform came to fruition only after the Crimean War had proven yet another medical disaster for the British. With the French medical service destroyed after Napoleon's defeat and the British unwilling to learn from their experiences in the Peninsula and at Waterloo, the stage was set for yet another medical catastrophe when both countries once again stumbled into war.

THE CRIMEAN WAR

The Crimean War represented one of the great medical disasters of all time. Every major combatant entered the war with either an obsolete military medical system or, as in the Turkish Army's case, no military medical system at all. A war in which only four major offensive ground engagements were fought, the Crimean conflict was characterized by continuous artillery bombardments and the terrible living conditions associated with long sieges and trench warfare that contributed to incredibly high rates of disease. The war saw the first use of the new conoidal bullet that Capt. Claude-Etienne Minié (1804–1879) developed. Along with the introduction of the rifled musket barrel that the Russian Army used extensively, this new ammunition increased the infantry's range and killing power by a factor of seven.[69] The new weapon produced battle wounds that were as much as thirty times larger than the size of the residual track of the penetrating projectile because the soft lead bullet broke apart upon impact. The improved rifle's killing and wounding power was demonstrated in November 1854 at the Battle of Inkermann, where it caused 91 percent of the British casualties.[70] While Russian and French forces used the new rifle, British forces remained armed with the Brown Bess smoothbore, muzzle-loading musket that fired round lead balls with a range of only 120 yards.

The medical statistics of the war were tragic. The French contingent numbered 309,268 men but only 500 medical officers. British forces comprised 97,864 troops with 448 medical officers, and the Sardinian contingent fielded 21,000 men with 88 surgeons. Despite the generally backward state of Russian military medicine at this time, the Russian Army deployed the largest military medical contingent with 1,608 medical officers and 3,759 feldshers for a force of 324,478 men. Turkish forces numbered 35,000 men but had no military medical support at all.[71] The casualty rate from wounds and disease, when taken as a percentage of the forces deployed, was among the highest in history. For the Russians, of the 92,381 wounded, 14,671 men died; of the 332,097 sick, 37,454 succumbed to their illnesses; and 21,000 were killed in action.[72] The French Army lost 8,250 men to hostile fire, 39,868 wounded, 4,354 died of wounds, 196,430 sick, and 59,815 dead from disease. The British suffered 2,255 killed in action, 18,183 wounded, 1,847 died of wounds, 144,390 sick, and 17,225 dead from disease.[73] The Crimean War saw the highest battle losses per 1,000 men per annum (Russians) and the highest disease loss rate per 1,000 men per annum (French) than any previous war in recorded history.

Disease and infected wounds were the two largest causes of death among the armies. The germ theory of infection was still unknown, and the poor sanitary conditions in the few available military hospitals produced extremely high rates of wound infection and death. Among the British wounded in the Scutari hospital in Istanbul, for example, the mortality rate for amputees averaged nearly 30 percent.[74] Of every 100 men admitted to military hospitals among the French forces, 42 percent died, or a hospital mortality rate equivalent to that of the Middle Ages.[75] The disease rate per 1,000 men per annum was 253.5 for the French, 161.3 for the British, and 119.3 for the Russians. This proportion compares to a similar rate of 110 per 1,000 men in the Mexican War, 65 for the Civil War, and 16 in World War I.[76]

Florence Nightingale (1820–1910) and her trained nurses arrived in November 1854 after the Battle of Balaklava, and they introduced basic standards of hygiene and sanitation in the British military hospitals. Nightingale reported a hospital mortality rate at Scutari of 41 percent. As a result of her efforts, the rate dropped to 2 percent by the end of the war.[77] She is often credited with starting the first female nursing corps in the Western armies. In fact, the credit for this innovation belongs properly to the Russians. The Russian grand duchess Elena Pavlovna (1807–1873) urged the czar to send trained female nurses to the Crimea so they could assist Nikolai Ivanovich Pirogov (1810–1881), Russia's great surgeon general. A large nursing corps was deployed in Russian military hospitals almost a year before Nightingale and her nurses arrived in British military hospitals.[78] That the Russian Army suffered fewer losses to disease and infection than the French did may be attributed, to some extent, to the former's introduction of basic hygiene and sanitary conditions in its military hospitals earlier than the French did.

England

The start of the Crimean War found the British medical structure essentially as it had been in 1815.[79] Despite McGrigor's best efforts to institutionalize his reforms, the medical service had been allowed to deteriorate after Waterloo. No fewer than seven independent governmental authorities had some responsibility for operating the British medical service. The two major authorities were the Army Medical Department, then headed by a senior physician with no military experience, and the Ordnance Department, presided over by an appointed nobleman. They did not include any purveyors to purchase supplies or any apothecaries in the system at all; indeed, these positions had gone unfilled since 1830.[80] The medical service had only twenty-six clerks housed in a small London office to manage the entire medical department.[81] The British military medical service had sunk to such a low position that the only medical regulations governing its operations consisted of a small pamphlet drawn up years before that outlined the rules for managing a thirty-bed hospital in peacetime. In addition, the army lacked any standard sanitary regulations.[82] Less than a year before the outbreak of war, the British made minor reforms in the administrative system and placed authority for the military medical service under a single administrative office, but this move produced no significant change in medical capabilities.

Of the 225 medical officers serving in the British Army's medical service at the beginning of the war, only 52 had medical degrees, while the rest had surgical diplomas.[83] The quality of the military surgeons' medical training was close to what it had been a half century earlier at Waterloo. Curiously, most British military physicians and surgeons were of Irish and Scottish descent.[84] Doctors from these areas lacked civilian opportunities as a consequence of class discrimination, so many entered the military to gain position and experience. Although the number of military physicians eventually grew to approximately a thousand during the war, it was never sufficient to handle the extensive casualties. British authorities argued, however, that the ratio of 1 medical officer to 77 men under Lord Raglan (1788–1855) was better than the ratio in the Peninsular War when British forces had 1 medical officer for every 145 men. It was also noted that the French had only 276 medical officers compared to the British 406, even though the French Army was twice the size of Raglan's force.[85]

The British ambulance corps was woefully inadequate. Although a few prototypes of the Larrey-type ambulance evacuation wagons had been produced, their number was far too small to provide adequate support. Moreover, these few vehicles arrived late behind the deploying army, and since the quartermaster did not give the corps horses, drivers, or carpenters to assemble the wagons, they had to leave the vehicles in Varna. Each regiment was issued eight stretchers but no litter corps to bear them. Any available men for stretcher duty had to be drawn from the line regiments, a situation that often led to mustering the regimental band members, the recovering sick and wounded, and whatever few men the regimental commander cared to spare. When the army proposed hiring local Turks and Bulgars as stretcher bearers, London denied the option as too expensive. As the casualty death rate mounted, however, the War Office ultimately provided for raising a Hospital Conveyance Corps to act as stretcher bearers. To keep costs down, the corps recruited from old pensioners and low-status personnel whose only virtue was their willingness to work for low wages. This small corps arrived in Varna in July during a cholera epidemic and was immediately incapacitated by the disease. Because the British failed to plan for medical support, they never succeeded in establishing a regularized system of ambulances or stretcher bearers during the war. Instead, the physicians had to go into the line and treat the wounded in the trenches where they fell.

To move the wounded and sick to hospitals, the British improvised and had the navy ferry casualties from the Crimea to the two major base hospitals three hundred miles away in Turkey. Conveying the casualties from the line to the ports remained a major difficulty throughout the war, and the poor means of overland transport caused many deaths. The navy had plenty of ships to accommodate the casualties once they arrived in port, but it had no organized system for loading them. As a consequence, the wounded and sick often lay in the rain for one or two days until placed aboard. Further, only a handful of ships were modified to house and care for casualties. Most often no trained medical personnel and few medical supplies were on board. Overcrowding also became a problem. One ship, the HMS *Kangaroo,* was equipped to carry 250 casualties but packed aboard more than 1,500 sick and wounded on a single trip.[86] Loss rates among the sick and wounded of 20 percent were common, and soldiers arrived at the hospital days after being wounded still in their dirty, mud-covered uniforms and with their wounds untreated.[87] Only in the last year of the war did the British medical service establish regularly scheduled steamships for ferrying the wounded from the front to the general hospitals in the rear.

The general hospitals, however, were little more than pestholes. The largest hospital, at Scutari, had no beds, so patients lay on the floor with the same clothing or blankets they had brought with them from the front. It did not have a kitchen to prepare food, and its two thousand patients were expected to make do with only twenty bedpans. The British did not even create a corps of hospital orderlies until the end of the war. It took the arrival of Nightingale and her nurses to improve the basic sanitary conditions of the British general hospitals. Their simple sanitary procedures, such as providing bedding, changing sheets, wearing hospital gowns, and regularly washing the physical plant, drastically reduced the rate of death from disease and infected wounds.

Dr. John Hall (1795–1865) oversaw the British medical system in the Crimea. His medical staff of fifty-six men included a director of hospitals, forty surgeons and assistant surgeons, a medical storekeeper, and fourteen noncommissioned officers. The regimental medical system, in place for more than a century, remained intact for all its faults. The regiment's medical assets stayed in the hands of the field commander, however, and medical personnel had no authority to coordinate medical care between regiments. The regimental hospital, also a relic of earlier days, was equipped with only twelve beds with blankets and sheets, a medical chest, and a pannier of medical supplies for the horse carriage. The bell tents could only be closed from the outside, and the treatment of most casualties occurred on the ground.[88] Most trained physicians served in the general hospitals, leaving the regiments with the least trained personnel to deal directly with the wounded. From the start, the number of casualties overwhelmed the regimental system, and it never recovered its ability to deal adequately with the wounded.

The poor organizational structure of the British military medical service in the Crimea was equaled by the generally poor medical treatment it offered. Dr. Hall had strong suspicions about chloroform and believed that the pain associated with surgery served to heighten the body's ability to fight and survive amputation and infection. Although he did not prohibit it, Hall issued a warning on the use of chloroform that the younger surgeons took to mean that they ought not administer it regularly. The best trained and more experienced surgeons still widely used chloroform, but Hall's directive kept the supply service from making chloroform a priority item to stock.[89] Accordingly, chloroform was always in short supply, and the British missed an opportunity to standardize anesthesia's use in battlefield surgery. Generally, the medical establishment also was strongly opposed to using chloroform. As late as 1857, the Crimean Medical and Surgical Society, an organization formed among surgeons who had seen service in the Crimea, warned against the general use of anesthesia.[90]

The medical horrors of the Crimean War provoked such a public outcry in the press and in Parliament that some reforms were attempted. Most, however, were not implemented in time to improve medical treatment during the war. In 1855, the medical service formed a corps of hospital orderlies consisting of nine companies of seventy-eight enlisted men to staff the general hospitals. After the war the corps became the Medical Staff Corps and a permanent part of the medical service.[91] An inspector general's postwar report led the British for the first time to establish a regular strength and resource table for medical assets. From then on, a medical corps of 280 men would be authorized for every division of 10,000 men. Unfortunately, the report did not address the formation of a stretcher or ambulance corps, and none was established on a permanent basis until the Second Boer War. In 1860, the first British military medical school to train military surgeons was established at Fort Pitt, and a system of regular medical reports was instituted throughout the army. In 1874, the regimental system, including its hospital system, was abolished to make way for new, larger fighting formations. The new hospital system, copied from the American experience in the Civil War, was organized around divisional units. In 1878, the army brought medical officer pay, privileges, and ranks into line with the rest of the service, but it still denied medical officers the privileges of command and needed the permission of their field commanders to gain control over medical resources. In 1890, the medical corps was placed on the same social and military level as the corps of engineers, and in 1898 its designation was changed to the Royal Army Medical Corps.[92]

France

The French medical corps was outdated, disorganized, and still suffered from the organizational and political effects of the army's defeat at Waterloo. The political suspicions accompanying the Restoration compounded these problems, and the destabilization of the Revolution of 1848 and the rise of Napoleon III (1808–1873) followed. The turmoil of 1848 provoked widespread street fighting, and the French medical corps was pressed into service to treat the casualties with two significant results. First, French surgeons gained experience in using chloroform and standardized its use in the medical service. When the Crimean War broke out, the French administered chloroform as a matter of course and did so, they claimed, in thirty thousand operations during the war.[93] Second, the political authorities recognized that the military medical service needed reform. In April 1848, the service began allowing its officers to exercise independent command of their own personnel and resources. The French were the first to take concrete steps to create an independent and autonomous military medical service. Unfortunately, when Minister of War Gen. Alphonse Henri d'Hautpoul (1789–1865) reversed these reforms a year later, the French medical service plunged into another period of disorganization.

General d'Hautpoul's actions almost destroyed the service. He ordered that surgeons, physicians, and pharmacists be recruited exclusively from the graduates of civilian training institutions, so the French Army dismantled its military medical educational establishment. To prepare civilian medical personnel for military service, d'Hautpoul directed that they must take a one-year course in military medicine at the École d'Application de la Médicine Militaire at Val-de-Grâce. A year later, the French medical service equalized the status of physicians and surgeons by prescribing essentially the same refresher training for both, but it made no effort to assimilate these disciplines into the military's ranks.[94]

The wars of Napoleon III all resulted in major medical disasters. Under d'Hautpoul's medical system, the French entered the Crimean War with an acute shortage of medical officers, physicians, and surgeons. Before the war, the medical recruitment system had failed badly, and once the war broke out, it flunked completely. Few civilian medical personnel could be convinced of the value of military service, resulting in a precipitous decline in both numbers and quality. Between 1853 and 1855, of the eighty medical officer recruits required to fill out the ranks annually, the service attracted fewer than fifteen a year to take the examination. More damaging, of these, only four per year passed.[95] During this period, the French Army in the Crimea expanded by ten battalions of infantry, enlarging the cavalry and artillery forces and creating an Imperial Guard. The French medical service never deployed sufficient medical personnel to serve this increased force. Moreover, of the 550 medical officers that served in the Crimea, eighty-three officers, or 15 percent, lost their lives.[96]

The medical disaster in the Crimea had even further negative consequences for the French medical service. The few remaining physicians after the war quickly left military service for calmer lives. Although the French created a new medical school at Strasbourg to train their replacements, it attracted few students. The service reduced the number of surgeons assigned to each division to four, but most regiments had only a single surgeon, who was usually an untrained assistant, or none at all. The ambulance system, never fully staffed, was allowed to decay to even smaller numbers. When war broke out with Italy in 1859, medical talent was in such short supply that in place of the required 150 physicians and 150 surgeons, the medical service had to make do with 200 untrained medical students to serve as assistant physicians in the regiments.[97]

The Battle of Solferino (1859) demonstrated that the French had learned nothing from their medical experience in the Crimea. The medical service was short of physicians, surgeons, nurses, dressings, ambulances, hospitals, surgical instruments, rations, anesthesia, and general transport. Henri Dunant, an eyewitness to the battle, found the slaughter and neglect of the wounded and sick so appalling that in 1862 he published *Un Souvenir de Solferino* (*A Memory of Solferino*), portraying the horror to the world. His work provoked a conference of the national Red Cross societies in Geneva in 1863 that led, in 1864, to the founding of the International Committee of the Red Cross and to fourteen nations signing the first Geneva Convention regulating the treatment of the wounded and conferring noncombatant and neutral status on the medical personnel of the national armies. The convention also adopted the red cross as the international symbol of the military medical services.

The Red Cross convention prompted France to create a Society for the Aid of Wounded Soldiers. When war broke out with Germany in 1870, the French medical service still was as ill prepared as it had been for the last war. French soldiers carried no first aid kits, and the medical service had no litter bearers, few ambulances, and no organized ambulance transport services attached to the regiments. Medical help to the soldier essentially stopped when he was dumped behind the regimental aid station, for no organized method existed to systematically move the wounded to interior hospitals. The medical supply storehouses were located too far to the rear to move supplies rapidly; however, within a few weeks, they ran out of medical supplies completely. The lack of a reserve pool from which to draw replacements compounded the shortage of physicians and surgeons. Because the French had also forbidden the use of inoculation, more than 200,000 soldiers contracted smallpox during the course of the war.[98] The high death rates from wounds, infection, and disease prompted one commentator to refer to the period as "the most grievous in the history of French demography in the 19th century."[99]

The French Society for the Aid to Wounded Soldiers obtained its first experience in providing ambulance and medical personnel to troops in battle with some considerable success. By the end of the war with Germany in 1870, however, many commonly recognized that the French medical service needed reform. In 1878, the International Congress of Military Medicine held in Paris passed a resolution calling for the creation of an autonomous medical service to guarantee better control over medical assets in wartime. A governmental commission was appointed to study the problem but adjourned a year later with no results. It required ten years' worth of coverage in newspapers and journals to convince the French legislature finally to vote, in 1882, to create a semiautonomous military medical service. In 1889, the French became the last major Western power to adopt an autonomous military medical service for its armies. They created a new medical school to train military physicians, and they improved and organized recruitment. At last the medical personnel had control over their own resources, but they were still greatly restricted in their control and authority over the support resources needed to make the medical service perform adequately. This state of affairs continued until 1914 where, once again, the French entered another major war with a less than adequate medical service to treat its casualties.

Russia

If the medical care provided to the armies of France and England was poor, it was poorer still in the Russian Army. The Russian military medical corps entered the nineteenth century considerably behind the medical services of Europe because the medical profession in Russia was chronically underdeveloped. The country had only a few facilities for training physicians and surgeons, and their graduates were not attracted to a normal military career, which required twenty-five years of service. Consequently, the czarist armies relied heavily on barber-surgeons. Although the service made some efforts to train these feldshers, most of the medics assigned to military units were only marginally competent. In 1805, the Russian Army had only 74 feldshers assigned to the army and 388 to the navy.[100] The official army title for them was *tsiriulnik* (barber), a title that reflected their low status.

At the outbreak of the Crimean War, however, Russia was able to produce sufficient numbers of barber-surgeons to fill out most field units. Indeed, as noted earlier, the Russian Army had the largest ratio of medical men to force, with 1,608 officers and more than 3,759 feldshers serving in the Crimean War.[101] Despite these numbers and Russia's internal lines of communication in the theater of operations, the quality of medical support provided to the Russian Army was dismal. What few hospitals existed were makeshift affairs and had high mortality rates from infection. Few provisions had been made for adequate beds and linen and none for an ambulance service. Transport was accomplished with whatever available wagons could be obtained on the spot, and the wounded were regularly transported while unprotected in foul weather. At the Battle of Sevastopol (1854–1855), the nearest aid station was sixteen miles away, and the trip in the open wagons took seven days.[102]

As mentioned previously, the most famous Russian surgeon to serve in the Crimea was Nikolai Pirogov. Well educated and having traveled extensively in Germany and the West, Pirogov had seen military duty in the Caucasus campaign in 1849 and was the first European military surgeon to use etherization in surgical procedures on battle casualties.[103] Pirogov served two years in the Crimea as a battle surgeon, was an observer in the Franco-Prussian War and the Turko-Russian conflict, and developed renown as Russia's greatest surgeon.[104] He published two major works on military surgery, *Introduction to General Military Surgery* and *Principles of General Military Field Surgery* (1865), that are both regarded as classics. He was also a strong campaigner against large hospitals, which he viewed as cesspits of disease from overcrowding and poor sanitation. Instead, he recommended the use of pavilion hospitals along the model of those first used in the American Civil War.

Only two medical highlights emerged from the medical disaster of the Crimean War. First, the French surgeons' widespread use of chloroform and the Russians' use of ether convinced the rest of the world that anesthesia was an important and effective aid to field surgery. Although the British were slow to adopt its use, anesthesia became standard military medical procedure in the Union Army during the Civil War. A second important medical advance was the debut of plaster of Paris in splints. Antonius Mathijsen (1805–1878), a Dutchman, published his work on using plaster for bandaging broken bones in 1852. He may have called it plaster of Paris because in Paris in 1765 Antoine Laurent Lavoisier (1743–1794) had shown that a 95 percent solution of calcium sulfate with the right amount of water would crystalize and harden.[105] Until plaster of Paris, physicians immobilized fractured limbs with a bandage stiffened with freshly made starch and cardboard, but the technique had little military use, since the starch took twenty-four hours to harden. While the evidence is less than clear, it seems likely that while in the Crimea, Pirogov was the first surgeon to use plaster of Paris splints in a military environment.[106]

THE MEXICAN WAR AND THE AMERICAN CIVIL WAR

Protected by its oceans, the United States remained little affected by the frequent wars in Europe. Accordingly, its military medical establishment had fewer opportunities to develop in response to actual field experience. The army was dismantled at the end of the American Revolution, and by 1802 the medical corps had only two surgeons and twenty-five mates. These few assets were assigned to garrisons and frontier posts and not the regiments. By 1808, the number of surgeons increased to seven and surgical assistants to forty. With the start of the War of 1812, the army found itself critically short of medical staff. Although additional medical personnel were obtained through the contract system, the number of medical officers was never sufficient to provide adequate medical care.[107] The medical corps thus fell back on the old practices of the Revolution. Lacking an ambulance corps, the medical corps sent what few wagons it could obtain to search the battlefield and the woods to find the wounded. There were no hospitals. Temporary shelters called "Indian houses" were built after each battle, and the wounded were treated there.[108] Requests to establish an ambulance corps were ignored, and with the cessation of hostilities the army once again dismantled its medical service.[109]

The medical system of 1812 suffered most from the army's failure to provide a central authority responsible for creating and deploying medical assets. In 1818, Congress authorized the appointment of a surgeon general to head the medical corps, establishing for the first time an administrative organization for the medical department. Dr. Joseph Lovell (1788–1836), the first American surgeon general, served until 1836. At the start of the Mexican War in 1846, the American Army of 7,000 men included a medical corps consisting of a surgeon general and 71 medical officers. Congress increased the number of medical officers to 115 for the regular forces and 135 for the volunteers. The army had grown to about 100,000 men, proving even these increased medical assets inadequate.[110] No provisions were made for an ambulance corps, although a few Larrey-type ambulances were used, and the old practice of begging available wagon transport from the quartermaster prevailed. Regimental hospitals used a few tents to provide primary medical care to the wounded; however, they were usually understaffed and inadequate to deal with the numbers of casualties. General hospitals were few and still created on an ad hoc basis. Both types of hospitals lacked stewards, nurses, cooks, adequate supplies, and trained physicians. Once again, the American Army suffered a medical disaster.

Of the 100,182 combatants committed to the Mexican campaign, 1,458 were killed in action and 10,790 died of disease. Statistically, the Mexican War was the deadliest from disease ever fought by an American force. Per 1,000 men per annum, mortality from disease averaged 110 men compared to a rate of 65 for the Civil War, 27 for the Spanish-American War, and 16 for World War I.[111] The single positive medical contribution of the Mexican War was that an American military surgeon used ether anesthesia for the first time in combat. After the war, the American military medical service was once again reduced in strength, and no significant reforms were achieved.

Thirteen years later, no one was prepared for the magnitude of slaughter that accompanied the American Civil War. It was the first modern war insofar as the integration of the productive capacities of the Industrial Revolution with the military effort was complete. The magnitude of combat engagements was the largest in history to that time, and the exponential increase in the weapons' killing capabilities, especially the improvements in the rifle, produced rates of casualties beyond the imagination of commanders and military medical personnel. In a five-year period, the combatants fought 2,196 engagements.[112] A total of 620,000 men perished, 360,000 in the Union Army and 260,000 in the Confederate Army.[113] Some 67,000 Union troops were killed outright, 43,000 died of wounds, and 130,000 were disfigured for life, often with missing limbs. In the Confederate forces, 94,000 men died of wounds.[114] For the Union Army, the minié ball caused 94 percent of all wounds, artillery shell and canister led to nearly 6 percent, and the sabre and bayonet accounted for 922 wounds, of which only 56 were fatal.[115] Thirty-five percent of the wounds were to the arms, 35.7 percent to the legs, and wounds to the trunk and head accounted for 18.4 percent and 10.7 percent, respectively.[116]

In a statistical sense, the Civil War was the most horrible war ever fought. The chance of a Civil War combatant *not* surviving the war was 1 in 4 compared to 1 in 126 for the Korean War. Of the Union dead, 3 of every 5 died of disease; in the Confederacy, 2 of every 3. Tables 8, 9, and 10 provide statistical summaries of the official casualty data for the Union Army.

Table 8. Special Causes of Death in the Union Army

	Officers	Men
Killed in action	4,142	62,916
Died of wounds	2,223	40,789
Died of disease	2,795	221,791
Accidental deaths	142	3,972
Drowned	106	4,838
Murdered	37	483
Killed after capture	14	90
Suicide	26	365
Executed by U.S. authorities	X	267
Executed by the enemy	4	60
Sunstroke	5	308
Other known causes	62	1,972
Causes not stated	28	12,093
Total	9,584	349,944
Total, Officers and Men—359,528		

Source: Official Records, *Medical and Surgical History of the War of the Rebellion* (Washington, DC: Government Printing Office, 1870).

Table 9. Wounds and Sickness in the Union Army

Wounds

Of the 246,712 cases of wounds reported in the Medical Records by weapons of war, 245,790 were shot wounds and 922 were sabre and bayonet.

Sickness

Of 5,825,480 admissions to sick report there were:

Cases	Conditions	Deaths
75,368	typhoid	27,050
2,501	typhus	850
11,898	continued fever	147
49,871	typho-malarial fever	4,059
1,155,266	acute diarrhea	2,923
170,488	chronic diarrhea	27,558
233,812	acute dysentery	4,084
25,670	chronic dysentery	3,229
73,382	syphilis	123
95,833	gonorrhea	6
30,714	scurvy	383
3,744	delirium tremens	450
2,410	insanity	80
2,837	paralysis	231

Source: Official Records, *Medical and Surgical History.*

One reason for the staggering increase in the number and seriousness of the men's wounds was the introduction of the new Springfield .58-caliber rifled-barreled firearm capable of propelling a minié ball at 950 feet per second to an accurate range of 600 yards. It used heavy, soft lead bullets that were unjacketed. The bullets flattened out upon impact, producing terrible wounds and carrying pieces of clothing into the wound itself. When the bullet nicked a bone, the weight and deformation of the projectile shattered the bone or severed it completely from the limb. Traumatic amputation or compound fracture was the most common result. Incredibly, the infantry continued to use the old tactic of massing forces to concentrate their firepower, which the old, inaccurate and limited-range musket necessitated, and made their

Table 10. Amputations in the Union Army (29,980 Reported Cases)

	Cases	Deaths	Percent Fatality
Fingers	7,902	198	3
Forearm	1,761	245	14
Upper arm	5,540	1,273	24
Toes	1,519	81	6
Leg	5,523	1,790	33
Amputation at thigh	6,369	3,411	54
Amputation at knee joint	195	111	58
Amputation at hip joint	66	55	83
Amputation at ankle joint	161	119	74

Source: Official Records, *Medical and Surgical History.*

formations vulnerable to long-range rifle fire. Moreover, the need to move the lines over greater frontages than ever before also increased the dispersal of the wounded to unprecedented levels, placing a greater premium on the ability to locate, treat, and evacuate the wounded. The Civil War medical officer faced problems of wound management that were unique for the time, and he was as unprepared to deal with them then as he had been in previous wars.

The improved kinetic power of the rifle bullet made amputation the most common battlefield operation during the Civil War. Of the 174,200 gunshot wounds to the arms and legs suffered by Union soldiers, 29,980 required amputation.[117] Confederate soldiers suffered 25,000 primary amputations (meaning as soon as possible after wounding) and the Union Army 20,993.[118] More limbs were lost in this war than in any other conflict fought by the United States, including World Wars I and II, Korea, Vietnam, Iraq, and Afghanistan. The old debate about primary versus secondary amputation reappeared. Within two years, experience had shown that the soldier's chances of survival increased with primary amputation. The mortality rate for primary amputation was 26 percent compared to 52 percent for secondary amputation.[119] Interestingly, however, 26,467 wounds of the extremities complicated by injury to the bone were treated "by expectation" (leaving the wound alone to heal itself) with a mortality rate of only 18 percent, which was much lower than the rate for either primary or secondary amputation.[120]

In the first year of the war, hemostasis was achieved mostly through the tourniquet and cautery, but both methods were dangerous to the patient. As the minimally trained surgeons gained more experience, however, they more commonly used ligature and pressure dressings to control bleeding. One of the war's beneficial medical effects was that it gave thousands of surgeons experience in ligature, a training they could practice in civilian life. The common practice, however, was to leave the ends of the ligature long and extending outside the body. These loose ends proved to be excellent avenues for infection, producing septic conditions that led to secondary hemorrhage. The mortality rate for such secondary infections was 62 percent.[121] The usual array of infections—tetanus, hospital gangrene, and various streptococcus infections—were ever present. In the early days, the mortality rate in some hospitals was as high as 60 percent. As surgeons gradually began using debridement and bromine solution applications, the mortality rate from wound infection fell to 3 percent near the end of the war.[122]

The Union blockade caused shortages of medical supplies that forced Confederate surgeons to develop alternatives that proved beneficial in fighting wound infection. Both sides cleansed wounds with sea sponges kept in buckets of water near the operating table. Used repeatedly after being squeezed in the dirty water, these sponges were major sources of disease transmission. A shortage of sponges in the South forced Confederate surgeons to use cotton rags instead. Since the rags were recycled, cleaned, boiled, and ironed, they served as relatively sterile wound dressings. The same was true of the bandages. With bandages in short supply, practitioners used raw cotton, but to manufacture the product, it was necessary to oven bake the cotton, producing a sterile bandage. While Northern surgeons used unsterile harness-maker's silk for ligatures and sutures, silk was not available to the Southern surgeons, who used horsehair for the same purposes. To make the horsehair sufficiently pliable for surgical use, they had to boil it. By happy accident, the boiling process produced sterile sutures.[123] Nonetheless, wound infection, especially in the general hospitals, remained a major problem. William W. Keen (1827–1932), who served as a surgeon in the Army of the Potomac, noted, "It was seven times safer to fight all through the three days of Gettysburg than to have an arm or leg cut off . . . and be treated in a city hospital."[124]

Military surgeons of the Civil War used chloroform and ether anesthesia on an unprecedented scale. Military physicians used no fewer than eighty thousand applications of anesthesia. Official records show that anesthesia was used in 8,900 operations within general hospitals, of which 6,784 involved chloroform and 811 involved ether alone. In 1,305 cases, they used a combination of ether and chloroform. Remarkably, only thirty-seven deaths were attributed to anesthesia.[125] They also made advances in immobilizing limbs, with plaster of Paris widely used for this purpose. Having studied in Europe, Dr. Gordon Buck (1807–1877) brought the technique to America, and the first application to immobilize a limb was accomplished in 1855. Dr. Nathan Little is generally credited with introducing the technique to the military medical community during the Civil War.[126] In 1863, Union surgeon John Hodgen (1826–1882) introduced the famous Hodgen splint, which is still used today in fractures of the lower femur.

Drug application during the war was quite primitive because physicians of the period knew little about the specific effects of drugs. Except for calomel (mercurous chloride), which was so heavily prescribed that Surgeon General William Hammond (1828–1900) forbade its use as dangerous, most drugs did little harm if little good. The most indispensable and well-known drugs included morphine, opium, and quinine. Morphine was usually dusted directly on the wound and occasionally injected hypodermically. The hypodermic syringe appeared in the 1850s, but only 2,093 syringes were issued to the Union Army during the war. That their use had any medical significance is unlikely. Yet, Silas Weir Mitchell (1829–1914) noted that at the army hospital for nervous diseases, Turner's Lane Hospital in Philadelphia, more than forty thousand doses of morphine were given hypodermically to patients in a single year.[127] A significant addiction problem resulted from the Union Army's wide use of opium pills and other addictive opium-based prescriptions. Records show that *ten million* opium pills were administered to patients during the war, along with 2,841,000 ounces of other opium-based preparations, such as laudanum, opium with ipecac, and paregoric. By contrast, only 29,828 ounces of morphine sulfate were administered.[128] While not all addicts in the country were former soldiers, the United States had 200,000 drug addicts by 1900.[129]

A number of antiseptics were widely used, including potassium permanganate, sodium hypochlorite, bromine, iodine, turpentine, and creosote. Lister had not yet made his important discovery regarding antisepsis, and none of these preparations were used in wound treatment. They were, however, commonly used as deodorants in hospitals and did have the unintended effect of providing better sanitary conditions in the hospital wards.

As in all past wars, disease was the most common killer of Union and Confederate soldiers. Both armies were armies of volunteers, and in the early years of the war the armies performed little more than perfunctory medical examinations of their recruits. A normal day's load for physicians examining recruits was between forty and fifty examinations a day. The quality of recruits, often motivated by patriotic fervor and the enlistment bounty, was less than desirable. In 1861, a Union Sanitary Commission report noted that three-quarters of the soldiers who had been discharged from the Union Army were so physically unfit that they should never have been allowed to enlist in the first place.[130]

Most recruits came from largely rural populations. Their isolated locations had prevented them from developing immunities to a wide range of childhood diseases. Once they were brought together in the close quarters required of military life, many fell ill.[131] Their poor physical conditions and few immunities were compounded by generally poor nutrition from military rations and the general stress of military life. Scurvy was endemic, and outbreaks of cholera, typhus, typhoid, and dysentery took a generally heavy toll.[132] Although tetanus mortality was high—89–95 percent—relatively few cases of tetanus arose because most battles did not occur in the richly manured soil of overworked farmland. Most cases of tetanus were contracted in field hospitals, when barns and stalls served as temporary surgical hospitals and aid stations.[133] Disease killed approximately 225,000 men in the Union Army and 164,000 in the Confederate ranks. It is estimated that disease killed five times as many men as were slain by weapon fire.[134]

The Union Medical Department was totally unprepared for war. Its head, Surgeon General Thomas Lawson (1789–1861), was a sick and dying man who economized on expenditures by refusing to purchase medical books for the military. The small 26,000-man army was scattered along the frontier and had no military medical service to speak of. The regular army in 1860 had only thirty surgeons and eighty-three assistant surgeons, and twenty-four of them resigned to serve with the Confederacy.[135] Medical supplies consisted of a few incomplete surgical kits and clinical thermometers. The country had no general hospitals, and the largest post hospital, located at Fort Leavenworth, Kansas, had only forty-one beds.[136]

There was no ambulance service. In the 1850s, Secretary of War Jefferson Davis (1808–1889) had ordered two military officers, one of whom was Capt. George B. McClellan (1826–1885), to prepare a study of the lessons to be learned from the Crimean War. McClellan's report included a section on ambulance trains and medical supplies and recommended creating an army ambulance corps. A committee was appointed to accept designs for medical transport vehicles, but by 1860, the army had rejected all the designs and had not created an ambulance corps.[137] For the war's first two years, neither side had a systematic way to evacuate the wounded. After the disaster at the First Battle of Bull Run (July 1861), where vehicles had to be commandeered from the streets of Washington to move the wounded, individual field commanders improvised what little medical transport they could. Toward the end of the Peninsula campaign, an army corps of thirty thousand men had an ambulance transport system sufficient for only a hundred casualties. At the Battle of Wilson's Creek (August 1861), the wounded could not be moved for six days owing to the lack of ambulances. In November 1861, Gen. Ulysses S. Grant (1822–1885) and his forces at Belmont, Missouri, had to abandon their wounded because they did not have ambulances.[138] Ambulance transport in the Confederacy was even worse. In 1863, Confederate medical officers reportedly had only thirty-eight ambulances in the entire Army of the Mississippi. As the war continued, the situation worsened. In 1865, not a single ambulance could be found in the combat brigades of the armies of West Virginia and East Tennessee.[139]

Meanwhile, the appalling medical conditions of the Union Army provoked a public outcry, much as similar conditions had provoked public outrage among the British during the Crimean War. In 1861, Dr. Henry Bellows (1814–1882), a Unitarian minister from New York, led a committee that created the U.S. Sanitary Commission, which made recommendations to improve medical treatment. Its first suggestion was to fire Surgeon General Lawson and replace him with Dr. William Hammond. Upon assuming his position, Hammond appointed Dr. Jonathan Letterman (1824–1872) as surgeon general of the Army of the Potomac. Making several contributions to the Union's medical service, Letterman quickly set about reorganizing the system and creating an ambulance corps.

Letterman's ambulance corps was built around the Larrey model, and each army corps had its own dedicated medical transport assets. Each division, brigade, and regiment had its own medical officer responsible in a direct chain of command to the corps medical officer, who was responsible for coordination at all levels. The chief surgeon within each division controlled the ambulance corps, and he assigned all details regarding parking, roll call, stable call, veterinary services, and police duty to a line officer of the division. Each regiment received three ambulances and a complement of drivers and litter bearers, and each division had its own ambulance train of thirty vehicles. The ratio of ambulances to men averaged 1 to 150.[140]

Letterman established a trained corps of ambulance drivers and litter bearers and gave them a distinctive uniform and insignia. He specified that only medical personnel could remove the wounded from the battlefield, a regulation designed to reduce the manpower loss that normally resulted when soldiers left the line to transport their wounded comrades to the aid station. Ambulance wagons were removed from the quartermaster's control and were to be used only for medical transport. Ambulances traveled in the front of the column to ensure they would be easily reached once the battle commenced. The first test of Letterman's ambulance system came at the Battle of Antietam Creek (September 1862). Union forces suffered ten thousand wounded scattered over a six-mile area, but the system reached and evacuated most of them within thirty-six hours. Three months later at Fredericksburg (December 1862), the system worked so well that the wounded piled up at the aid stations faster than they could treated.[141] Within twelve hours, all of the nearly ten thousand Union wounded had been located and cleared through the aid stations.

Letterman's field ambulance system would not have worked as well as it did had it not been integrated into a larger network of casualty evacuation linking the field hospitals to the general hospitals in the rear. They also used the excellent Northern railway network to move casualties from collection points behind the battlefields to the general hospitals. The hospital cars varied in quality from first-class heated passenger coaches to unheated boxcars with little more than straw on the floors. By the end of the war, the Northern railways had transported 225,000 sick and wounded men from the battlefields to the general hospitals.[142]

The Union medical service also used coastal steamers and river steamboats to transport the sick and wounded. The Union contracted these hospital ships from civilians and initially gave the quartermaster corps control of them. Later in the war, the medical corps assumed control of these assets and used them exclusively for medical purposes. In 1862, the Union Army contracted for fifteen steamboats for use on the Mississippi and Ohio Rivers and seventeen ocean-going vessels for use along the Atlantic coast. In the last three years of the war, 150,000 casualties had been transported by boat to general hospitals.[143] The first systematic use of the hospital ship was at the Battle of Fort Henry in February 1862 when the *City of Memphis* transported 7,000 casualties to hospitals along the Ohio River.[144] The army purchased its first ship, the *D. A. January*, to serve as a hospital ship, and the crew saw its first action after the Battle of Shiloh in April 1862. The ship had a 450-bed hospital, bathrooms, laundry, baking and cooking facilities, and a full complement of surgeons and nurses. By the end of the war, the *January* had transported 23,738 patients on the Ohio, Missouri, and Illinois Rivers. The mortality rate among its wounded passengers was only 2.3 percent, better than most land-based hospitals of the day.[145] The first naval nurses in America were the Catholic Sisters of Mercy, who served aboard the first U.S. Navy hospital ship, the USS *Red Rover*, and tended the wounded after the siege of Vicksburg.[146] The ship also had African American women nurses aboard.

Letterman's field ambulance system proved so successful that in March 1862 Surgeon General Hammond recommended that all Union armies adopt it. The army high command dragged its feet for two years before Congress in March 1864 forced it to institute the system for all Union commands. It was only by the end of the war that the system was fully implemented. The United States had gradually developed a military medical system adequate enough to treat the casualties that a modern war produced only to see it demobilized with the rest of the army less than a year after the war ended. With the army returning to garrison and frontier duties, a mass casualty system was no longer needed.

Letterman also changed the structure of the field hospital system by turning the old regimental hospitals into frontline aid stations, or the equivalent of the modern battalion aid clearing point. Treatment of the wounded at these aid stations was limited to controlling bleeding, bandaging wounds, and administering opiates for pain. Limiting the functions of these aid stations enabled the medical personnel to hold the slightly wounded close to the front for their possible return to duty. Behind the aid stations, Letterman placed mobile surgical field hospitals. Controlled by division, the most competent medical personnel were assembled at these hospitals to perform major operations. These hospitals were the critical link, missing for most of military medical history, between the frontline aid stations and the rear area general hospitals. Behind these mobile field hospitals were the general hospitals, and the field ambulance corps, the railways, and hospital ships tied the whole system together. Letterman was also concerned about the manpower loss due to hasty and needless evacuation. To prevent it, all medical officers were ordered to hold the less severely injured at their respective hospitals. Letterman instituted systematic inspections of all patients to screen those held for possible return to duty before deciding what patients to evacuate.[147]

Letterman's third major contribution to the Union medical service was the establishment of medical supply and equipment tables for medical units. Until this reform, the service obtained medical equipment and supplies from the quartermaster through the usual military supply system. Under the pressure of war, however, medical units rarely received what they needed. Letterman arranged supply tables equipping all units from corps through regiments with "basic loads" of medical provisions. Each unit was supposed to carry supplies for thirty days. A purveyor accompanied the army and was responsible for continually replenishing medical supplies. With each medical unit requiring specific amounts of supplies, the purveyor could now plan in advance to fill the requirements of each unit. For the first time, an army had developed a relatively modern medical supply service that worked well under field conditions.[148]

Most units in the Union Army were volunteer units that the states created. The state governors then commissioned the great number of surgeons and physicians that served in the war to provide medical support to state regiments. With few standardized licensing procedures for medical certification, it was not surprising that competency was a problem. Few of the physicians entering the state regiments had any surgical training. Indeed, the educational training of a physician or surgeon at this time entailed only one year of formal schooling and one year as an apprentice to a practicing doctor. Many of the "medical schools"—including Harvard University at the time—were little more than diploma mills.[149] For reasons that remain unclear, all medical schools in the South, with the exception of the University of Virginia, were closed shortly after the outbreak of war, thus depriving the Confederate armies of a vital source of trained medical talent.[150] As the war wore on, however, many of the marginally competent physicians and surgeons on both sides became excellent practitioners as a consequence of their battlefield experience.

About 13,000 physicians and surgeons served with the Union forces. Of these, Congress appointed about 250 regular army surgeons and assistant surgeons to serve as staff and administrators. Congress commissioned approximately 547 Surgeons of Volunteers, also called "brigade surgeons," to assist the corps of regular army surgeons. Governors appointed some 3,882 regimental surgeons and assistants to provide medical support to state regiments. Most saw service in the regiments, aid stations, and mobile field hospitals. The army hired 5,532 contract civilian surgeons to staff the general hospitals in the major cities. These physicians and surgeons often divided their time between private practice and military service. An additional 100 doctors staffed the Veteran Reserve Corps to provide aid to the disabled, and 1,451 surgeons and assistants served with the 179,000 black troops in 166 regiments.[151] One of the Union surgeons, Dr. Mary Edwards Walker (1832–1919), a graduate of Syracuse Medical College, served in the army as a nurse until finally appointed as an assistant surgeon. She became the first woman in American history to hold such a position.[152] She was also the first to earn the Congressional Medal of Honor for her wartime service at Fredericksburg and Chickamauga, among other duties.

The general hospitals—designated as such because they treated the wounded regardless of what unit they were from—were located in the major cities along well-established water and rail routes. By 1862, a building program was undertaken in the North to provide hospital facilities for the rapidly growing lists of casualties. A year later, the Union Army had established 151 general hospitals with 58,715 beds. Two years later it had 204 such hospitals with a capacity of 136,894 beds.[153] These hospitals ranged in size from small to 100-bed units, which the South commonly established next to railway crossings, and to the large Mower General Hospital in Philadelphia with 4,000 beds. The largest hospital on either side was the 8,000-bed Chimborazo Hospital in Richmond. With 150 single-story pavilions organized into five divisions, each with forty to fifty surgeons and assistant surgeons per division, it was the largest military hospital ever built in the Western world.[154]

The range of injuries that military medical practitioners confronted prompted the development of hospitals specializing in specific medical conditions. There were special hospitals for orthopedics and venereal diseases, and the famous Turner's Lane Hospital in Philadelphia acquired a worldwide reputation for its expertise in nervous disorders. St. Elizabeth's Hospital in Washington became the world's first military hospital for combat psychiatric cases.[155] It had long been recognized that large hospitals were conducive to infection and disease and that better ventilation and isolation reduced these problems. The pavilion-style hospital evolved as the best design for reducing infection and improving ventilation and isolation. These hospitals consisted of a series of long single-story buildings, each isolated from the next but connected by corridors. High ceilings with vents at the top and sufficient windows provided adequate ventilation. Normally connected to the central semicircular corridor, these sixty-patient building units were sometimes unconnected, providing excellent isolation for specific disease wards. The pavilion hospital design is generally credited to Dr. Samuel Moore (1813–1889), the Confederate surgeon general, who supposedly obtained the idea from British hospitals used in the Crimean War.[156] More accurately the design is much older and generally reflects the arrangement that the Romans utilized.

Both armies in the Civil War used female nurses, a precedent that the Russians first set and the British soon followed in the Crimean War. The special place of women in Southern culture militated against allowing women to work in military hospitals; consequently, female nurses were not used on a large scale. In the North, however, 3,214 nurses served in military hospitals under the control of Dorothea Dix (1802–1887), who had been appointed as the Union Army's superintendent of women nurses.[157] An even larger female corps of cooks, cleaners, and general attendants—some of whom were African American—supported this nursing corps. Large numbers of Catholic Sisters of Mercy, Sisters of St. Joseph, and Sisters of the Holy Cross also served in this capacity. Dix did not trust Catholics but found that because the sisters were accustomed to discipline and obedience, they made excellent workers.[158] Having gained valuable experience in treating the sick, all three of these religious orders remained in the hospital business after the war. Clara Barton (1821–1912), one of Dix's regular nurses, went on to found the American Red Cross.

The prevalence of facial injuries encountered during the war stimulated the emergence of the new medical subdiscipline of plastic surgery. Civil War surgeons performed six reconstructions of the eyelid, five of the nose, three of the cheek, and fourteen of the lip, palate, and other parts of the mouth.[159] Dr. Gordon Buck, while serving as a contract surgeon for the Union Army, performed the first total facial reconstruction in history.[160] Another Civil War surgeon, Joseph J. Woodward (1833–1884), became the first person to link the new technology of the camera to the microscope and published the first microphotographs of disease bacteria in 1865. In 1870, while working for the newly formed Army Medical Museum, Woodward became the first person to take microphotographs, using artificial illumination.[161] Woodward is also credited with the independent discovery of using aniline dyes to stain tissues for microscopic analysis.[162]

A comprehensive history of the Confederate medical service is yet to be written. The great Richmond fire of 1865 destroyed almost the entire archive of the Confederacy's medical records. For the most part, however, the Confederate medical service was organized and operated almost as a copy of the Union system, although shortages of personnel and equipment nearly crippled it from time to time. The total number of medical officers in the Confederacy was 3,236—1,242 surgeons and 1,994 assistant surgeons. There were 107 officers in the naval medical corps, including 26 surgeons and 81 assistant surgeons.[163] The Confederate general hospital system was every bit as good as what operated in the North. Chronically short of ambulance wagons in the first few years of the war, the South made greater and more efficient use of steamboats and rail to transport their wounded. Early in the war

(1861), Surgeon General Moore established high qualifications for those wishing to enter the medical service and, in a truly revolutionary step, examined those physicians already in the service for competency, forcing significant numbers to resign.[164] Shortages of quinine and chloroform plagued the South until the end, and Confederate disease losses might have been reduced had they embarked upon a smallpox vaccination program earlier in the war. The South recognized dentistry as a separate medical discipline and encouraged its growth. As secretary of war before hostilities broke out, Jefferson Davis had tried to convince the U.S. Army to establish a separate dental corps but failed. The South had a much more comprehensive dental care program than did the North, which contented itself with shipping to the artillery toothless soldiers who could no longer bite the end from their cartridge packets.[165]

Gen. Thomas J. "Stonewall" Jackson (1824–1863) introduced one of the more significant military medical contributions of the South when in 1862, he ordered all Union medical officers held by his command to be released and, henceforth, treated as noncombatants. By June of that year, both Robert E. Lee and McClellan agreed to a similar practice. Medical personnel were no longer subject to capture and, if taken, were supposed to be allowed to treat their wounded and immediately released. All medical personnel held in Union and Confederate prison camps were freed in 1862, and exchanges of captured medical personnel continued until the end of the war. Jackson's actions had anticipated the Red Cross regulations dealing with medical personnel that the first Geneva Convention adopted a few years later.[166]

With the cessation of hostilities, the Union Army and its military medical service were demobilized. By the end of 1866, the Union Army had been reduced to a force of only 30,000 men.[167] The army and its skeleton medical corps were scattered among 239 military posts stretching from Alaska to the Rio Grande. By 1869, the entire medical service comprised no more than 161 medical officers, and the frontier posts were forced to rely on civilian contract surgeons, which increased to 282.[168] Although a young doctor could make more money in military service than he could in the first few years of his own practice, the shortage of military doctors remained a chronic problem. One reason was that the army maintained much higher entrance and training requirements than were generally found for civilian physicians.[169]

In 1862, Surgeon General Hammond ordered the establishment of the Army Medical Museum in Washington, D.C., to collect and study artifacts and information relevant to military medical care. In 1865 when John Shaw Billings (1836–1913) became director of the Library of the Surgeon General's Office of the Army, he soon built it into the largest military medical library in the world, and the collection remains so today.[170] After the war, Congress established a pension system for disabled soldiers that was far more generous and comprehensive than anything seen in Europe.[171] The pension system was chosen over an asylum system of permanent care because it provided the disabled soldier with more freedom and mobility.

A number of significant advances in military medicine resulted from the Civil War. For the first time an accurate medical record system was established that made it possible to track casualty records for every soldier. One consequence was the U.S. government's publication of the massive six-volume *Medical and Surgical History of the War of the Rebellion* (1870–1888), which remains the standard against which all such works are judged. The army also developed the first effective military medical system for mass casualties, complete with aid stations, field and general hospitals, ambulance and theater-level casualty transport, and the staff to coordinate it. It was the best military medical system ever deployed and remained a model for other countries for decades. The introduction of the pavilion hospital was so effective at reducing disease mortality that it became the standard design for military and civilian hospitals for the next seventy-five years. Wide use of anesthesia, primary amputation, the splint, and debridement of necrotic tissue were the first effective doctrines for wound management. Thousands of physicians learned these techniques through hard experience and carried them into their civilian practice, elevating the general level of medical care available to the nation. Effective sanitary measures, especially in hospitals, reduced disease and death. The advent of microphotography made the American military medical establishment receptive to the discoveries of Pasteur and Lister when they appeared a few years later. Nurses were used on a wide scale for the first time. The terrible slaughter of the Civil War ironically marked one of the most progressive periods in the development of military medicine until the twentieth century.

THE INVENTION OF MILITARY PSYCHIATRY

Fear and psychiatric debilitation are constant companions in war. Battle is one of the most threatening, stressful, and horrifying experiences that man is expected to endure. Even in relatively small engagements, the participants often suffer a wide range of psychiatric conditions that, if pressed by events, lead to mental collapse.[172] Severe emotional response to battle is neither a rare nor an isolated event. One of the most outstanding medical developments of the Civil War was the emergence of the neurological profession in America and, along with it, the beginning of military psychiatry as a major subdiscipline of military medicine.[173] Military psychiatry dates from the Civil War when neurologists made a systematic attempt to link damage to the brain to emotional behavior, but it did not become a separate discipline until the Russo-Japanese War of 1905.

Psychiatry was still in its infancy at the time of the Civil War, but neurologists recognized that soldiers could become debilitated from purely emotional forces. At that time, the discipline focused on the physiology of the brain and attempted to link disruptions of that physiology to behavioral disorders. Fewer than a dozen mental hospitals existed in the United States, but none served patients who developed mental disorders in war. Care of the mentally ill rested with the handful of superintendents of these mental asylums. The movement for humane treatment of the mentally ill that began in France fifty years before was only beginning to take root in the United States.[174] The military itself had no psychiatrists and continued to take the traditional view that soldiers who broke in battle were cowards or had "weak" characters. By 1860, American military psychiatry had not come very far since the Revolution, and the discipline was considerably behind developments in Europe.[175]

Almost immediately after the outbreak of the Civil War, medical officers had to deal with the problem of psychiatric casualties. The War Department had rejected the offer by a group of superintendents of insane asylums to treat the problem on the battlefields, and treatment of psychiatric casualties fell to army physicians and surgeons. Their experience gained with psychiatric cases led to the birth of neurology in the United States and hardened further the tendency of medical practitioners of the day to regard soldiers' mental problems as caused by damaged physiology of the brain. The Turner's Lane Hospital in Philadelphia treated what were called "nervous diseases" during the war, but even the neurologists had to admit that a range of disorders that afflicted the soldiers had no sound physiological explanation. At the doctors' urging, the Government Hospital for the Insane in Washington, D.C., admitted the psychiatric casualties to specific wings in 1863. The men preferred to call it St. Elizabeths Hospital, after the land on which it was built.

The most common psychiatric condition that military physicians had to confront was "nostalgia," a cluster of symptoms resulting from emotional fatigue that made it impossible for the soldier to continue to fight. Nostalgia was marked by excessive physical fatigue, an inability to concentrate, an unwillingness to eat or drink that led at times to anorexia, feelings of isolation and frustration, and a general inability to function in a military environment. Swiss armies first reported the condition in 1569, and Swiss military physicians described it again in 1678.[176] German physicians of the same period called the condition *heimweh* (homesickness), French military doctors termed the same symptoms *mal du pays,* and the Spanish, who noted their soldiers' suffering an outbreak of nostalgia in Flanders during the Thirty Years' War, called it *estar roto* (literally, to be broken).[177] Even then military doctors recognized that the source of the symptoms was emotional and not physical, noting that "imagination alone can cause all this."[178] Nostalgia again was recognized and widely reported during the eighteenth century among the armies of France, Italy, Germany, and Austria. In one instance, a unit of Scottish Highland troops in 1799 succumbed to the condition almost to a man. To trigger the onset of symptoms, the report noted, the Highlanders only needed to hear the sound of the bagpipes. Nostalgia was reported among Napoleon's troops at Waterloo, during the retreat from Moscow, and in the Egyptian campaign, where it became so serious among the officer corps that it threatened to cripple the army.[179]

During the Civil War, autopsies performed on nostalgia patients confirmed that besides producing emotional turbulence, nostalgia was capable of producing physiological symptoms of disease. Tragically, nostalgia itself was often fatal, especially if a wound or lack of nutrition weakened the soldier's general resistance. When it did not kill, nostalgia often drove the soldier insane. In the first year of the Civil War, military physicians diagnosed 5,213 cases of nostalgia, or 2.34 cases per thousand.[180] By the end of the war, almost 10,000 cases had been diagnosed among Union soldiers. In addition, physicians diagnosed a range of illnesses that are now known to stem from emotional turbulence and included "exhausted hearts," paralysis, severe palpitations (called "soldier's heart" at the time), war tremors, self-inflicted wounds, and various states of nostalgia.[181] Military doctors diagnosed the more severe psychiatric conditions as "insanity"—today the condition is termed "psychosis"—and it accounted for 6 percent of all medical discharges granted by the Union Army.[182] Physicians also identified a number of cases that they diagnosed as "feigned insanity," a condition in which emotional turbulence produced severe symptoms for which a physiological cause could not be found. These conditions included lameness, blindness, deafness, local paralysis, and lower back pain.[183] Today, military psychiatrists call these conditions "conversion reactions." Psychiatric symptoms became so common among Union soldiers that field commanders pleaded with the War Department to provide some form of screening to eliminate recruits susceptible to psychiatric breakdown.

In 1863, the Union Army instituted the world's first military psychiatric screening program for recruits. It proved no more helpful than it would later in World War I, and the number of psychiatric cases continued to increase.

Meanwhile, only a handful of physicians in the country—the superintendents of civilian mental asylums—had any experience in dealing with psychiatric patients, but none of these doctors saw military service during the war. Accordingly, military physicians were often at a loss when treating cases of insanity. With a long historical precedent in the armies of Europe, their particularly cruel solution in the first three years of the war was simply to muster out those soldiers diagnosed as suffering from severe psychiatric problems. Union and Confederate soldiers with psychiatric symptoms were escorted out of the main gates of their respective army camps and turned loose to fend for themselves. Others were put on trains with no supervision, the name of their hometown or state pinned to their tunics. Others were left to wander about the countryside until they died from exposure or starvation or were arrested for committing crimes. By 1863, the number of insane or shocked soldiers wandering around the country was so large that the public demanded an end to the military's practice of expulsion. That same year, the military began sending psychiatric cases to the hospital for the insane in Washington.

As noted earlier, the Union Army had discharged nearly ten thousand soldiers suffering from nostalgia by the end of the war. The number suffering from "epilepsy" and forms of hysterical paralysis was probably twice as large, while those discharged for "general insanity" reached several thousand. Although the problem of psychiatric breakdown among soldiers reached major proportions by the war's end, not a single article or book on the subject was published in the postwar years.[184] The General Hospital for the Insane closed its military psychiatric facilities, and the government made no effort to involve the doctors who treated civilians with mental illness in helping the psychiatrically wounded. The veterans' problems were conveniently forgotten, and except for the advances in neurology, battle shock and psychiatric debilitation were no longer of concern to the military. The failure to learn from this experience returned to haunt the American Army when it took the field again in World War I.

THE FRANCO-PRUSSIAN WAR

By the first quarter of the nineteenth century, surgery had attained the general status of a legitimate branch of medicine in the United States, France, and England. The old barber-surgeons' guilds had largely disappeared. In Russia and Germany, this development did not occur until after mid-century; thus, in Russia, with some exceptions, surgery and military surgery remained largely in the hands of the feldshers. In Germany, surgery was still regarded as a low-status craft that barber-surgeons practiced in the military. The general status of medicine in the larger society was also low; however, surgery found a home in the universities, where it was practiced by medical researchers, academics, and scientists. The beneficial result of this situation was that as being researchers and academics first, surgeons in the universities tended to be more strongly grounded in the sciences, where the rigors of empirical proof and scientific investigations had long traditions. When the opportunity came to transfer these skills to military medicine, German surgeons were better prepared to assimilate and integrate new knowledge than were their counterparts in other countries.[185]

Until the 1830s, German medicine was mired in the Hegelian period of its development, and debates centered on the philosophy of science with little in the way of empirical emphasis. After 1848, German science and medicine began its transition toward systematic realism, with a strong emphasis upon data collection and observation. The old academic habits of rigorous method and proof moved German medicine rapidly in the direction of an exact science.[186] As a consequence, German medicine was much more receptive to demonstrated evidence than were the medical professions in the rest of Europe. For instance, German physicians and surgeons were the first to accept Lister's practice of antiseptic surgery. Once the idea of antisepsis caught on, the Germans' thoroughness propelled them to be the first to introduce steam sterilization, to use surgical face masks and gowns, and to invent the sterile operating room.[187] By 1870, German medicine had established itself among the foremost scientific medical establishments in the world. By the 1880s, the medical world had adopted German as its official scientific language because its linguistic precision lent itself perfectly to the new science.[188]

This well of scientific talent continued to reside in the universities and research institutions until after 1866 and the Austro-Prussian War, with the result that military medicine remained generally behind that of other countries. The political fragmentation of the German state also presented significant barriers to utilizing German medical talent in the armies, for the old *länder* (state) regimental system made it difficult to form a professional national army. With national unification under Otto von Bismarck (1815–1898), these political barriers disappeared. Moreover, the creation of a national army raised the status of any association with the military, making a military career attractive to physicians. The reserve system, designed to rapidly fill out the standing army, created expanded social opportunities for medical academics to obtain commissions in the reserve regiments. When these regiments were called to national service, as in the Franco-Prussian War, the best German physicians and surgeons in the country went along with them.[189] Overnight, the German soldier became the recipient of the best military medical care in the world.

In the eighteenth century, military medical care had never been a matter of great concern for Frederick the Great. Between his death and the outbreak of the wars of the French Revolution, the German military medical system, along with much of the rest of the military establishment, had ossified.[190] The press of the French wars, however, demonstrated the need for reform, and Johann Goercke (1750–1822), who served as surgeon general from 1797 to 1822, infused a new spirit into the German medical service.[191] Goercke's battlefield experience convinced him to improve the medical service, and he spent two years studying medicine in the leading centers of Europe before attempting reforms. In 1795, he founded the Pépinière in Berlin to train military medical officers and established a reporting system for evaluating the competency of medical personnel. To attract talent to military service, he convinced the king to establish a pension for military medical officers. The Pépinière graduated 1,359 medical officers for service in the army between 1795 and 1821, when it became the Frederick Wilhelm's Institute.[192] Goercke also obtained funds to create mobile field hospitals, but they did not become established until after the German defeat at Jena in 1806. By 1813, however, the German Army operated three general hospitals of twelve hundred beds each, one reserve hospital with three thousand beds, and nine mobile field hospitals of two hundred beds each. To support this system, thirty-eight military reserve hospitals were created in cities and towns.[193] Although Goercke had introduced a small number of field ambulances as early as 1795, probably copying the French experience, by the time of Waterloo the army only had three ambulances left. The Prussian medical corps during the Napoleonic Wars had developed a well-trained litter bearer corps that was equipped with two-wheeled carts and distinctive badges and scarves for the personnel, but without a mobile ambulance system to transport casualties, the medical service still was rudimentary at best.[194]

Although some changes in the German medical service helped provide sufficient numbers of trained medical personnel to the army in wartime, the real stimulus for reform came with the experience of the Austro-Prussian War. For the first time the German Army used breech-loading rifles and artillery on a large scale. The Austrians, meanwhile, were equipped with the old smoothbore muzzle-loading cannon firing case shot, while their infantry carried the muzzle-loaded Lorenz rifles with .57-caliber rounds. The Prussian Army numbered 669,076 men, of which 2,286 were medical officers and 1,909 hospital assistants. Also seeing service were 3,420 apothecaries.[195] Medical support was organized around the army corps, not the regiment. It is unclear how the Germans hit upon this idea, but they probably copied it from the Americans' experience in the Civil War.[196] Each army corps was provided with a medical train of three hundred men and an ambulance corps of one hundred men. The Prussians had twenty-seven corps hospitals, ten light field hospitals, and six general hospitals to treat casualties. Behind them were four reserve medical depots far to the rear. The system could accommodate forty-seven thousand casualties.[197]

Although the Prussian system was adequately staffed, its performance proved to be less than acceptable to the German high command. The Prussian Army inflicted more battle casualties upon the enemy than it suffered itself, but its sickness and disease death rates were higher. The army endured epidemics of cholera, typhus, and dysentery at higher rates than the Austrians did and averaged a manpower loss from illness of approximately 2.5 percent.[198] Moreover, the death to wound ratio averaged between 11 and 12 percent, or much higher than expected, and the percentage of men with disease who were permanently invalided was also higher than expected.[199] Shortly after the hostilities ceased, the German Army totally reorganized its medical service and created an independent military medical corps for the first time in German history.[200]

A few years later, the German medical corps performed so well in the Franco-Prussian War that it became the model that the British military medical system followed when it introduced reforms almost immediately after the war.[201] The German hospital system remained almost structurally the same as it had been in 1866, but it had made great improvements in hygiene and sanitation. Most important was its first large-scale use of Listerian methods of antisepsis.[202] The results were remarkable, and after the war Lister toured Germany as a hero, even while his innovations were still being debated in England and France.[203] The Germans also made great improvements in their field ambulance system and assigned trained litter bearers to each regiment. A reserve litter company rushed stretcher bearers to those regiments that were particularly hard pressed. Special liaison teams whose task it was to manage the flow of vehicles from the field hospitals to the general hospitals coordinated the increased use of field ambulances.[204] The medical service made extensive use of the American-style medical wagons that Dr. Letterman introduced in the Civil War, with their two tiers of ambulance beds, medical laboratory, and supplies of drugs and equipment.[205]

The smooth flow of wounded to the aid stations and collecting points behind the battle augmented the German medics' ability to provide treatment to the wounded soldier more rapidly than any other army had previously accomplished. Each German soldier was provided with his own sterile first aid kit, which included an elastic Esmarch bandage,[206] sterile lint, and other bandages. When medical personnel reached a soldier, the equipment they needed to stem bleeding and prevent shock was thus readily at hand. Utilizing special units of noncommissioned officers as corpsmen trained in the tourniquet's use also reduced death from blood loss and shock. Among the Germans' most interesting innovations were the medical cards that the soldiers wore around their necks. The field medics used these cards to record the soldiers' injuries and condition. It provided the surgeon with a much-needed source of information that also saved time.[207]

As casualties flowed to the rear, the German Army's railway corps provided a crucial link in evacuating casualties to general and reserve hospitals. Each army corps had its own medical railway unit to coordinate and oversee the wounded's evacuation, with two hundred rail cars equipped with mattresses, straw, and nursing personnel who were organic to its organization. Those soldiers who were unable to travel were held at battalion aid or temporary barracks hospitals until their conditions stabilized. Railway medical personnel evacuated the most seriously wounded on a priority basis. Every hour or so, an average of fifty railway cars pulled out of German stations bound for rear area hospitals.[208]

The innovations of the German medical system greatly reduced the death rate. Using antiseptic surgery, curiously forbidden by the French, drastically reduced the surgical mortality rate from infection. Systematic vaccination, a procedure the French also chose not to employ, resulted in a smallpox casualty rate four times lower than what the French suffered.[209] German Army doctors outnumbered their French counterparts almost 4 to 1, and the French ambulance corps was decidedly primitive by German standards. The French were still using hired labor to drive their field ambulances and saw the usual results. While the German system handled thousands of casualties smoothly, more often than not the French system was overwhelmed in the first few hours of battle. Even their rear area hospitals were inadequate to the task of handling the casualty load. The German system worked so well that for the first time in modern history, a war was fought where the number of casualties caused by hostile fire was greater than the number of soldiers lost to disease.

Perhaps no century in history saw more progress in the development of military medical care than the nineteenth century. The quality of care provided to a soldier during any period depended upon two factors—the quality of medical knowledge available to the military practitioners and the degree of organizational sophistication within an army to actually deliver medical care to the soldier lying injured on the battlefield. The nineteenth century witnessed the emergence of anesthesia, antiseptic surgery, and bacteriology as the three most important innovations in medical knowledge contributing to the improvement of military medicine. As rudimentary as these innovations were when compared to the degree to which they have developed in modern times, they were nevertheless revolutionary. Without them, many of the medical advances of the present day would not have been possible. In a sense, they were true conceptual revolutions that laid the basis for much of modern medicine.

Not a single major European army began the nineteenth century with an independent and well-developed medical system that could systematically deliver the medical knowledge of the day to the wounded soldier. By the end of the century, however, every army had such a system. Some, such as the Germans and Americans, gained extensive firsthand experience in handling mass casualties. Others either lacked this experience, as they fought only small colonial wars (British), or failed to learn from their experience with mass casualties (French and Russians). At the very least, however, although some armies failed to staff their medical services with adequate men and equipment during peacetime, the idea that any successful army required a medical service had set deep roots in all the armies of the world. Events might prove that existing arrangements for medical care were inadequate for a given war, but never again would a major power send an army into the field without providing some sort of medical care system.

The Franco-Prussian War of 1870 was the last major war of the century and produced the now commonly high casualty rates inflicted by modern weapons. Marking the last quarter century were small-scale colonial wars, often in medically hostile environments—for example, the Boer War and Spanish-American War—in which sickness and death by disease played greater havoc than injuries from weapons did. At the same time, medical advances in the etiology of disease contagion served as the starting point for a new approach in which it was more important to discover the mechanism of disease transmission than to discover the cause of the disease itself. Often after an initial period of terrible experience with disease epidemics among troops in the field, armies began to pay serious attention to preventing disease before an epidemic occurred. This approach led to great upgrades in military hygiene, beginning with improvements in the health and quality of the soldier himself. Advances in bacteriology, in turn, led to advances in immunology, and the list of diseases for which inoculations were available increased.

Military medicine had reached a point in its development at which it stood on the brink of a new frontier where the soldier could expect to survive most of the rigors of the battlefield unless his body was torn apart by flying metal. The focus on military sanitation, disease, and hygiene, coupled with the fading memories of mass casualties produced in previous wars, led to a reduction in the number and type of resources available to the peacetime armies. At the same time, few military thinkers truly appreciated the lethal possibilities inherent in the technological improvements that had occurred in weaponry since 1870. Not a single army in the world had changed its tactical thinking very much since the last major war. Because the colonial wars had been short and cheaply fought, the strategic doctrine of the day held that the next war, even if fought among the major powers in the European heartland, would also be short lived, with victory going to the side that could most rapidly mobilize and deploy its reserves. When the shots fired in the streets of Sarajevo echoed through the chancelleries of Europe, events proved just how wrong these strategic thinkers' assumptions had been.

NOTES

1. McGrew, *Encyclopedia of Medical History*, 14.
2. Hypnotism, popularized by Franz Joseph Mesmer, became known as mesmerism. Another earlier anesthetic technique that military surgeons used includes placing a metal helmet on the patient's head and striking it with a wooden hammer to render the patient unconscious.
3. J. Antonio Aldrete, G. Manuel Marron, and A. J. Wright, "The First Administration of Anesthesia in Military Surgery: On Occasion of the Mexican-American War," *Anesthesiology* 61, no. 5 (November 1984): 585.
4. Samuel Guthrie, an American, was the inventor of chloroform. He also invented the percussion cap that increased the rate of fire of Civil War muskets.
5. Although first used in obstetrics, chloroform was widely held to be dangerous because it reduced the pain that was "natural" to childbirth. It was further believed that chloroform induced sexual fantasies when administered to women. These objections came to an end when Queen Victoria was administered chloroform in childbirth in 1853.
6. John A. Shepard, "The Smart of the Knife: Early Anesthesia in the Services," *Journal of the Royal Army Medical Corps* 131, no. 2 (June 1985): 109–12.
7. Ibid.
8. Aaron M. Schwartz, "The Historical Development of Methods of Hemostasis," *Surgery* 44, no. 3 (September 1958): 608.
9. Ibid.

10. Ibid., 609.
11. Chamberlain, "History of Military Medicine," 248.
12. Robert Wagner and Benjamin Slivko, "History of Nonpenetrating Chest Trauma and Its Treatment," *Minnesota Medical Journal* 37, no. 4 (April 1988): 301.
13. Theodore E. Woodward, "The Public's Debt to Military Medicine," *Military Medicine* 146 (March 1981): 172.
14. Chamberlain, "History of Military Medicine," 249.
15. Peter Aldea and William Shaw, "The Evolution of the Surgical Management of Severe Lower Extremity Trauma," *Clinics in Plastic Surgery* 13, no. 4 (October 1986): 556.
16. Ibid.
17. McGrew, *Encyclopedia of Medical History*, 34; and Crissey and Parish, "Wound Healing," 4.
18. Forrest, "Development of Wound Therapy," 271.
19. Kirkup, "History and Evolution," 284.
20. Wangensteen et al., "Some Highlights," 108.
21. Lewis N. Cozen, "Military Orthopedic Surgery," *Clinical Orthopaedics and Related Research* 200 (November 1985): 52.
22. Ibid.
23. Inspector General Hercule Sieur, "Tribulations of the Medical Corps of the French Army from Its Origin to Our Own Time," *Military Surgeon* 64, no. 6 (June 1929): 843.
24. Ibid., 851.
25. Garrison, *Notes on the History*, 162.
26. A. G. Chevalier, "Hygienic Problems of the Napoleonic Armies," *Ciba Symposium* 3 (1941–1942): 975.
27. Colin Jones, *The Charitable Imperative: Hospitals and Nursing in Ancien Régime and Revolutionary France* (London: Routledge, 1989), 228.
28. After the battle of Marengo in 1800, France signed a treaty with Austria and England in 1802. Napoleon was regarded in France as a peacemaker, and the military hospitals were dismantled. Shortly after the demobilization of the hospitals began in 1803, the War of the Third Coalition broke out. Napoleon won so quickly at the battle of Austerlitz that the defects of the dismantled military medical system were not appreciated, and the dismantlement of the hospitals was allowed to continue.
29. Garrison, *Notes on the History*, 169.
30. A similar outbreak of ophthalmia among French troops in Syria six hundred years earlier had crippled the army and forced a retreat. Given the prevalence of hospitals dedicated to treating blind Crusaders during the Middle Ages, it seems reasonable that ophthalmia presented a serious disease threat to these armies.
31. Garrison, *Notes on the History*, 166.
32. For cold injury rates in all the wars from the Napoleonic Wars to World War I, see Charles Schechter and Irving A. Sarot, "Historical Accounts of Injuries Due to Cold," *Surgery* 63, no. 3 (March 1968): 535.
33. Blaine Taylor, "Some Medical-Historical Aspects of the Later Napoleonic Wars, 1812–1815," *Maryland State Medical Journal*, December 1978, 27.
34. Launcelotte Gubbins, "The Life and Work of Jean Dominique, First Baron Larrey," *Journal of the Royal Army Medical Corps* 22 (1914): 188.
35. Sieur, "Tribulations of the Medical Corps," 855.
36. Wangensteen et al., "Wound Management," 224.
37. Chevalier, "Hygienic Problems," 979.

38. Wangensteen et al., "Some Highlights," 224.
39. Lyman A. Brewer, "Baron Dominique Jean Larrey (1766–1842): Father of Modern Military Surgery, Innovator, Humanist," *Journal of Thoracic and Cardiovascular Surgery* 92, no. 6 (December 1986): 1097.
40. E. Robert Wiese, "Larrey: Napoleon's Chief Surgeon," *Annals of Medical History* 1 (July 1929): 444.
41. These wagons were called *ourgons*.
42. Wiese, "Larrey."
43. Taylor, "Some Medical-Historical Aspects," 27.
44. David M. Vess, "French Military Medicine during the Revolution," PhD diss., University of Alabama, 1965, 118–19. This outstanding research work deserves to be published.
45. F. M. Richardson, "Wellington, Napoleon, and the Medical Services," *Journal of the Royal Army Medical Corps* 131, no. 1 (1985): 9–10.
46. Wiese, "Larrey," 44.
47. Garrison, *Notes on the History*, 164.
48. Chevalier, "Hygienic Problems," 976.
49. Richard L. Blanco, "The Development of British Military Medicine, 1793–1814," *Military Affairs* 38, no. 1 (February 1974): 5.
50. Robert M. Feibel, "What Happened at Walcheren: The Primary Medical Sources," *Bulletin of the History of Medicine* 42 (1968): 64.
51. Taylor, "Retrospect of Naval and Military Medicine," 622.
52. Garrison, *Notes on the History*, 167.
53. Taylor, "Retrospect of Naval and Military Medicine," 622.
54. Garrison, *Notes on the History*, 167.
55. Taylor, "Retrospect of Naval and Military Medicine," 622.
56. Ibid.
57. Blanco, "Development of British Military Medicine," 9.
58. G. A. Kempthorne, "The Medical Department of Wellington's Army," *Journal of the Royal Army Medical Corps*, February–March 1930, 214.
59. Richard L. Blanco, *Wellington's Surgeon General: Sir James McGrigor* (Durham, NC: Duke University Press, 1974), 117–19.
60. Kempthorne, "Medical Department," 214.
61. J. M. Matheson, "Comments on the Medical Aspects of the Battle of Waterloo, 1815," *Medical History* 10 (1966): 205.
62. Blanco, *Wellington's Surgeon General*, 147.
63. A. Campbell Derby, "The Military Surgeon—Not Least in the Crusade," *Canadian Journal of Surgery* 28, no. 2 (1985): 183.
64. M. K. H. Crumplin, "Surgery at Waterloo," *Journal of the Royal Society of Medicine* 81, no. 1 (January 1988): 38. Also by the same author, see "Vascular Problems at the Battle of Waterloo," *European Journal of Vascular Surgery* 137, no. 1 (April 1987): 137–42.
65. Crumplin, "Surgery at Waterloo," 40.
66. Ibid.
67. Blanco, *Wellington's Surgeon General*, 147.
68. Peter Alexander Young, "The Army Medical Staff: Its Past Services and Its Present Needs," *Edinburgh Medical Journal* 4 (1898): 17.
69. Robert L. Reid, "The British Crimean Medical Disaster: Ineptness and Inevitability?," *Military Medicine* 140 (June 1975): 424. Another important work based on original sources is

Joseph O. Baylen and Alan Conway, eds., *Soldier-Surgeon: The Crimean War Letters of Dr. Douglas A. Reid, 1855–1856* (Knoxville: University of Tennessee Press, 1968).
70. Reid, "The British Crimean Medical Disaster," 424.
71. Garrison, *Notes on the History*, 171.
72. Ibid.
73. Ibid.
74. Reid, "The British Crimean Medical Disaster," 424.
75. G. H. Rice, "The Evolution of Military Medical Services from 1854 to 1914," *Journal of the Royal Army Medical Corps* 135, no. 3 (1989): 149.
76. Reid, "British Crimean Medical Disaster," 422.
77. Owen Wangensteen and Sarah D. Wangensteen, "Letters from a Surgeon in the Crimean War," *Bulletin of the History of Medicine* 43, no. 4 (July–August 1969): 376–79.
78. George Halperin, "Nikolai Ivanovich Pirogov: Surgeon, Anatomist, Educator," *Bulletin of the History of Medicine* 30, no. 4 (July–August 1956): 351.
79. Rice, "Evolution of Military Medical Services," 148.
80. G. A. Kempthorne, "The Medical Department in the Crimea," *Journal of the Royal Army Medical Corps* 53, no. 55 (August 1929): 132.
81. John Sweetman, "The Crimean War and the Formation of the Medical Staff Corps," *Journal of the Society for Army Historical Research* 53, no. 214 (1975): 113.
82. Kempthorne, "Medical Department in the Crimea," 138.
83. Reid, "British Crimean Medical Disaster," 422.
84. Nelson D. Lankford, "The Victorian Medical Profession and Military Practice: Army Doctors and National Origins," *Bulletin of the History of Medicine* 54 (1980): 513–14.
85. Sweetman, "Crimean War," 114.
86. Reid, "British Crimean Medical Disaster," 423.
87. Kempthorne, "Medical Department in the Crimea," 138.
88. W. A. Eakins, "Thomas Crawford: Regimental Medical Officer in the Crimea, 1855," *Ulster Medical Journal* 51, no. 1 (1982): 47–48.
89. Shepard, "Smart of the Knife," 112.
90. Ibid., 113. The fact that bleeding remained a common practice during the war did little to help speed the recovery of the wounded. Lord Raglan ordered twelve thousand leeches to be sent from Myrna for this purpose. They all arrived in tightly sealed jars, quite dead.
91. Sweetman, "Crimean War," 118.
92. Chamberlain, "History of Military Medicine," 240. See also P. S. London, "An Example to Us All: The Military Approach to the Care of the Injured," *Journal of the Royal Army Medical Corps* 134 (1988): 83–85.
93. Ian Fraser, "The Doctor's Debt to the Soldier," Mitchiner Memorial Lecture, Royal Army Medical College, June 8, 1971, 63.
94. Sieur, "Tribulations of the Medical Corps," 211.
95. Ibid., 212.
96. Ibid.
97. Ibid., 217.
98. Ibid., 219.
99. Ibid., 220.
100. Samuel Ramer, "Who Was the Russian Feldsher?," *Bulletin of the History of Medicine* 50, no. 2 (1976): 213.
101. Garrison, *Notes on the History*, 171.

102. Halperin, "Nikolai Ivanovich Pirogov," 351.
103. Ibid., 350.
104. Ibid., 354.
105. Fraser, "Doctor's Debt to the Soldier," 63.
106. Ibid.
107. Wolfe, "Genesis of the Medical Department," 840.
108. Grissinger, "Development of Military Medicine," 322.
109. Wolfe, "Genesis of the Medical Department," 23.
110. Grissinger, "Development of Military Medicine," 324–25.
111. Thomas R. Irey, "Soldiering, Suffering, and Dying in the Mexican War," *Journal of the West* 11, no. 2 (1972): 285.
112. Stewart Brooks, *Civil War Medicine* (Springfield, IL: Charles C. Thomas, 1966), 74.
113. F. William Blaisdell, "Medical Advances during the Civil War," *Archives of Surgery* 123, no. 9 (September 1988): 1045.
114. Ibid.
115. Brooks, *Civil War Medicine*, 74.
116. Ibid.
117. Ibid., 99.
118. Aldea and Shaw, "Evolution of Surgical Management," 558.
119. Brooks, *Civil War Medicine*, 100.
120. Ibid.
121. Blaisdell, "Medical Advances," 1049.
122. Ibid.
123. Willis G. Diffenbaugh, "Military Surgery in the Civil War," *Military Medicine* 130 (1965): 491.
124. Aldea and Shaw, "Evolution of Surgical Management," 558.
125. Brooks, *Civil War Medicine*, 95.
126. Robert F. Weir, "Remarks on the Gunshot Wounds of the Civil War," *New York State Journal of Medicine* 82, no. 3 (1982): 392.
127. David T. Courtwright, "Opiate Addiction as a Consequence of the Civil War," *Civil War History* 24, no. 2 (1978): 104–5.
128. Ibid., 106.
129. Ibid., 101.
130. Brooks, *Civil War Medicine*, 8.
131. Stanley B. Burns, "Early Medical Photography in America: Civil War Medical Photography," *New York State Journal of Medicine* 80, no. 9 (August 1980): 1447.
132. McCord, "Scurvy as an Occupational Disease," 590.
133. John F. Fulton, "Medicine, Warfare, and History," *Journal of the American Medical Association* 153, no. 5 (October 1953): 180.
134. Brooks, *Civil War Medicine*, 106.
135. Taylor, "Retrospect of Naval and Military Medicine," 615.
136. Brooks, *Civil War Medicine*, 41.
137. Miller J. Stewart, *Moving the Wounded: Litters, Cacolets & Ambulance Wagons, U.S. Army, 1776–1876* (Johnstown, CO: Old Army Press, 1979), 26.
138. Ibid., 33.
139. Ibid., 36.
140. Taylor, "Retrospect of Naval and Military Medicine," 617.

141. Stewart, *Moving the Wounded*, 182.
142. Brooks, *Civil War Medicine*, 37.
143. Estelle Brodman and Elizabeth B. Carrick, "American Military Medicine in the Mid-Nineteenth Century: The Experience of Alexander H. Hoff, M.D.," *Bulletin of the History of Medicine* 64 (Spring 1990): 71.
144. Brooks, *Civil War Medicine*, 37.
145. Brodman and Carrick, "American Military Medicine," 72.
146. Philip A. Kalisch and Beatrice J. Kalisch, "Untrained but Undaunted: The Women Nurses of the Blue and the Gray," *Nursing Forum* 15, no. 1 (1976): 21–22.
147. Chamberlain, "History of Military Medicine," 248.
148. Reasoner, "Medical Supply Service," 17–18.
149. Burns, "Early Medical Photography," 1447.
150. Brooks, *Civil War Medicine*, 24.
151. Burns, "Early Medical Photography," 1450–57.
152. Brooks, *Civil War Medicine*, 28.
153. Blaisdell, "Medical Advances," 1048.
154. Brooks, *Civil War Medicine*, 46.
155. Ibid.
156. Ibid., 47.
157. Kalisch and Kalisch, "Untrained but Undaunted," 24–25.
158. Blaisdell, "Medical Advances," 1046.
159. Richard B. Stark, "The History of Plastic Surgery in Wartime," *Clinics in Plastic Surgery* 2, no. 4 (October 1975): 511.
160. Ibid.
161. Leonard D. Heaton and Joe M. Blumberg, "Lt. Colonel Joseph J. Woodward (1833–1884): U.S. Army Pathologist-Researcher-Photomicroscopist," *Military Medicine* 131, no. 6 (June 1966): 534.
162. Burns, "Early Medical Photography," 1463.
163. Ibid., 1464.
164. Frank R. Freeman, "Administration of the Medical Department of the Confederate States Army, 1861–1865," *Southern States Medical Journal* 80, no. 5 (May 1987): 632.
165. Gordon E. Dammann, "Dental Care during the Civil War," *Illinois Dental Journal* (January–February 1984): 14–15.
166. Burns, "Early Medical Photography," 1464–65.
167. Peter D. Olch, "Medicine in the Indian-Fighting Army, 1866–1890," *Journal of the West* 21, no. 3 (1982): 32.
168. Ibid.
169. Ibid., 34.
170. Grissinger, "Development of Military Medicine," 338.
171. As noted in chapter 2, for example, the British did not have a comprehensive pension system even after the Crimean War.
172. For more on the general subject of military psychiatry, including its history and development, see the following from Richard A. Gabriel: *No More Heroes*; *Soviet Military Psychiatry: The Theory and Practice of Coping with Battle Stress* (Westport, CT: Greenwood Press, 1986); *Military Psychiatry: A Comparative Perspective* (Westport, CT: Greenwood Press, 1986); and *The Painful Field: The Psychiatric Dimension of Modern War* (Westport, CT: Greenwood Press, 1988).

173. Albert Deutsch, "Military Psychiatry: The Civil War," in *One Hundred Years of American Psychiatry*, ed. J. K. Hall, G. Zilboorg, and H. A. Bunker (New York: Columbia University Press, 1944), 367.
174. Dorothea Dix was a major force in encouraging humane treatment for the insane in the United States.
175. Germany and Russia were the home of nosological biological psychiatry, and Russian neurologists serving in the Crimean War were the first to take systematic notice of psychiatric casualties. This interest was continued after the war and eventually resulted in the first military medical system for dealing with psychiatric casualties on the battlefield during the Russo-Japanese War of 1905.
176. Donald Lee Anderson and Godfrey Tryggve Anderson, "Nostalgia and Malingering in the Military during the Civil War," *Perspectives in Biology and Medicine* 28, no. 1 (Autumn 1984): 156. See also George Rosen, "Nostalgia: A 'Forgotten' Psychological Disorder," *Psychological Medicine* 5 (1975): 340–41.
177. Gabriel, *No More Heroes*, 57.
178. Rosen, "Nostalgia," 342.
179. Gubbins, "Life and Work of Jean Dominique," 188. Larrey treated the disorder by offering officers suffering from nostalgia bribes and better food if they would remain at their posts.
180. Deutsch, "Military Psychiatry," 377.
181. Ibid., 370–72; and Weir, "Remarks on Gunshot Wounds," 393, for the tendency to confuse psychiatric symptoms with malingering.
182. Ibid., 377.
183. Ibid., 372.
184. Ibid., 384.
185. McGrew, *Encyclopedia of Medical History*, 323.
186. Halperin, "Nikolai Ivanovich Pirogov," 348.
187. Aldea and Shaw, "Evolution of the Surgical Management of Wounds," 599.
188. Halperin, "Nikolai Ivanovich Pirogov," 348.
189. Fraser, "Doctor's Debt to the Soldier," 65.
190. After the Prussian defeat at Jena in 1808, the army was reformed under the direction of Gerhard von Scharnhorst, who invented the prototype of the German general staff system that became the hallmark of German military efficiency for the next hundred years.
191. Garrison, *Notes on the History*, 168.
192. Ibid., 163.
193. Ibid., 169.
194. Stewart, *Moving the Wounded*, 18.
195. Fielding H. Garrison, "The Statistics of the Austro-Prussian War ('7 Weeks'), 1866, as a Measure of Sanitary Efficiency in Campaign," *Military Surgeon* 41 (1917): 711.
196. The German Army, along with others, sent observers to the respective sides in the Civil War. These observers prepared staff reports on various aspects of the war.
197. Garrison, "Statistics of the Austro-Prussian War," 711–13.
198. Ibid., 713.
199. Ibid.
200. Sieur, "Tribulations of the Medical Corps," 219.
201 Fraser, "Doctor's Debt to the Soldier," 65.
202. Lawson, "Amputations through the Ages," 225.
203. McGrew, *Encyclopedia of Medical History*, 23.

204. Sieur, "Tribulations of the Medical Corps," 219.
205. Valentine A. J. Swain, "The Franco-Prussian War, 1870–1871: Voluntary Aid for the Wounded and Sick," *British Medical Journal* 29, no. 3 (August 1970): 514.
206. Chamberlain, "History of Military Medicine," 246.
207. Swain, "Franco-Prussian War," 512.
208. Ibid.
209. Henry E. Sigerist, "War and Medicine," *Journal of Laboratory and Clinical Medicine* 28, no. 5 (February 1943): 535.

6

THE TWENTIETH CENTURY

The Emergence of Modern Military Medicine

As the twentieth century began, general and military medicine stood on the threshold of remarkable progress in their ability to save lives. The period witnessed the most important advances in disease prevention and surgical knowledge in human history. Medicine had become fully integrated into the larger web of general scientific exploration and discovery to where it finally stood as an equal partner in developing and sharing new scientific discoveries. This trend toward the integration of science and medicine, first begun by the Germans in the 1870s, has become the major characteristic of modern medicine in all developed societies. The walls between academic and scientific disciplines have largely crumbled, and the old prejudices between surgeon and physician have finally disappeared.

The advancement in medical knowledge and technique characteristic of postindustrial societies was already evident at the turn of the century and has resulted in the rapid application of these discoveries to military medicine. In turn, the press of war and the social organization of research increased the military medical establishment's ability to make contributions to general and specialized medicine that would have probably taken years to occur in peaceful times. For example, military doctors achieved almost all the early advances in immunization and the prevention of communicable disease.[1] The general mobilization of civilian medical resources for wartime use brought many new problems to the attention of the civilian medical establishment and at the same time provided its practitioners the opportunity and resources to address them through wartime service. Except for social rank, now no significant differences remain between military and civilian medical practitioners.

Moreover, neither medical establishment is able to generate significant new knowledge without quickly attracting the attention of the other.

As the century began, however, military medicine differed only marginally from what it had been in 1870. The great achievements in military health care and the organizational sophistication needed to deliver that care to the wounded were far from certain; indeed, the belief in the inevitable progression of science to produce social betterment is a relatively new phenomenon, dating only from the close of World War II. The wars that occurred in the early part of the twentieth century—Spanish-American War, Boer War, and Russo-Japanese War—experienced the same familiar failures that had reduced military medicine's effectiveness for a hundred years. Most of these failures can be attributed to the unwillingness of armies to take military medicine seriously as a means for salvaging manpower.

On the eve of World War I, the armies of Europe remained as unprepared to meet the challenge of saving lives on the battlefield as they had been for a hundred years previously. At the turn of the century, most medical service corps had officially existed for only a few years, none had sufficient manpower or supplies, military physicians lacked standing in their own armies, and surgeons continued to use techniques that most previous wars had demonstrated were ineffective. The rise of the industrial state and the integration of civilian populations into the armies serving as reserve forces, coupled with the increased destructive power of new weapons, convinced most governments that slaughter on the battlefield was an inevitable condition of modern warfare.[2] Although the progress in military medicine seems obvious today, as the nations of the twentieth century lurched from one war to another—the Boer War, Russo-Japanese War, World Wars I and II, Korean War, and Vietnam War—that development was always in doubt when each war began. Any progress must have surely seemed less certain for the wounded and dying than we see it today.

THE BOER WAR

The Boer insurrection in South Africa lasted from October 1899 to May 1902 and saw a Boer force of 87,000 mounted guerrillas confront a British Army of 450,000 men and 520,000 horses. In this war Mohandas Gandhi (1869–1948), then a young lawyer, served as a stretcher bearer, which the troops called "bodysnatchers," and Arthur Conan Doyle (1859–1930), the creator of Sherlock Holmes, was knighted for his service as a civilian contract physician serving with the British medical corps in 1900.[3] British casualties amounted to six thousand dead from enemy fire and another sixteen thousand dead from disease, mostly typhoid and dysentery. Four thousand Boer soldiers were killed, and twenty-six thousand Boer women and children died in British concentration camps of disease and starvation.[4] As in so many previous wars, disease was the primary killer of the armies. Only twenty-two thousand British soldiers were treated for wounds, injuries, and accidents during the thirty-one-month-long war, but twenty times that number were admitted to hospitals for disease. Seventy-four thousand British troops suffered from typhoid and dysentery alone, and eight thousand died from the former.[5] In the spring of 1900, the British Army halted at Bloemfontein, and during the single month of November, there were both five thousand disease cases and forty deaths a day in the hospital.

The British Army Medical Corps had officially existed for only a year before the war broke out, and it was critically short of personnel. Even so, it deemed the initial deployment of medical resources as adequate to support a force of two army corps and one cavalry division. Eight hundred and fifty medical officers were sent to staff seven "stationary hospitals" and three general hospitals located along the lines of rail communication.[6] In addition, 40 warrant officers, 240 sergeants, and 2,000 enlisted men were assigned to the medical corps.[7] Within a few months the military clearly saw that these assets were sorely inadequate and hired seven hundred civilian contract physicians and surgeons. As casualties mounted, the British medical corps continually augmented these numbers until, at war's end, 8,500 personnel were assigned to the medical corps, including 151 staff and regimental medical units, 19 bearer companies, 28 field hospitals, 5 sanitary disease hospitals, 16 general hospitals, 3 hospital trains, 2 hospital ships, and 3 advance and 2 base depots for medical supplies.[8] A total of twenty-one thousand hospital beds scattered over southern Africa were available, and eight hundred trained female nurses served these facilities.[9] The centuries-old problem of medical unpreparedness evident at the start of the war required more than a year before adequate medical assets were in place.

British field hospitals were placed as far forward as possible, being consistent with the Germans' doctrine of forward treatment that was proven in the Franco-Prussian War of 1870 and now adopted as standard practice in all armies. Stretcher bearers transported the wounded from the field to regimental aid posts, and from there, bearer companies moved casualties to the field hospitals. Although the wounded received attention at the regimental aid station, the service sent the severely wounded soldiers directly to the field hospitals, which were equipped with bell tents and performed much of the major and emergency surgery. A field hospital could accommodate a hundred casualties.[10] Behind the field hospitals and located at intervals along arterial roads and primary rail lines were the stationary hospitals. These hospitals also had a hundred-bed capacity and were deployed forward as the army moved. Behind the stationary hospitals were the rear zone general hospitals, each of which had 520 beds.

A number of difficulties accompanied this structural arrangement. Although each brigade had a field hospital, there were no clearing points for triage and sorting casualties for evacuation to the rear. The gap between field and stationary hospitals proved as troublesome as it had been to the Americans in the Civil War. The Germans had improved on the American model used in the Franco-American War by creating mobile clearing stations at points between the field hospitals and the rear area hospitals. Surprisingly, the British had not adopted the idea. Near the end of the war, however, British medical units began to establish clearing stations at railheads for triage, stabilization, housing, and eventual evacuation by trains. In 1907, these new units were officially incorporated into the British medical service.[11]

One reason why the field hospitals assumed the load of emergency surgery was that transporting the wounded to rear medical stations was chaotic.[12] The lines of communication were incredibly long, with the Boer theater of operations extending eleven hundred miles from north to south and six hundred miles east to west. Moreover, it was a war of mobility as small units ranged over wide areas, operating independently and often working without medical support. Transportation of any kind was scarce and vulnerable to attack, conditions that made it difficult for medical supplies and replacement personnel to reach the front regularly. Although designed for mobility, the field hospitals proved too cumbersome to move rapidly. Ambulance transport used two-wheeled Maltese carts and cape carts, four-wheeled wagons, and ox trek wagons, none of which was equipped with springs. They overturned easily on rough roads and provided such a rough ride that many of the wounded died en route. The troops refused to ride in them, as American troops had in the Civil War.

A lack of coordination between the litter bearer companies and the field hospitals made transporting the wounded even more difficult in the war's early days. Although twenty-four hundred men were assigned stretcher bearer duty, their litter companies were attached to brigades and under military command of the division and not the hospital.[13] After collecting the wounded and conveying them to the field hospitals, these companies returned to their line units and often marched off with the advancing brigade, leaving the field hospital deluged with casualties who needed evacuation to the rear but without the personnel or vehicles to accomplish this duty. The litter companies and the field hospitals eventually developed better coordination, but it was not until 1905 that the British finally combined the two into a single unit under the command of a medical officer in the medical corps chain of command.

The Boers had no formal medical support system when operating as guerrilla bands; yet they solved the problem of evacuating their wounded very well. The Boers went into battle in pairs, often with brothers or other relatives assigned as buddies. If one was wounded, the other was responsible for ensuring that the wounded man was saved from capture and transported on horseback to receive medical attention. Given the general scarcity of medical support usually available to insurgency units in these types of wars, the system worked as well as could be expected.

The Boer War presented a number of new challenges in the surgical treatment of the wounded; however, amputations, the scourge of all wounded since time immemorial, and high mortality rates were relatively rare. In the Crimean War, for example, 73 percent of those who underwent amputation died. Of those treated conservatively, 72 percent died. In the Civil War the rates were 53.8 percent and 49.9 percent, respectively. On the German side in the Franco-Prussian War, the rates were 65.6 percent and 28.7 percent, despite the wide use of Listerian methods of antisepsis, while on the French side, the amputation mortality rate was 90.6 percent.[14] Almost no amputations were attempted for small-caliber gunshot wounds in the Boer War, even when they involved damage to the bone. Wounds caused by shrapnel or grenades generated the few amputations that were attempted. Whereas in the Crimean War no cases of knee joint wounds in which amputation was attempted survived, in the Boer War none died.[15]

This remarkable record was owed less to the quality of British medical practices than to other objective factors. Both sides in the Boer conflict used the new high-velocity rifles first adopted in 1888. The 7mm, thirteen-gram bullets were much lighter and smaller than the soft-lead bullets of earlier wars that often weighed between a half and a full ounce. The new bullets had protective metal jackets that considerably reduced the bullet's tendency to deform upon impact and carry bits of clothing into the wound. Finally, improved powder propelled these projectiles at twenty-four hundred miles an hour, decreasing the probability that the bullet would lodge in the body rather than pass through it. These rifles made often small and clean wounds that only rarely produced extruding tissue. Further, their bullets were likely to nick a bone or pass completely through it rather than shatter it. These new rifles are often described as "humane" weapons in the military literature of the day, but these weapons had the unanticipated effect of introducing multiple wounds—a new problem to military medicine—when a bullet passed completely through its victim and wounded another soldier.

Another advantage was that sepsis was not a major problem in the Boer theater of operations. The area was only thinly inhabited, with few domestic animals to pollute the soil and no long tradition of farming with constant applications of manure to the soil. The soil itself was dry and sandy, rainfall was slight, and the hot, strong winds that blew over it prevented the growth of surface vegetation or any decaying vegetable and animal matter. These conditions reduced the probability of contaminating a wound, while the dryness and heat aided healing.

One consequence was that British doctors quickly adopted conservative techniques for treating gunshot wounds. They generally did not probe wounds, and their standard practice was to apply antiseptic dressings and immobilization, allowing the wound to heal by secondary intention. British soldiers also carried first aid dressings in pouches that contained gauze dressings impregnated with a solution of corrosive sublimate.[16] After application, they covered the dressing with a waterproof jaconet. Experience demonstrated, however, that the waterproof covering prevented exposing the wound to the hot, dry climate, and keeping it moist only increased the chances of infection. The army eventually ordered the men not to apply these waterproof jaconets to their wounds.

British Army doctors were delighted that conservative wound management resulted in low rates of infection and high rates of successful healing. After the war, conservative treatment became the standard wound doctrine of the day. Unfortunately, British surgeons did not comprehend that their success was primarily because of the unique conditions of high-velocity wounds and that South Africa's general climate was beneficial to healing. When the conservative approach was tried during the first years of World War I, it resulted in disaster. Unlike the Boer War, more than 60 percent of wounds in the First World War were caused not by high-velocity rifles but by shrapnel, which did far more damage. Moreover, the soil conditions of Flanders—damp, wet, and richly manured for centuries—were far more hostile to healing and produced high rates of wound infection. Because of their experience in the Boer War, the British also forgot about debriding wounds, which the Germans had first used extensively in 1870. Thousands of wounded soldiers died of infection as surgeons uselessly treated their wounds based on the lessons they had learned in the Boer war.

British physicians in the Boer War made frequent use of the new X-ray machine that Konrad Röntgen invented in 1895. American doctors had first utilized it in wartime during the Spanish-American War. Although more accurate than other "bullet detectors" of the day, the machine was cumbersome, so the army only installed them in rear area hospitals. The use of glass plates, which often broke in transit, instead of photographic film also posed a supply problem. Knowing the machine was available, doctors in field hospitals did not probe for the gunshot victim's bullet, preferring instead to evacuate the casualty to a hospital equipped with the machine. Hundreds of casualties thus arrived in the rear with bullets still inside them and their surface wounds healed over. The ability of the X-ray to locate bullets without disturbing the wound further reinforced the medical service's doctrine of conservative treatment.

More than in any other previous war, military surgeons in the Boer War paid close attention to the problem of surgical shock. For the first time, doctors extensively used the water bed, a system of tubes through which heated water was pumped to warm the patient and prevent shock. Although not used as extensively, they also administered transfusions of saline solution as a means of resuscitation and stabilization. Doctors did not do blood transfusions since they were regarded as dangerous and provoked systemic reactions. Scientists had not yet invented the technique of blood cross matching or discovered the anticoagulants necessary to ensure a proper flow of blood through the tubes connecting the donor with the patient.

The British record in preventing disease during the Boer War was outstandingly poor. Although the medical corps was now an officially established branch of the military, the army often regarded its sanitary officer as the most useless man in the service. Over the objections of the medical service, his post was officially abolished prior to the outbreak of the war.[17] Sanitary regulations existed, but it was beyond the medical officer's authority to enforce them. Field sanitation then depended upon the unit commander, who often ignored the issue. As one officer noted regarding sanitation, "Tommy doesn't understand it, and his officers regard it as just a fad."[18] The troops frequently did not receive any training in personal hygiene. With little water to wash mess kits, the practice of washing them in sand or not at all became common. The men did not routinely clean the wooden water barrel carts and individual service water bottles, so they became breeding grounds for bacteria that caused intestinal diseases. The line commanders' general refusal to require that water supplies be boiled resulted in 100,000 of their men being hospitalized for bowel infections before war's end. The general sickness rate from all diseases during the war was 958 men per 1,000 per year.[19]

Typhoid was a major cause of disease for British troops. Of the mean annual deployed force of 208,000 men, 10 percent per annum were admitted to hospital with typhoid, with a 1.5 percent per annum death rate.[20] Immunization for typhoid was known at the time but was new to medical practice. Dr. Almroth Wright (1861–1947), professor of pathology at the Army Medical School at Netley, England, developed a prototype antityphoid vaccine in 1896.[21] The Plague Commission had granted permission to test the vaccine on Indian troops in 1898, and four thousand Indian soldiers were vaccinated with generally good results. During the Boer War, however, the War Office authorized typhoid vaccination only on a voluntary basis. Because of the often violent, though temporary, reaction to the injection, only 5 percent of the troops submitted to vaccination.[22] The old canard, still heard among troops today, that certain kinds of injections affect virility probably did much to reduce the popularity of vaccination. The British medical service's failure to pay adequate attention to sanitary measures resulted in fourteen thousand soldiers' deaths from disease compared to only six thousand killed in action.[23]

By contrast, the American experience with typhoid was better. In the Spanish-American War, typhoid killed 1,580 men while only 243 died in action.[24] American doctors were aware of the German and British experiments in typhoid vaccination, and medical officers were sent to the European laboratories to investigate their progress. Using the initial results as a base, an American Army doctor, Maj. Frederick F. Russell (1870–1960), modified the vaccine, and the first American attempt at vaccination for typhoid was tried in 1904. In 1909, the surgeon general ordered that the vaccine be tried on American troops. After administering twenty thousand vaccinations and observing the results, the American Army introduced compulsory vaccination for typhoid for all American recruits in 1911. Typhoid practically disappeared in the peacetime army.

The formal establishment of the medical corps in the British Army's bureaucracy accorded it new influence with which to improve medical care for the soldier. To their great credit, the medical officers took the lessons of the Boer War seriously. Between 1901 and 1914, these officers brought about significant reform. The army medical school was transferred to London, where it could be in the center of medical advances developed in universities and teaching hospitals. They raised the general standards of training and practice for medical service officers. A school of sanitation was opened at Aldershot in 1906 to train regimental officers and noncommissioned officers for service in sanitary detachments that were now regularly assigned to each combat brigade. All troops were required to receive regular instruction in field sanitation and hygiene, and for the first time, to gain promotion, all officers had to pass regular examinations in sanitation. Immediately prior to World War I, Col. William Horrocks (1859–1941) of the Medical Corps had invented a sand filtration and chlorine process for decontaminating water for field use. His process was widely adopted, and portable water carts with the sterilizing apparatus were allotted to each field unit.

The British Army's problem of casualty evacuation was addressed in 1906 when it combined the litter bearer companies with the field hospitals and placed them under the command of a medical officer. In addition, three field ambulances were allotted to each division, with one held in reserve. To fill the gap between the field hospitals and the stationary hospitals, the service introduced the clearing hospital, or the forerunner of the casualty clearing station. It served as the pivot around which the field medical service operated. It received casualties and sick personnel from the field ambulances; conducted triage, stabilization, and sorting; and then oversaw the wounded's transport to the rear. To increase its mobility, it was located as far forward as possible and its load lightened. Although the idea was revolutionary, the failure to provide the casualty clearing hospital with its own transport to carry out its multiple missions proved a serious shortcoming when it first saw battle in World War I. Finally, the British Army created a Home Hospital Reserve with members of the Red Cross, reserve medical officers, and other ranks to expand the regular field medical force in time of war. Since most of these reforms had been implemented a few years prior to World War I, the British were relatively well prepared for what awaited them in Flanders' fields.

THE RUSSO-JAPANESE WAR

The Russo-Japanese War of 1904–1905 had its roots in Japan's emergence on the world stage as a major power in international politics. In 1871, scarcely forty years since Adm. Matthew Perry (1794–1858) opened Japan to Western influence, the entire structure of the Japanese state was reorganized along modern industrial lines. Shunting the old aristocracy aside, the new nationalist political order established a modern political, economic, and military infrastructure more appropriate to a great power. Desperately short of expertise in modern technology, the Japanese sent hundreds of military officers abroad to study war and industry. Most of its young army officers were trained in Germany, which had recently completed a successful war against France. Japan sent most of its naval officers to England, then the foremost naval power in the world, although some attended the U.S. Naval War College. Within a decade, Japan had created a modern ground army modeled after the German Army, including its general staff system, and equipped it with the latest weapons. By 1904, Japan was ready to challenge Russia for a place in Asia and the Far East and to signal its emergence as a world power.

When the war started in February 1904, the Russian Imperial Army had 1.1 million men in uniform compared to 180,000 for the Japanese. The Russian ready reserve totaled another 2.4 million men, while the Japanese could muster only 200,000 men in ready reserve and another 200,000 in second-echelon reserves. Many forget that the Russo-Japanese War featured major land actions that were larger than those fought at Gettysburg, Waterloo, and Borodino. The Battle of Liaoyang in August 1904 was second only to Battle of Sedan in terms of the numbers of men thrown into action. Six months later, at the siege of Mukden, the Russian forces numbered 275,000 infantrymen, 16,000 cavalry, and 1,219 pieces of artillery, or the largest field army that any nation had assembled in more than five hundred years.[25] The Japanese threw 200,000 men against the Russian force. A Japanese field division comprised 11,400 infantry, 430 cavalry, 36 artillery guns, and 5,500 noncombatants, many of whom were in the medical corps.

This war saw the first large-scale use of the hand grenade and the introduction of the trench raid. While both sides carried the bayonet, only the Russians used it extensively in close combat.[26] Of the 709,587 Russians who saw action, 146,000 were wounded and 4.2 percent of them died.[27] The Japanese lost 43,892 killed in action and 145,527 wounded, of which 9,054 died, a wound mortality of 6.2 percent. This rate is comparable with a died-of-wounds rate of 6.1 percent for U.S. forces in World War I and 4.5 percent in World War II.[28]

From a medical perspective, the worst battle was the siege of Port Arthur (1904–1905). The Russians' ability to cover the slopes with rifle and artillery fire made the Japanese recovery of their wounded almost impossible. The wounded on both sides crawled around for days without rescue or medical attention until they died. At night, Japanese litter bearers crept from the trenches to rescue their wounded, often only to meet Russian medical teams on the same mission. The Russians were suspicious of Japanese casualties' feigning death and assigned armed men to their medical teams. They routinely shot Japanese wounded lying next to Russian casualties, and firefights broke out between the guards accompanying the rescue teams.[29]

The Russians' habit of throwing food and personal waste outside their trenches, especially in the summer months of the siege, coupled with thousands of rotting corpses created serious health problems. The stench in the Russian trenches above Port Arthur was so strong that the men put up cloth strips soaked in camphor and carbolic acid in the trench dugouts to kill the odor. Japanese artillery often fell on Russian dressing stations and hospitals. When the seven-month siege finally ended in January 1905, the Japanese had suffered 57,780 men killed and wounded.[30] As the Japanese medical officers moved into the city of Port Arthur, they found thousands of Russians suffering from scurvy and typhoid.[31]

The Russo-Japanese War was the first major war in history in which the number of men killed by bullets and wounds exceeded the number of soldiers who died from disease. The Japanese forces had 162,556 casualties from all diseases, of which 11,992 died. Official Russian sources put the number of Russian deaths from disease at 7,960, but the number is probably not reliable, given the generally poor quality of Russian medical care.[32] While the Russian Imperial Army may indeed have lost more men to bullets than to disease, military physicians in the West studied the Japanese performance more, and the Japanese received great credit for their remarkable achievement in limiting disease casualties. Historically, in battle, an average of four to five soldiers had been lost to disease for each one lost to hostile fire. During the Russo-Japanese War, approximately 8 percent of the Japanese Army died from enemy fire and only 2 percent died from disease, thus reversing the historical pattern.[33] The Japanese performance in military medicine became the envy of the world, and military medical officers from the Western nations flocked to Japan to learn how it was done.[34]

Japan

The modern phase of Japanese medicine began in 1870 when thirteen Japanese students were sent to Germany to study medicine. In 1877, Japan opened a medical school at the Imperial University and staffed it with German professors. As Japanese students returned from medical study abroad, they were integrated into the teaching faculty, and by 1900 the medical school's faculty was almost entirely Japanese. For several more years, however, the language of medical instruction in Japan continued to be German.

The formative period of Japanese medical study abroad coincided with the findings of Louis Pasteur and Joseph Lister gaining prominence in Germany and German medical researchers, most notably Robert Koch, finally confirming the bacteriological nature of infectious disease. The Germans' emphasis on germ theory and the prevention of disease strongly influenced the Japanese students, who taught it in Japanese medical schools upon their return to Japan. Thus, Nagano Sendai was placed in charge of a national program of disease prevention upon his return from Germany. Dr. Baron Kitasato Shibasaburō (1853–1931), who had been a student of Koch's in Berlin, introduced the widespread use of bacteriological analysis to Japan and discovered the tetanus bacillus and its first antitoxin. Later, Dr. Masanao Goto established a series of national and military quarantines to prevent the introduction of disease by troops returning from overseas.[35] From the beginning, Japanese military medicine had a strong emphasis on disease prevention that had no real counterpart in the West.

The real triumph of Japanese military medicine in the Russo-Japanese War came in the area of military hygiene and disease prevention. In Japan's war with China in 1894, one of every nine Japanese soldiers suffered from some form of infectious disease. The Imperial Japanese Army in that war suffered 12,052 cases of dysentery, 7,667 cases of cholera (with a mortality rate of 61 percent), and 41,734 cases of malaria in a field army half the size of that employed in 1904. In addition, almost a third of the navy became sick with beriberi, a vitamin deficiency–related disease.[36] With a small army of less than 200,000 men, a disease rate of these proportions almost crippled its combat power. The Japanese military medical establishment took steps to prevent a similar situation from occurring in the next war.

A key aspect of the Japanese preventive effort to control disease was ensuring that adequate means be available to achieve this goal. The National Sanitation Bureau undertook to produce sufficient drugs to tackle the problem of disease prevention and treatment. Under its auspices, the bureau oversaw the production and shipment to the army of 55,000 bottles of diphtheria antitoxin serum, 125 bottles of erysipelas antitoxin, 300 bottles of typhoid antitoxin, and 2,500 bottles of tetanus serum. It provided 450,000 capillaries for tetanus vaccination, each capable of vaccinating five persons.[37]

The success of the preventive medicine program is evident from the following data. During the Russo-Japanese War, the Japanese Army suffered 162,556 casualties from sickness, but only 10,565 suffered from infectious diseases, such as cholera, typhoid, and dysentery. Most of the sick suffered from noninfectious diseases, with 24 percent of the total sick suffering from beriberi. Of the infectious disease cases, only 4,557 died.[38] In total, less than 1.2 percent of the entire field force of about 600,000 men died from disease. This result contrasted sharply with the usual 25 percent that had succumbed to diseases in various armies of the world over the previous two hundred years. In addition, 35 percent of the Japanese field force was never admitted to a military hospital during the entire course of the war, and 45 percent of the wounded were eventually returned to active duty.[39] Japanese military medicine was extraordinarily successful in conserving Japanese military manpower.

The Japanese Army used the system of medical support and casualty evacuation that the Germans had copied from the U.S. Civil War system and then introduced in their war with France in 1870. The Germans had improved it by filling the gap between the field and base hospitals with a medical unit that functioned as a clearing station, and the Japanese also used this type of unit. Volunteer and Red Cross units in the Japanese armies functioned entirely under the army medical chain of command, while the Russians followed the Crimean War practice of allowing them independent status. The Japanese Red Cross never had independent status. It was created as a military auxiliary and was used exactly that way. The Japanese Red Cross had 1.25 million members located throughout the twelve Japanese military districts. During the war, it provided 3,852 nurses and staffed the army hospital ships. Eighty-two medical detachments were sent to the front, and the Red Cross provided thousands of litter bearers.

The Japanese casualty servicing structure placed the battalion aid and main dressing stations well to the front, either in the trenches or in a close-by ravine. The battalion collecting stations provided emergency first aid, while the dressing station somewhat more thoroughly examined the casualty and tried to stabilize his condition. Six regimental surgeons along with a number of attendants staffed each dressing station.

Behind the division-level dressing station was the field hospital, where temporary hospital treatment was provided. With a chief surgeon, eight assistant surgeons, and sixty enlisted men to act as nurses, the field hospital was the first point in the system where an operating table was available, and much emergency surgery was performed here. Behind the field hospitals were "stationary" hospitals, where more extensive care could be provided. These stationary hospitals, however, were expected to move with the army on short notice. When ordered to move, the usual practice was to divide the hospital contingent and leave behind the wounded to be cared for by the next echelon. The Japanese established base hospitals at key rail points to prepare casualties for evacuation to reserve hospitals in Japan.

The medical service also operated twenty-seven hospital ships to transport casualties to the homeland.[40] These ships were originally merchant ships that had been converted for medical use and outfitted with operating rooms, electric lights, plenty of light and ventilation, and bacteriology and chemistry laboratories. Female navy nurses cared for the wounded. Each hospital ship could accommodate about two hundred patients. The Japanese Navy established major naval hospitals in Sasebo, Kure, Tokosuka, and Maizuru. These hospitals were of pavilion design and had separate sections for patients suffering from wounds, contagious diseases, or psychiatric conditions.

Another innovation copied from the Germans was the provision of a sanitary detachment at the division level. Despite its name, the detachment's primary function was to act as a clearing station. Staffed by nine surgeons and sixty enlisted nurses, it had two litter bearer companies of two hundred men who were equipped with their own stretchers.[41] The unit's litter-carrying capability was greatly enhanced by hiring or dragooning Chinese coolies for this task. This divisional unit operated on the battlefield at all levels, moving casualties from the battalion and dressing stations back to the division's field hospitals. They were also capable of performing emergency surgery to stabilize the patient.

Japanese surgical practice followed the then current thinking on conservative treatment of wounds that had become popular through the British experience in the Boer War.[42] Most of the wounded in the Russo-Japanese War also suffered injuries from the new high-velocity, lightweight jacketed bullets that had made their appearance a decade earlier. Shells and hand grenades injured only one-seventh of the wounded.[43] Thus, the Japanese instructed their soldiers and medical personnel not to touch a wound unless it was absolutely necessary to do so. Soldiers received instructions in advanced first aid and how to apply sterile first aid pouches and bandages. Each company was assigned a number of "instructed men"—enlisted soldiers who were especially skilled in advanced first aid, bandaging, and stopping hemorrhage—to serve as combat medics. Their goal was to stop bleeding and keep the wound as sterile as possible. Within the medical chain itself, surgery was permitted on the battlefield only to the degree that it was absolutely necessary to stop hemorrhage. Otherwise, emphasis was on stabilizing and rapidly evacuating patients to rear hospital facilities, where surgery could be performed under antiseptic conditions. During the sixteen days of fighting around Mukden, the division hospital performed only five amputations.[44] While each division hospital was equipped with an X-ray machine, personnel only rarely used it since they did not anticipate that the surgeons at the division level would need the information. Japanese medical doctrine reasoned that a soldier was at greater risk from infection than from the injury itself.

The Japanese medical corps was structured and utilized as an integral part of the military command apparatus. Its chief held the rank of lieutenant general and was a member of the general staff. Each field army also had a surgeon general who held the rank of major general. Unlike most armies of the West, Japanese medical officers held full command rank and status in their armies and were regarded as essential personnel to the fighting effort.[45] In the field, the medical corps had its own parallel chain of command and had effective control of medical matters at all levels. Combat priorities might lead a line officer to override his medical officer's recommendations, but he did so at great risk since the medical officer reported the incident up through his own independent chain of command, ensuring that the line officer's decision would soon be brought to the attention of his commander.

The Japanese Army became the first army in history to require that the combat operations field order routinely include a plan for medical support.[46] The fact that all officers, regardless of assignment, were required to take staff courses in hygiene and medical care and that field hygiene was a subject for examination in the naval and army academies also testifies to the importance that the army placed upon medical support. Further, the Japanese medical officers earned the line officers' respect by bearing the burden of battle. At Mukden, for example, fourteen medical officers were killed or wounded.[47]

The emphasis placed on military hygiene and preventive medicine led the Japanese to staff their medical system with sufficient numbers of medical personnel at all levels. The Japanese never experienced a shortage of doctors or medical supplies at any level of command during the war. The ratio of doctors to patients was approximately 1 to 100, and the ratio of nurses to patients was 1 to 5. The Japanese had twelve major hospitals in Japan itself, each with five attached branches in the military districts. By war's end, the rear area hospital system had 58,263 available beds.[48] As the war progressed, Japan drew upon its supply of 45,000 physicians and surgeons for wartime duty, and almost 10 percent of the army's manpower resources were assigned to the military medical system. The success of the Japanese system led most Western nations to adopt this 1 to 10 ratio as the basis for assigning medical personnel in their own armies, if only for planning purposes.[49]

The Japanese Army was the first to establish a successful medical supply service, originally designed around the German system. The Japanese soon introduced major innovations to their system, and chief among them was establishing the medical supply system as an independent section of the medical corps. Each level of the medical support structure had its own supply section, which was responsible for providing and moving medical supplies. Once in the theater of operations, these supplies moved through the medical supply system's own dedicated transport. Rear area supplies moved in regular army ships and trains but in a planned, allocated space specifically for medical supplies. The Japanese utilized prepositioning of supply amounts based on tables of consumption calculated at various levels of combat activity, an innovation that Dr. Jonathan Letterman introduced during the Civil War. The provisioning of medical supplies was very efficient, and the Japanese Army did not report a single case of a medical unit finding itself short of necessary medical supplies.

The Japanese success in reducing death and illness due to disease was also attributable to their excellent field hygiene system. Their disastrous experience in the China incident of 1894 taught them that one of the most important roles of the medical officer was disease prevention, and the Japanese created an excellent military hygiene program for their armies.

The army had an official hygienic code that was promulgated among all ranks. Each line officer was responsible for continuously educating the men and enforcing hygiene practices in the field. Through their own chain of command, the medical officers immediately reported any line officers who failed to accomplish their duty. Every division hospital had a bacteriological unit whose job was to diagnose illness and to ensure that steps were taken to prevent the further outbreak of diseases. All units down to the battalion level were issued equipment for testing water supplies, and water testing was a command responsibility. The standard practice was to boil drinking water, and troops never ventured into the field without adequate supplies of boiled water. Division medical officers were assigned to lower units on patrols to test and mark wells, and a medical briefing was standard procedure prior to undertaking combat operations in unfamiliar areas. Foraging and scouting parties routinely brought along a medical officer to make assessments. Medical officers were also responsible for cleansing newly captured positions so their troops would not be exposed to diseases left by the enemy. The Japanese utilized the most advanced system for enforcing field hygiene measures that the world had ever seen to that time.

The Japanese solider had good personal hygiene habits. Daily bathing, a regular routine in peacetime, was practiced whenever possible, as was daily shaving and ensuring that the soldier kept his hair short. The men themselves regularly laundered their own uniforms, although fumigating ovens were provided at division level for cleansing the uniforms of disease patients. On average, the Japanese soldier was also younger than the Russian soldier and carried a lighter load in the field.[50] The extensive use of coolies, forced or hired from local populations, and the greater availability of rail transport also kept the soldier's load light. Used to a light diet of rice and vegetables, the Japanese soldier adjusted better to the hot weather than the Russian did; indeed, even Russian commanders were impressed by how little the Japanese succumbed to sunstroke and heat exhaustion.[51]

The Japanese Army also practiced excellent field discipline to reduce venereal disease and alcohol problems. No camp followers were permitted, and only a small coterie of licensed vendors was allowed near the army. The only place to obtain alcohol—a scourge of the Russian ranks, especially in hot weather—was in canteens located fifty miles behind the Japanese lines. The soldier was provided with cigarettes, handkerchiefs for personal cleanliness, toothbrushes, soap, rice paper fans with which to cool himself, and writing paper. He was also allowed to fish to supplement his diet with protein.

One of the most important factors reducing disease was the Japanese cultural practice of cremating their dead. At the start of the war, the Japanese prepared individual funeral pyres, but the shortage of wood on the Liao-tung Peninsula quickly led to the dead being cremated in groups of five or six. Individual cremation was reserved for high-ranking officers. Immediate cremation of the dead removed a potentially dangerous source of disease contagion.[52]

The emphasis on disease and infection control was also present in the hospitals that treated the wounded. Japanese surgeons preferred to operate without rubber gloves, but strong antiseptic control of all elements of the surgical process kept the wound infection and hospital death rates to a minimum.[53] All hospitals had hand-washing basins scattered throughout the wards and corridors, and the doctors and nurses washed their hands in disinfectant before they entered a ward. The staff kept the wards spotlessly clean, and all human and medical waste was burned every day. Latrines were covered and disinfected every day, and mosquito netting was provided for each bed. These measures' effectiveness in reducing infection and disease is evident from the record of Toyama Hospital, which treated 15,759 patients after the Battle of Mukden from April through June 1905: it lost only 41 patients in this period to infection and disease.[54] At Daley Hospital, within the war zone itself, 222,000 casualties were treated during the war, and only 3,150 died, or a hospital death rate of 1.4 percent.[55]

One of the more interesting aspects of the Japanese military medical system during this period was the field evacuation system. For most of history, the seriously wounded found being transported to rear area hospitals on springless vehicles was the bane of their existence. The Japanese, however, did not use any vehicles to transport the wounded. Instead, thousands of litter bearers organized into bearer companies carried all the wounded in stretchers through each stage of the casualty servicing structure from the front line to rear area hospitals behind division level, or a distance of approximately five miles.[56] No estimate is available indicating how many seriously wounded men reached medical treatment alive because of the gentle nature of this type of transport, but it must have been substantial.

The Japanese medical structure that made its debut in the Russo-Japanese War was the most sophisticated medical service that any army had used until that time in history. The Japanese willingness to examine the medical services of the West and to improve upon them proved a major resource for conserving the manpower of their small nation for war. For the first time in history, the emphasis on disease and infection prevention allowed the Japanese to bring the latest advances in bacteriology to bear on military operations and to achieve incredible results. For at least two hundred years prior to the Russo-Japanese War, armies lost 25 percent of their field forces to disease and infection. The Japanese, however, lost less than 2 percent of their force to these causes. Moreover, their various hygiene procedures were so effective that more than a third of the field army went through the entire war without ever reporting sick.

Russia

The Russian medical system in this war was unchanged in its essentials from what the Imperial Russian Army used in the Crimean War. As in Russian society, the status of physicians and surgeons in the military was far lower than in any army of the West. Contract physicians and feldshers, the latter of questionable medical training, provided most of the medical care. Russian doctors in military hospitals were not usually billeted with line officers and had to sleep on the floor between the patient's beds. General Ezerski, the chief inspector of hospitals at Sha-Ho, was not a medical officer but a former police chief. The status of Russian medical officers was so low that doctors who did not wear their swords in the wards while attending patients were disciplined. Even the diagnosis of disease was biased by status pressure. Because the line officers considered an outbreak of dysentery as reflecting poorly on their commands, they often forced doctors to classify dysentery cases as influenza.[57]

The old practice of having line officers command medical units, abandoned in most Western armies after the Crimean and American Civil War, was still in effect in the Russian Army, as was the habit of relying on the quartermaster to supply transport for moving casualties. The Russian Army had no official ambulance corps and still depended on troops from the firing line to carry casualties back to the dressing stations, as it had in the Crimea. As Wellington had noted in the Peninsular War, when several soldiers carried a wounded comrade to the rear, their absence negatively affected combat power on the firing line. Using the same methods during this war left Russian combat power seriously depleted at critical points in numerous battles.[58] Without ambulance vehicles assigned to the medical service to evacuate casualties, the army expected that soldiers would use empty supply wagons. They carried the wounded over the rough Manchurian roads and trails in small springless carts (*dvukolks*) that had been shipped to the army to move supplies. As in the American Civil War and the Boer War, the rough treatment the wounded suffered while being transported in these "avalanches," as the troops sometimes called them, caused a considerable number to die.

In Port Arthur, some Russian hospitals were large, spacious buildings. Most, however, were makeshift affairs with little medical equipment. The medical staff in Port Arthur comprised 136 surgeons and apothecaries, 15 medical students, 17 army officers used as inspectors, 11 priests, 46 clerks, and 112 female "nurses," who were actually girlfriends and family members of the officers.[59]

The condition of the Russian field hospitals was dreadful. Soap, mattresses, and bedpans were in critically short supply, and infection and dysentery were universal problems. A description of conditions in a Russian field hospital in Port Arthur noted that patients "lie side by side on the floor, on the bedboards, underneath them, just as they were placed when they came in. . . . Faces are shapeless, swollen and distorted, and upon the yellow skin are large blue bruises. Inside, in spite of the musty and sickening stench, the cold is intense. On all sides is filth, nothing but filth, and on it and among it crawl millions of greasy gray lice."[60] The traditional Russian fervor for religion, however, led the army to assign priests as medical assistants to every regiment. These priests were required to make regular visits to the sick and wounded in the hospitals. Although they were short of medical supplies, the physician who did not have an adequate supply of religious icons to give to the wounded and bolster their faith was subject to discipline by military authorities.[61]

The chronic shortages of boots, greatcoats, blankets, and food exacerbated the terrible conditions under which the Russian soldier had to fight. Nutrition was poor, and while scurvy was only a minor problem among the Japanese, it was endemic among the Russians. The problem of scurvy worsened when the corrupt medical corps officers took the best food for themselves and their families. When the siege of Port Arthur ended, Japanese medical officers found that 32,400 members of the Russian garrison were suffering from scurvy.[62]

Because of the chronic shortage of salt and poor field discipline, Russian forces also suffered a high number of sunstroke and heatstroke casualties. Only the black Chinese variety of salt was available, and the Russians couldn't stomach it. Sugar, fresh fruits, and canned meats were unobtainable. The only item in great supply seems to have been vodka, which the troops and officers consumed in large quantities. The medical officers seem to have made no effort to ensure a supply of potable water for the garrison, and no water-testing apparatus was available. Japanese officers found that almost every well was infected with typhoid. The Russian Army did not have official hygiene regulations, formal field hygiene instructions for the men and officers, or sanitary officers or detachments posted with the troops. The Russian Army was a medical disaster waiting to happen, as it had been a half century earlier in the Crimean War.

The terrible conditions of combat and prolonged artillery bombardment produced a large number of psychiatric casualties and men with self-inflicted wounds. Line officers often made midnight raids on hospitals and evacuation trains, seeking to recover "malingering" soldiers who could be forced back into the line. The problem of psychiatric casualties reached alarming proportions. Curiously, the army was prepared to deal with this area of military medical concerns.

The Russian military had encountered significant numbers of psychiatric casualties in the Crimean War. A large number of British soldiers had also been driven insane by the tremendous firepower of indirect artillery barrages.[63] Unlike the British, however, Russian military doctors remained interested in the phenomenon of battle shock after the war ended. Evidence of psychiatric casualties in the American Civil War and the Franco-Prussian War further stimulated their interest. In the Russo-Japanese War, the Russian Army became the first in modern history not only to determine that mental collapse was a consequence of the stress of war but also to regard it as medical condition. It was also the first army to try to treat psychiatric casualties, and in so doing, the Russians laid the foundations of modern military psychiatry.

Russian Army physicians diagnosed and treated approximately two thousand casualties during the war that they attributed directly to battle shock; however, the number of soldiers complaining of psychiatric symptoms was much larger. These numbers increased so much as the war progressed that field medical facilities were unable to handle the psychiatric casualty load. Many psychiatric casualties were evacuated to the rear through normal medical channels and turned over to the Russian Red Cross for institutionalized care. The number of cases reached such proportions that they eventually overwhelmed even these resources. The Russian experience with these myriad psychiatric casualties provided the first modern example of "evacuation syndrome." When soldiers realized that "insane" soldiers were being relieved of combat duty, the number of psychiatric casualties increased dramatically, as soldiers unconsciously manifested psychiatric symptoms to escape the horrors of the front. Paradoxically, the Russian medical team's willingness to recognize and deal with psychiatric casualties is what produced even more psychiatric casualties among the troops.

The Russian Army was the first to place psychiatrists near the front line. Most of these psychiatrists, however, came from civilian mental hospitals and had little training in treating psychiatric casualties in a military environment. Psychiatric dispensaries staffed with psychologists, neurologists, a psychiatrist or neurologist who specifically dealt with brain injuries, a physician's assistant, and a complement of three feldshers were also established near the front lines. Western armies' dispensaries did not attain this degree of organizational sophistication for managing psychiatric casualties until 1917. The Russians also set up a separate chain of medical evacuation for psychiatric cases. It was the first time an army attempted to handle psychiatric casualties through a special medical evacuation channel, an innovation that became standard practice in the later years of World War I.

The Russians made a major contribution to military psychiatry when they introduced the principle of proximity, or the forward treatment of psychiatric casualties.

Experience had taught them that a number of psychiatric problems could be readily cured if treated rapidly within the battle zone. Experience in both world wars proved the Russians correct. Today the principle of forward treatment of psychiatric casualties remains the most basic principle of all military psychiatry.

The Russian Army was also the first to establish a central psychiatric hospital immediately behind the battle lines. Located in Harbin, Manchuria, this hospital recorded between forty-three and ninety psychiatric admissions a day. Only a few patients were quickly cured and returned to the front line. The rest remained in the hospital for fifteen days and were subjected to a variety of treatments. If recovery did not take place, a physician and a small staff of physician's assistants accompanied the psychiatric patients as they were evacuated by train to Moscow, a trip that often took more than forty days on the single-track railroad. By the end of the war, the army was operating several special trains exclusively for psychiatric patients that were equipped with isolation compartments, restraint rooms, and barred windows.

Of the 265 officers admitted to the Harbin hospital for psychiatric reasons, only 54 recovered sufficiently to be sent back to the fighting. The rest were moved to Moscow. Of the 1,072 enlisted soldiers treated at Harbin, only 51 recovered and returned to duty, while 983 were evacuated. Russian psychiatrists made significant advances in clinically linking battle stress with a number of somatic symptoms, and they developed diagnostic categories that were quite modern. During the Russo-Japanese War, the Russians established most of the psychiatric diagnostic categories that the Western armies later used during World War I. Russian psychiatrists recorded cases of hysterical excitement, confused states, fugue, hysterical blindness, surdomutism, local paralysis, and neurasthenia. Since Russian psychiatry had its roots in German biological nosological psychiatry, Russian doctors tended to define these symptoms in physiological terms and attribute their causes to damage in the brain. In 1905, 55.6 percent of Russian battle stress casualties were diagnosed as stemming from traumatic damage to the brain, an approach that gave rise to a similar diagnostic methodology in the West with the "shell shock" issue of World War I.[64]

By World War I, the Russian Army was the most experienced army in the world in dealing with clinical problems of battle stress. It was the first to specify categories of psychiatric problems in a military environment, the first to institutionalize forward treatment, the first to develop a theory of what caused battle shock, and the first to handle the problems of evacuation syndrome and secondary gain. The West mostly ignored these lessons until World War I when the Western armies, confronted with their own huge manpower losses for psychiatric reasons, finally attempted to develop methodologies for managing the problem. While the Germans quickly adapted to the new reality, the French, English, and American armies managed barely to put a psychiatric casualty servicing structure in place by the end of the war.[65]

From the perspective of the development of military medicine, the Russo-Japanese War was one of the most important wars in history. Both Japan and Russia developed and introduced major medical innovations to treat battle casualties and disease that set new standards for the armies of the world. Improving greatly upon the American and German models, the Japanese were the first to introduce a thoroughly modern military medical system that integrated all the major elements of casualty care and disease prevention into a complete command structure. The Japanese Army was the first to require a medical plan as part of the combat operations order, the first to place the chief of medical services in the general staff structure, the first to provide full rank and status to medical corps officers in combat theaters of operations, and the first to create an effective, independent medical supply service with its own transport. These organizational changes constituted major modifications to the medical corps and revolutionized its capability to attend to its mission.

Building on the German Army's initial efforts in 1870, the Japanese Army became the first modern army to thoroughly integrate modern science into the care and treatment of casualties. Its emphasis on disease and infection prevention by applying the lessons of bacteriology, vaccination, and antiseptic surgery resulted in an army losing fewer casualties to disease and infection than to enemy weaponry for the first time in two hundred years. The army's hygienic practices and field discipline far surpassed anything that modern history had ever seen, and it resulted in a level of manpower conservation that remained unsurpassed until the Vietnam War.

Given the generally backward state of Russian medicine and the almost pre-modern condition of the Russian military administrative structure, that the Russians made such major advances in the treatment of psychiatric casualties is surprising. It is no exaggeration to say that the Russian Army established the modern foundations of military psychiatry both organizationally and clinically. The conceptual foundations of modern military psychiatry remain unchanged in their essentials since the Russian Army introduced them in 1905. The principles of proximity, immediacy, and expectancy, known in the modern discipline by the acronym PIE, still undergird all methods of battlefield treatment of psychiatric casualties. While the discipline has since expanded the range of diagnostic categories, the original categories of mental disorder found on the battlefield remain as sound today as they were when the Russians first identified them more than a century ago.

When taken together, then, the Russo-Japanese War was a period of major innovation in military medicine. It was a time when modern military somatic and psychiatric medicine made its debut.

WORLD WAR I

The First World War was the most destructive conflict in history up to that time: the combatants mobilized 60 million men, killed 7 million of them, and wounded more than 19 million. Half a million soldiers underwent amputations. The introduction of smokeless powder propelled rifle and artillery projectiles at higher velocities and greater distances than ever before. Shrapnel and exploding artillery shot caused 70 percent of battle wounds and produced mutilations on an unprecedented scale.[66]

Military medicine witnessed a number of important medical advances in treating the wounded. For the first time diagnostic bacteriology conducted in mobile laboratories was available in frontline hospitals. Improvements to X-ray machines, making them lighter, allowed their use in forward surgical stations. Intravenous saline infusions in resuscitation became common, as did clinical thermometers, hemostatic forceps, hypodermic syringes, and better retractors and surgical lighting. The first field blood transfusion teams were introduced, and the casualty clearing station grew into the evacuation hospital and became a standard feature of the casualty evacuation system.

At the start of the war, the doctrine of conservative treatment and healing by secondary intention was widely used with disastrous results. The continued practice of limited debridement and secondary closure of severe shrapnel wounds that were contaminated by the richly manured soil of the battlefield led to high rates of amputation and infection, the latter almost always in the form of deadly gas gangrene. Wound mortality approached 28 percent in 1915, and the amputation rate ran as high as 40 percent for wounds of the extremities involving injuries to the bone.[67] First attempts to control infection involved using various antiseptics directly on the wound. Experience taught that this procedure was ineffective and often harmed healthy tissue. Military surgeons gradually relearned old lessons and used debridement on all major wounds. In addition, they continually irrigated wounds with Eusol (Edinburgh University Solution of Lime) and, eventually, Carrel-Dakin solution—a diluted antiseptic of sodium hypochlorite and boric acid—to aid draining. Mobile bacteriology laboratories attached to the various hospitals took daily bacterial smears to determine the bacteria count before doctors closed wounds and saved many lives.

As these surgical procedures were gradually implemented, the rate of wound infection fell dramatically. In 1917, the Battles of Messines and Passchendaele (also known as the Third Battle of Ypres) produced more than twenty-five thousand wounded, of which only eighty-four contracted gas gangrene.[68] By the end of the war, wound suppuration had become relatively rare. Signs in hospitals often included a statement by Alexis Carrel (1873–1944), the coinventor of the Carrel-Dakin solution: "Every wounded man who develops suppuration has the right to ask his surgeon to justify it." By war's end, overall wound mortality was 8 percent compared to 13.3 percent for the American Civil War and 20 percent in the Crimean War.[69]

Advances in wound surgery and reduced infection had the effect of decreasing the amputation rate, and as surgeons abandoned the traditional practice of prophylactic amputation for all compound fractures by 1917, the amputation rate dropped to less than 10 percent. Nonetheless, with half a million total amputations during the war, this area of surgery generated considerable interest and led to standardized surgical procedures, clinical definitions, prosthetic limb application, and the start of the science of rehabilitation. Sir Robert Jones (1857–1933), inspector of military orthopedics for the British Army, is credited with establishing seventeen rehabilitation centers of various types and introducing the first comprehensive approach to the rehabilitation of combat wounded attempted by an army.[70] More than four hundred surgeons gained training in the new science of orthopedics during the war.[71] Jones also advocated using the Thomas splint at all first aid posts when transporting men with compound femur fractures, reducing the mortality rate from this injury to less than 20 percent.[72]

Attempts to control shock in treating the wounded received major attention. Surgeons were aware that low blood pressure triggered shock, and they first tried intravenous saline replacements after the Battle of the Somme in 1916 but had disappointing results. In the same year, forward area surgeons tried to conduct blood transfusion by the direct method. Dr. J. Roussel is credited with making the first successful battlefield blood transfusion during the Franco-Prussian War. He drew upon the work of James Aveling, who invented a rubber bulb syringe to pump blood more quickly from the donor to the recipient. The French, Austrian, Belgian, and Russian armies adopted Roussel's "transfuseur" apparatus at the turn of the century.[73]

Blood transfusions were not common before World War I, but sufficient numbers were performed for researchers to determine its major problems. The donor's blood tended to clot before it could be infused into the recipient's system. Various anticoagulants, such as sodium phosphate, were first used as early as 1869. Attempts were also made to remove the blood's fibrin, but this process had the undesirable effect of removing other valuable components. The introduction of the Kimpton-Brown waxed tubes in 1917 to reduce clotting in the transfer apparatus helped only slightly.[74] Antiseptic control of bacteria helped reduce the danger of infection, and in 1909 Karl Landsteiner (1868–1943), working from his discovery of blood groups, developed a classification of blood types to reduce the probability of reactions from transfusion.

By the start of World War I, Albert Hustin (1882–1967) had shown that sodium citrate was an effective anticoagulant; thus, for the first time, it became possible to store blood for future use. Coupled with type matching and waxed transfer tubes, these advances made blood transfusions practical. Although transfusion remained a major procedure that was as complex as the surgery itself, the British and American armies established the first transfusion resuscitation teams and assigned them to special shock centers. These teams could be moved quickly in anticipation of major casualties and often deployed forward to the field hospitals. The war ended before transfusion could be applied on a large scale, but the value of field transfusion units was clearly established. During the interwar period, practically every major medical service established these teams for use in the next war.

Trench warfare produced large numbers of facial wounds, and more than three thousand of the eight thousand Allied personnel who suffered facial wounds died.[75] At the beginning of the war, no trained surgeons had specialized in treating maxillofacial injuries and no books on the subject of general plastic surgery were available.[76] Military surgeons were so inexperienced in this area that they often transported their patients who had facial injuries in the supine position, one that blocked their airways and killed them. The British government's initial effort to help those suffering from maxillofacial injuries was to contract civilian artists to create and paint realistic masks that the disfigured could use to hide their injuries.[77] In time, however, the British established special hospitals to treat these casualties, and significant numbers of plastic surgeons were trained to staff them. The British started the first maxillofacial injury hospitals, but the Americans' entry into the war in 1917 stimulated greater interest. By June 1917, the Americans had established four hospitals to handle maxillofacial injuries and are generally credited with introducing the team approach to reconstructive surgery that became standard in World War II.

Although military medicine had made great strides in disease treatment, the richly manured soil of Flanders caused high rates of tetanus infection in the early years of the war. Advances in tetanus antitoxin vaccines produced a more effective vaccine that saw its first large-scale military use during the war. Tetanus had a mortality rate of 89–95 percent in the Civil War, and shortly before World War I when the first anti-tetanus vaccines were available, the mortality rate was still between 40 and 80 percent.[78] In 1914, 32 percent of British wounded contracted tetanus. With the introduction of new vaccines and the practice of giving a wounded man a tetanus shot as soon as possible, the rate of tetanus infection dropped to 0.1 percent by war's end.[79] Even so, the mortality rate of those who contracted tetanus remained between 20 and 50 percent. Advances in tetanus antitoxins, the introduction of regular inoculations in the interwar period, and the widespread practice of debridement and secondary closure of wounds reduced tetanus deaths to almost zero by the end of the war. Among U.S. forces in World War II, of the 10.7 million men who served, only eleven known cases of tetanus were recorded.[80]

Advances in disease prevention and treatment were evident in World War I's low rates of death to enteric fever, plague, smallpox, cholera, and typhus. New typhoid vaccines drastically reduced typhoid rates. In the Spanish-American War, 20 percent of the soldiers contracted typhoid, but typhoid afflicted only 0.04 percent of the American Army in World War I.[81] While scientists had made some advances in the treatment of dysentery and malaria, these two diseases remained major problems. Trench foot (emersion foot) disabled thousands of soldiers on both sides, and trench fever, caused by parasites in the fecal matter of the louse, produced more than 200,000 casualties on the Allied side.[82] Allied troops suffered 115,361 casualties to frostbite during the war. For the most part, however, establishing professional military medical services in the major armies paid big dividends as medical officers used their expertise in disease control and prevention. Except for the worldwide influenza epidemic of 1918, disease claimed far fewer men in World War I than had been the case in other wars.

Germany

The German Army was the most medically prepared of all the combatants of the First World War. The organizational model of its field medical care that had been unveiled in the Franco-Prussian war—complete with its first aid kits, forward surgery, casualty clearing stations and transport system, the integration of rear area hospitals into a complete system linked by rail, and the first large-scale introduction of Listerian methods of antiseptic and aseptic surgery—remained in place in 1914. The Germans' penchant for planning—a product of that other German invention, the general staff—meant that sufficient medical personnel, supplies, rolling stock, and plans for moving the wounded had been put in place ten years before the war.[83] Furthermore, Germany was the only nation that had established plans and facilities for rehabilitating the wounded and disabled.

After 1870, German medicine became totally integrated into the larger scientific community. Accordingly, German military medicine was able to muster the full range of scientific and technical expertise drawn from the intellectual resources of the entire nation. On the eve of the First World War most other nations had not fostered this degree of integration; however, by war's end, the German pattern was characteristic of all the major combatants' military medical establishments. Meanwhile, German casualties amounted to 1,531,048 killed in action, and of a total number of 19,461,265 men admitted to the hospital for all causes, 155,013 died from disease. The total mortality of the German Army was 1,686,061, or a wound mortality of approximately 8.6 percent.[84]

Russia

Of all the major combatants, the Russian Army, whose general health and social condition had begun to collapse even before the war, endured the worst medical situation. The available statistics of Russian losses indicate that their disease rate was the highest of all combatants. A total number of 5,069,000 are recorded as having been hospitalized for disease. Of these cases, 21,093 had contracted typhus, 97,522 typhoid, 75,429 remittent typhoid fever, 64,364 dysentery, 30,810 cholera, 2,708 smallpox, and 362,756 scurvy.[85] A German medical team sent to Russia in July 1916 reported that every division set aside a hundred beds at the corps hospital to care for the victims of scurvy.[86] The state of Russian preventive field medicine was terrible, and its troops suffered huge losses from diseases that had ceased to be serious medical problems in other armies. The official Russian figure of only 130,000 soldiers dead from disease, therefore, is probably not reliable.

Based on the only recognized statistical study, Russian forces lost 664,890 men killed in action with 18,378 dead from wounds within their units; that is, medical personnel never reached them for evacuation. An additional 300,000 soldiers died in hospital from their wounds. The Russians suffered a total of 3,748,000 men wounded, suggesting a mortality rate of approximately 8 percent.[87] Another 1.4 million disabled men were discharged into a society wracked by revolution and lacking all facilities for rehabilitation.

France

The French medical service remained the only example of a major army whose medical officers were not part of an independent medical service and were under the command of line officers. Moreover, the general staff's attitude regarding field hygiene had not changed since the last century. The men had little interest in hygiene and provided no training; responsibility for hygiene remained with unit commanders, unimpeded by the medical service. As a result the French Army suffered 50,000 cases of typhoid in the first three years of the war. When American units were assigned to former French training areas, they were horrified to find that almost all the water supplies were polluted by typhoid.[88]

Without an independent medical supply service, the French medical officers had to secure the quartermaster's written permission for all supplies and vehicles. The chief surgeon of the army was relegated to the second line staff and separated from the general staff by thirty miles, indicating that the army had made no attempt to integrate a medical plan into the overall battle plan. Consequently, units often moved away from their hospitals and medical support without the hospitals being made aware of the redeployment.[89]

The French Army attempted to mobilize its civilian reserve physicians and surgeons for war only to discover that it possessed no complete list of their names and addresses. More than half of the medical personnel mobilized declined to serve as officers, resulting in a great waste of trained medical talent.[90] The number of physicians and surgeons that the general staff had originally estimated as required for war turned out to be quite insufficient. Indeed, the army needed more than double the planned number of medical assets to handle the high casualty rates.

The organizational structure remained a shambles throughout the war. The chief surgeon had only a small staff to support an army operating over a thirty-five-mile front that was a hundred miles deep. At the beginning of the war, the chief surgeon did not have his own transport. The general staff first echelon had to approve any requests for personnel, equipment, reinforcements, and even the deployment of medical resources to field units first, making coordination with events on the battlefield an impossibility. The French began the war short of medical equipment. Its table of organization strength for medical assets, which had been drawn in 1910, remained unchanged. Only ten army corps had sufficient surgical material to supply their field ambulances, and the hospital trains were more like boxcars than trains suitable for casualties.[91] Because these trains were not under the medical officers' control, trains were not only underutilized but also faced incessant delays and overcrowding at assembly points.

Troops assigned to medical detachments still reported to their line officers and not to the medical officers. Detachments of wagon drivers and litter bearers were under the orders of the logistics and transport officers and not the chief surgeon of the hospital. No medical officer, including the director of the medical service, could order a change in the disposition of medical personnel without the army corps commander's approval.[92] The medical officer was even forbidden to send troops to the forward dressing stations to relieve them during an influx of heavy casualties. The service's inability to move medical assets to the areas with the greatest casualties and lack of reliable manpower for the ambulance service produced delays in reaching and evacuating the wounded. Although the medical officers finally obtained some control over their own personnel by 1915, the problem of directing personnel assets persisted until the end of the war.

The quality of medical talent, including that of physicians and surgeons, was poor.[93] Few of the medical students who had served their one year of military service before the war had attended their required training sessions. Reserve doctors often failed to attend as well. Once pressed into service on the battlefield, most found their skills inadequate to their responsibilities. It did not help that in hard-pressed sectors, line officers stripped the hospitals of their medical personnel, including physicians, and pressed them into service as combat soldiers. Of all the major combatants in World War I, with the possible exception of Russia, the French Army presented the poorest example of a military medical service.

Great Britain

In August 1914, the British Army had 100,000 men on the continent resisting the German advance toward Mons, Belgium. By 1918, more than 4 million British soldiers had seen action in the war. More than 700,000 of them were killed, were missing, or had died of their wounds; 2 million more were wounded—or a hundred times more men than in the Boer War—and 6 million men had been hospitalized at one time or another for disease or illness. At the Battle of the Somme in 1916, 316,000 men were admitted to the field ambulances, with 24,675 carted away in the first twenty-four hours of the battle. In France alone, the British Army Medical Corps attended 129,675 wounded and sick officers and 2,525,350 men of other ranks.[94]

At the outbreak of war, the regular army and reserve components of the British medical service had only 20,000 men. By 1918, 13,000 officers and 154,000 enlisted men had seen service in the medical corps. Medical assets deployed in the war included 235 field ambulances, 127 sanitary detachments, 78 casualty clearing stations, 48 motor ambulance convoys, 63 ambulance trains, 4 ambulance flotillas, 38 mobile hygiene and bacteriological laboratories, 15 mobile X-ray units, 6 mobile dental labs, 18 advanced depots of medical supplies, 17 base depots, 41 stationary hospitals, 80 general hospitals, and 77 hospital ships. In 1914, the British had only 18,000 hospital beds spread throughout the empire. By 1918, the number of hospital beds had expanded to 637,000, with more than half of them located in England.[95]

The static nature of trench warfare made moving the wounded easier. Although motor transport for casualties was introduced in 1911, the army staff vetoed using these vehicles for medical transport because it maintained the roads were already overburdened with more important supplies. Once again, the British attempted to use empty trucks and wagons of the supply train for double duty as casualty transport. The time required to load and unload the casualties disrupted combat supply timetables, so the army decided to equip the medical corps with its own wagons and motor transport operating on its own schedules. The sequence of evacuation ran from the stretcher bearers at the regiment and its medical officer, who, in turn, passed his casualties to the advanced dressing station and then to the main dressing station.

In its major innovation in the structure of medical care, the British placed their casualty clearing hospitals behind the main dressing station. This clearing unit was developed from the prototype that had been first attempted on a small scale during the Boer War. Originally it had been intended to serve as a drop point that would allow the field ambulances to "clear" themselves before returning to the front line, but the large number of World War I battle casualties changed their nature and function completely. Casualty clearing hospitals were located barely beyond the range of the most intense artillery, or about seven miles from the front. Six medical officers and eighty orderlies sorted and stabilized the casualties before passing them down the line.[96] These stations could handle two hundred patients on stretchers, but they were not supplied with beds.[97] The clearing station had only marginal surgical equipment available since the unit was not designed to undertake major operations. Each station was attached to a division and had its own horse and lorry transport that the division quartermaster supplied.

As the burden of casualties grew, the casualty clearing stations expanded so that they could receive, stabilize, ship, or post a thousand casualties a day.[98] Their staffs increased to include medical surgical specialists, anesthesiologists, and special medical teams for serious surgery. They added two hundred beds per station, which became the main providers of field surgery in the forward area. In 1917 at the Third Battle of Ypres, for instance, surgeons performed 61,500 operations with anesthesia at the clearing stations.[99]

The litter bearers at regiment who served as the first line in the casualty evacuation system faced many obstacles. While the British planned to use two men to carry a stretcher, the explosive artillery disrupted the farmlands' irrigation and stream patterns where battles were fought, and the extensive network of trenches soon produced a year-round sea of mud. Often moving a single litter required as many as seven men. Even in relatively safe rear areas, the medical service used a mix of no fewer than eighty-three types of special transport—including stretchers, motorized lorries, mules, and sledges—compounding the problem of medical evacuation.[100] Medical units often designated combat soldiers to move their wounded comrades to the rear, but the British commander of the western front Gen. Douglas Haig (1861–1928) attempted to stop the practice because it drained combat power at the front. The average time elapsed from wounding to evacuation to a field hospital was five hours and then ten hours to the evacuation hospital. A number of factors slowed medical evacuation. Because of the sweeping machine gun and artillery fire, men wounded in the trenches could only be safely evacuated at night, often causing a delay of twelve hours. Men were told that if they were wounded in no-man's-land to crawl to the open shell craters and wait there until darkness, when "scavenger teams" would search for them. Finally, the mud, generally poor road conditions, and harassment fire falling in the rear exposed ambulance convoys to destruction.[101] Sometimes hand-carried litters transported the wounded the entire distance from the front to the field hospital.[102]

The United States

The American Expeditionary Force sent 2,039,329 men to combat duty in France, and of these men, about twenty-eight divisions, or 784,000 soldiers, engaged in battle. The total mortality of American soldiers in the western theater of operations was 75,658, of whom 34,249 were killed in action, 13,691 died of wounds, 23,937 died of disease, and 3,681 died of suicide, drowning, homicide, and other accidents.[103] Among American medical officers in France, 46 were killed in action; 212 were wounded, of whom 22 died; 101 died of disease; 9 died from accidents; and 7 were missing.[104]

During World War I, the American Army expanded twelve-fold from its peacetime strength. In June 1917, the medical department of the army had 443 medical officers, 146 medical reserve officers, and 4,670 enlisted men assigned to it,[105] but it had no real organization and mostly old equipment. By war's end, the medical corps had grown to 30,591 officers—of whom 989 were regular officers and 29,062 temporary active duty officers—and 264,181 enlisted men, for a total strength of 294,772 men. In addition, 8,587 nurses served on active military duty.[106] In France, the U.S. medical service provided 261,403 beds to service 193,448 patients—99,405 sick and 94,043 wounded. Stateside, 69,926 patients occupied another 121,883 available beds. The total beds, 383,286, were twice that available to the Union forces during the Civil War.[107] By November 1918, the American medical service had evacuated 129,997 men via twenty-one hospital trains and had transported another 197,708 on hospital trains that the French made available.[108] U.S. forces had sent some 6,875 motorized ambulances to France along with fifty medical barges operated on French inland waterways. Three hundred and thirty-three hospitals had been constructed by the U.S. government and military, with ninety-one of them located in the United States.[109]

The medical corps also provided other services, including administering psychiatric examinations to recruits. The high rates of psychiatric casualties had prompted field commanders to ask the medical corps to find some way of screening troops. The idea that some individuals were more prone to psychiatric collapse than others was adopted from the era's emerging racial and eugenics theories, which held that particular behavioral proclivities were characteristic of certain "races." This notion had already been established in criminology and psychiatric practice and had struck deep roots in Britain, Germany, and the United States. The medical corps administered 1,151,552 psychiatric examinations in an effort to screen the "unfit" from military service, but the screening had no effect at all on American rates of psychiatric casualties.[110]

The army medical corps also had the task of designing and producing gas masks. Until the task was turned over to the Chemical Warfare Service in June 1918, the medical corps produced 1,718,000 gas masks for soldiers, 154,000 masks for horses and mules, 502,000 breathing canisters, and 11,000 trench fans.[111] The introduction of gas warfare in the middle of the war was at first thought to present the medical corps with new challenges in treating gas casualties. It was soon discovered, however, that the effects of wind, temperature, terrain, and better training in the use of protective masks made delivering effective gas attacks very difficult. The number of physical casualties from gas proved remarkably small, while the number of psychiatric casualties (hysterical reactions and self-inflicted smearing of mustard gas residue on one's body) increased. In 1922 a British Army investigation concluded that most British "gas casualties" had in fact not been gassed at all or had inflicted the wounds upon themselves.

The casualty servicing structure of each regiment had a medical detachment of fifty-five officers and men. As this number proved inadequate, in times of heavy casualties the service commonly drew eight to twelve men from each combat company to assist the medical unit, usually as litter bearers. From the regimental aid post, the litter bearers from the ambulance company evacuated patients to the ambulance collecting stations, which were usually located at the most advanced points where motorized or horse-drawn ambulances could reach the casualties. The ambulance company headquarters was located about a mile from the fighting, and when a full ambulance passed through the headquarters' control point, an empty one headed to the front to replace it on the line.

As with the British units, American field hospitals were located immediately outside the range of artillery fire. Each division had four field hospitals, two of which deployed for immediate use with the other two held in reserve in the event that the division began to move. Only emergency surgery, stabilization, and resuscitation—wounds redressed, splints applied, pain relieved, nourishment given, and shock treated—were done in these field hospitals, and the patient prepared for movement to the rear. Shell-shocked soldiers suffering light to moderate symptoms were held at the field hospital for a few days. If they recovered, they were sent back to their units. Those men with persistent symptoms were eventually evacuated to psychiatric hospitals in the rear.

The evacuation hospitals were located on railway lines twenty to twenty-five miles to the rear. These hospitals were well equipped with physicians, surgeons, and female nurses. After surgery, hospital trains and motorized ambulances transported casualties to general hospitals. When the war of movement recommenced, the force never had enough ambulances to move casualties to the evacuation hospitals. At times the distance between the field hospitals and the evacuation hospital was fifty miles or more over poor roads. During the Meuse-Argonne offensive (1918), U.S. ambulance drivers made twenty-four thousand trips to the evacuation hospitals, averaging twenty-eight miles each way.[112] Each ambulance section had twelve ambulances, and two ambulance companies were assigned to each division. Even at the war's end, the number of ambulances was never adequate.

The American force lost 58,075 men from disease over the course of the entire war.[113] This figure is somewhat misleading, for the medical corps did a good job of controlling those diseases that had traditionally decimated armies of the past. There were, for example, only 1,055 cases of typhoid and paratyphoid with only 165 deaths. Diphtheria produced 4,860 cases but only 76 deaths. The 1,975 cases of dysentery resulted in 35 deaths; 950 cases of malaria, 2 deaths; 9,618 admissions for measles, 358 deaths; and 24 deaths from smallpox.[114] The greatest killers were influenza, which produced 167,141 admissions with 6,072 deaths, and pneumonia, which resulted in 20,445 cases and 6,481 deaths.[115] At the height of the influenza epidemic in November 1918, influenza patients occupied 193,016 hospital beds of the total 276,347 beds available.[116] Meanwhile, the introduction of the Lyster bag—a double-lined, spigoted canvas water bag that purified water with the addition of calcium hypochlorite—did much to reduce water-borne disease.[117]

The high rates of manpower loss to psychiatric casualties forced the American Army to confront the problem. Dr. Thomas Salmon (1876–1927) visited France to learn how the French and British handled their psychiatric casualties. These two armies evacuated psychiatric casualties in the normal medical chain, a practice that resulted in large numbers of troops being lost to the war effort. Seeking to avoid this situation, Salmon designed a system based on the proximity of treatment, the screening of casualties for psychiatric symptoms, and an expectation of the patient's return to combat. The American military began training doctors and support staff in military psychiatry and, by war's end, had 693 military psychiatrists in its ranks with 263 stationed in France.[118] Following the established Russian and German practice of forward treatment of psychiatric casualties, the Americans provided each division with a psychiatric section under the command of the division psychiatrist, and small psychiatric hospitals capable of handling thirty patients at a time were established near the front lines. Larger psychiatric hospitals were set up in the rear but still relatively close to the front. Approximately thirty-five men per thousand per year were admitted to these psychiatric facilities, with 40 percent returned to service.

WORLD WAR II

The Spanish Civil War, which ended six months before World War II began, was a testing ground for new weapons and tactics that the Germans and Soviets supplied to the respective sides. It also became a testing ground for military medical advances. Gaston Ramon (1886–1963) introduced a new tetanus vaccine at the Pasteur Institute in 1931 that received its first large-scale field test in the Spanish Civil War. For the first time that the new sulfonamides—sulfa drugs, or a new group of antibacterial drugs working by bacteriostatic action—were used in war. Both sides generally adopted the German methods of antiseptic and aseptic surgery, leading to the widespread use of antibiotics and new antiseptics. The war saw the medical services widely utilize mobile surgical teams, which the Allies later perfected in World War II, and combat blood transfusion using stored blood for the first time.[119] Overall these innovations in military medical care resulted in a drastic decline in the wound infection and amputation rates. Despite often primitive surgical conditions, only 342 of 42,000 wounded soldiers underwent amputations in the Spanish Civil War.[120]

During World War II, the British medical service treated 5 million patients, of whom 104,076 died of their wounds. Another 239,457 were wounded but survived.[121] More than a thousand British medical units were mobilized for the war, including 148 field and general hospitals in the overseas theaters and 88 at home, 36 casualty clearing stations, 141 field ambulances, 49 ambulance trains, 34 hospital ships, 42 medical supply depots, 50 surgical field units, 36 blood transfusion teams, 64 field dressing stations, 27 convalescent centers, 122 field hygiene units and sanitary sections, 71 antimalarial control units, and an unknown number of mobile laboratories and other specialized units.[122]

The British went to war with a medical structure essentially unchanged since World War I, but the new mobile tactics and distances that it had to cover during casualty evacuation required more mobile medical facilities. To solve the problem, they adopted the American idea of equipping the entire medical structure with motorized transport. They reduced the size of the casualty clearing stations and made the field ambulance units lighter but gave them more vehicles, created field dressing stations and mobile surgical teams and equipped them with enough surgical supplies to conduct a hundred operations without replenishment. They also introduced mobile neurosurgical, maxillofacial, and field transfusion teams. The Blood Transfusion Service quickly became an integral part of forward surgical units.

The British experience at the start of the war demonstrated that a casualty had to be transported 133 miles from the forward aid station to the casualty clearing station and another 236 miles to the general hospital.[123] This situation led to the creation of the advanced surgical center (ASC), which was located forward in the combat zone and designed to provide and rapid surgical care. Attached to a casualty clearing station or field dressing station, the unit was totally self-sufficient with complete facilities, personnel, and transport, including a field transfusion unit. The center could be quickly attached or detached from its parent unit and rushed to the point of greatest casualties. The advanced surgical centers dealt with all shock, penetrating abdominal wounds, chest wounds, amputations, femoral fractures, and major arterial injuries. They serviced approximately 15 percent of the total casualty load.[124]

New tactical units, such as airborne and commando outfits, required their own independent medical support, so the British developed special commando and airborne medical units. They trained twenty-five thousand special medical personnel for these sections, and the first air-droppable division medical component was used at Arnhem (1944).[125] The long distances that the casualty transports traveled placed a premium upon limb immobilization. At the Battle of Tobruk (1942), the British used the Tobruk splint with great success. Essentially an adaptation of the Thomas splint of World War I, the Tobruk splint incorporated a plaster shell with a traction pulley anchored to the splint's heel to allow constant traction on the fracture. Meanwhile, the first large-scale use of tanks and other armored fighting vehicles resulted in a high proportion of burn casualties. The early use of tannic acid for burn treatment proved ineffective and even damaging. Armored vehicle crews were later issued wound dressings made of sheets of gauze, which were impregnated with surgical jelly to which sulfanilamide had been added, and loose gloves made of waterproof silk that sealed at the wrist for hand burns. These efforts drastically reduced pain and infection from burns.[126]

World War II witnessed a number of major innovations in the soldier's medical care. Among the most important were the new antibiotics. Sulfonamides had been first identified in 1908 but did not appear as practical antibacterials until shortly after World War I. The military initially utilized them because of their effectiveness against venereal disease. Their successful application in surgical treatment in the Spanish Civil War led to their widespread use in World War II.[127] Alexander Fleming (1881–1955) discovered penicillin in 1928, and its gradual perfection by Howard W. Florey (1898–1968) and Ernst B. Chain (1906–1979) in the early 1940s led to the production of the most effective antibacterial wound agent that military physicians had ever used. The discovery in 1943 that large quantities of the drug could be made in cornstarch cultural mediums resulted in mass production and in the Allied armies' widespread use of the drug in 1944. Until 1943, production was barely sufficient to treat a hundred cases. By 1944, penicillin production escalated to 3 billion units a year.[128] By the Normandy invasion that June, the Allies had sufficient penicillin to treat all casualties.

Other significant medical advances in World War II were a better understanding of the causes of shock and the common use of blood transfusions. The first donor-originated, as opposed to cadaver-originated, blood bank was established at Chicago's Cook County Hospital in 1937. In the late 1930s, the British made efforts to store whole blood but had only limited success. In 1943, an American team working under the auspices of the U.S. National Research Council developed an effective preservative, and within a few months large quantities of preserved blood were shipped to troops overseas.[129] The team also developed a process for separating out fibrin and thrombin, valuable coagulants, and made them available to blood users in separate form. Early British experience with civilian casualties in the London air raids showed that the transfusion of blood was vital in preventing shock. It was not until the Battle of El Alamein in July 1942, however, that blood transfusions were attempted on combat casualties on a large scale.[130] The armies responded by creating field transfusion units that were regularly attached to the casualty clearing stations and often sent forward to the dressing stations. On average, every hundred casualties required sixty-three pints of blood.[131] Even larger quantities of plasma and blood products were needed.

Taken together, the short time from wounding to treatment, the standard practice of debriding and irrigating wounds, the bacteriological testing prior to wound closure, and the improved resuscitation due to available blood transfusions all worked to improve the casualty's chances of survival. In the Allied armies, 21 percent of the wounded were operated on within six hours of being hit–"the golden period"—but the bulk of the wounded, 47 percent, were operated on within the following six hours. Thus, 68 percent of the wounded received surgical treatment within the first twelve hours of being wounded.[132] Only 7 percent waited more than twenty-four hours for medical attention. The impact of such improved medical treatment in World War II was evident in the number of soldiers who reached medical treatment and later died of their wounds. Approximately 4.5 percent of the American wounded who reached treatment died of their wounds, down from 8 percent for American soldiers in World War I.[133] In terms of comparison, 19.5 percent of the Russian wounded in the Crimea and 22.1 percent of the French wounded died. In the Civil War, 14.1 percent succumbed to wounds. In the Franco-Prussian War, which saw the advent of antiseptic surgery, 11.5 percent of the German wounded died.[134] The death from disease rate of the American Army in World War II was less than 1 percent of what it had been for the Union Army in the Civil War. The only increase was in the amputation rate, which was 5.3 percent in World War II compared to 2.0 percent in World War I.[135] This jump reflects the more rapid and efficient evacuation system, which preserved the lives of the wounded until they received medical attention. In World War I, these same wounded would have succumbed long before they reached medical attention.

With the exception of the Soviets, who used essentially the same casualty servicing structure they had in World War I, most Allied armies in World War II organized their medical facilities the same way; thus, spending much time on detailed individual descriptions is not necessary. Some attention, however, is due the German medical service. For the most part, it was organized around the American model as practiced from its inception in 1870. It differed largely in triage, or the sorting of casualties for specialized hospitalization. As would a company medic in the American Army, the German medical officer rendered first aid in a *verwundetennest* (battalion aid station) in the extreme forward area. The wounded were then evacuated by litter to the *truppenverbandplatz* (regimental aid station), where an officer corresponding to an American battle surgeon attended the casualty. After stabilization and resuscitation, all wounded were evacuated to a *hauptverbandplatz* (main dressing station) established about four miles to the rear of the combat line. The *sanitäts kompanie* (medical company) of the division operated the unit and performed both clearing and hospitalization functions. It was assigned two operating surgeons but could be reinforced by six or eight more in times of casualty stress. Significant surgical procedures and major operations were performed at this level.[136]

The next unit in the chain of medical evacuation was the *feldlazarett* (mobile field hospital), which was designed to care for two hundred patients. Staffed by two surgeons, it dealt largely with head and chest wounds. Each German Army group was assigned a *kriegslazarett* (general base hospital), whose function was to hospitalize all patients who could not be returned to duty in a short time. In periods of heavy casualties, all serious patients were transported directly to the kriegslazarett, while the forward surgical units concentrated on treating only those soldiers whose wounds would allow them to return to the fight. In each division there was an *ersatz kompanie* (replacement company) that served as a replacement depot and reconditioning unit for lightly wounded men awaiting return to their combat units.[137] The entire structure was designed more to salvage manpower for continuing combat than anything else, and for the most part it did a credible job under very difficult combat circumstances.

Given that the German medical service was superior in the wars of 1870 and 1914, it is interesting to compare its reputation then with its performance in World War II. The difficult circumstances under which it had to operate during the war years accounts for some decline. What is most interesting, however, is that the quality of German medical care seems to have slipped far lower than anyone had imagined prior to the country's defeat in 1945. For example, an American military study after the war showed that the Germans apparently failed to incorporate developments in blood transfusion technology and had no regular blood banks to provide sufficient supplies of blood.[138] The Germans had not discovered the secret of storing blood and still administered almost all blood transfusions from donor to recipient.[139] More puzzling was the widespread belief among German doctors that blood should never be transfused in amounts greater than 1,000 cubic centimeters. If the soldier was not resuscitated by then, they neither made further attempts at resuscitation nor performed surgery.[140] Most shocking was that German doctors seemed to have practiced poor hygiene when inspecting wounded patients, routinely lacking gloves and not washing their hands between patient examinations. German military doctors came to believe that suppuration of wounds was a natural condition and lacking penicillin and facing critical shortages of sulfonamides, the wound infection rate must have been high.[141]

One consequence of the Nazification of the German officer corps was the substitution of political criteria for medical criteria when determining military assignments, including assignments to the medical service. Especially at the higher ranks of the medical service, political criteria predominated. Within the ranks themselves, the high number of casualties seems to have forced the Germans to reduce the training requirements for medical personnel. Many "graduate wonders," or poorly trained surgeons with little experience, found their way into the medical corps. For whatever reasons, one outcome of World War II was the decline of the German military medical service, a sad fate for a service that had been the envy of the military medical world for more than six decades.

THE KOREAN WAR

In the Korean War the U.S. military lost 8,769 men killed in action, and another 77,788 wounded were admitted to medical facilities for treatment. An additional 14,575 men were slightly wounded and "carded for record only" before being returned to their units.[142] Of the wounded, only 1,957 men died, for a wound mortality rate of only 2.5 percent.[143] Excellent preventive medicine also reduced disease rates considerably. Acute respiratory infections accounted for a fifth of all disease admissions, followed by ill-defined general symptoms of illness and then various parasitic diseases. The psychiatric admissions rate of thirty-six per thousand slightly exceeded that of World War II.[144] The success of sulfa and penicillin in preventing wound infection had become so common that young surgeons serving in the medical corps forgot the lessons of previous wars and, in the early days, failed to practice debridement and closed wounds prematurely. These oversights produced an initially high wound infection rate until the surgeons relearned the old lessons.[145] A total of 89,974 surgical operations were performed, an average of 1.2 operations per wounded soldier.[146]

Four major innovations in military medical care were introduced during the Korean War. Among the most important was the introduction of the mobile army surgical hospital (MASH) units, an outgrowth of the mobile field surgical detachments first introduced in World War II. A typical MASH unit had from sixty to two hundred beds and was staffed with special teams of surgeons. The unit was not positioned within the normal vertical medical evacuation chain; instead, it was placed next to the regimental collecting station and the division clearing station. The idea was to provide high-level surgical care as close to the battlefront as possible. The most serious surgical cases were filtered out of the normal vertical chain of evacuation and moved laterally to the MASH unit for immediate emergency surgical care. After treatment, it moved casualties directly to the evacuation hospital for further treatment and evacuation disposition.[147] With its complement of twenty-four medical officers and surgeons and forty-one nurses, MASH units sometimes served as many as twelve thousand surgical admissions a month.[148]

The army transported most of the wounded by vehicle. Curiously, U.S. forces ran short of proper ambulance vehicles throughout the conflict. The most common form of frontline casualty transport was the litter-jeep, which was capable of carrying four patients and was first used in World War II. Its virtues lay in its availability in sufficient numbers and its low profile, which made it a less inviting target on the roads. A major innovation was using the helicopter in medical evacuation for the first time, although the military's critical shortage of these machines prevented the helicopter from playing a major role. The early helicopters were light and could carry no more than two casualties in external pods attached to the landing skids. In normal practice these machines transported the seriously wounded from the regimental and division clearing points to the MASH units. They also carried cases requiring more sophisticated treatment to the evacuation hospitals. In only a few instances did helicopters pick up casualties on the battlefield, a practice that became common during the Vietnam War. The medical evacuation system in Korea worked relatively well. Fifty-eight percent of the wounded received medical care within two hours of being wounded, and 85 percent were treated within the first six hours. The median time between wounding and treatment was only 1.5 hours.[149] Fifty-five percent of the wounded were hospitalized within the same day of being wounded.[150]

A major medical advance arrived when battle surgeons could treat vascular injuries on a routine basis. Arterial repair was first tried in 1910, and the Russians reported their first large-scale series of attempted vascular repairs in the Balkan Wars of 1912–1913. In World War I, the Germans sought to undertake vascular repair in military hospitals, but the severity of the shrapnel wounds and the high infection rates halted progress in vascular surgery.[151] The increased use of high-speed projectiles and shrapnel in World War II produced a sharp rise in the number of arterial wounds. Arterial wounds accounted for only 0.29 percent of the wounds during the Civil War and only 0.4 percent in World War I. The rate of these wounds doubled in World War II to 1.0 percent and doubled again during the Korean War to 2.4 percent.[152]

Small numbers of vascular surgeons served during World War II, when the standard treatment for injuries to the major arteries was ligation (tying the artery itself in a small knot). But this technique produced only marginal results, with 49 percent of the ligated patients contracting gangrene and requiring eventual amputation. Thirty-six percent of the patients upon whom arterial repair was attempted had to undergo eventual amputation. Taken together, 62.1 percent of cases of arterial injury to the lower extremities eventually needed amputation.[153] When vascular surgeons first regularly operated in the frontline hospitals in Korea, they saw a dramatic drop in the amputation rate. In the early days of the war, the amputation rate from vascular injuries remained at the World War II rate of 62 percent. During the last eighteen months of the war, however, the amputation rate dropped to 17.7 percent and, finally, to 13 percent.[154]

Yet another advance in medical treatment was the great improvement in the management of shock. The ready availability of blood and transfusion helped greatly. Still, soldiers suffering from crushing injuries or prolonged shock often died of renal insufficiency while appearing to recover from their wounds. Doctors recognized this phenomenon during World War II, but no satisfactory treatment was available until the Korean War. A number of special medical units designed to treat acute renal insufficiency were placed near the MASH hospitals. The results of proper medical treatment were dramatic, and deaths due to renal failure declined by 50 percent.[155]

THE VIETNAM WAR

Between 1965 and 1970, 133,447 American wounded were admitted to medical facilities for treatment, of which 97,659 were admitted to a hospital.[156] In Vietnam, small arms automatic weapons fire produced about a third of the injuries, while fragmentation missiles—often from booby traps—produced most of the rest.[157] Burn injuries were frequent. Some resulted from explosions inside armored vehicles and bunkers, but more than half the burn injuries were accidental. Burn injuries were often accompanied by inhalation injuries, and wounds of this type produced 70 percent of the total burn fatalities.[158]

The official hospital wound mortality rate for the Vietnam War was 2.6 percent compared to 2.5 percent for Korea and 4.5 percent for World War II. These statistics are misleading, however, for they do not take into account how the excellent medical evacuation system successfully moved to hospitals seriously wounded men who would have died on the battlefield or at the battalion aid station in previous wars. A better way of understanding the medical care provided to the American soldier in Vietnam is to examine the "deaths as a percentage of hits ratio," that is, the number of wounded men who survived. Viewed from this perspective, in World War II this ratio was 29.3 percent, in Korea 26.3 percent, and in Vietnam 19.0 percent. Stated another way, in World War II for every soldier who died, 3.1 survived their wounds. In Korea, the figure was 1 to 4.1 and in Vietnam 1 to 5.6.[159]

The nature of counterinsurgency warfare in Vietnam produced a war of small units widely scattered over inhospitable terrain, a situation that forced a rethinking of the casualty evacuation system. The classic pattern of ground evacuation of casualties while passing them through five echelons of medical care could not work rapidly enough to save the wounded in Vietnam, where distance and terrain slowed ground evacuation to a crawl. The helicopter permitted the greatest flexibility of movement in evacuating casualties, and the complete control of the air by U.S. forces made it possible for helicopters to land very close to where the casualty was wounded. Once the casualty was aboard a helicopter, the pilot could bypass the battalion and regimental aid stations and take the casualty directly to a hospital equipped for major surgery. Casualties were routinely transported directly to a field hospital, evacuation hospital, or even a hospital ship offshore.[160] Hospital ships were used most often for surgical treatment of U.S. Marine casualties since the Marines came under the jurisdiction and control of the navy medical corps. Shipboard evacuation to hospital ships offshore for treatment of Marine casualties had been established during World War II when Marine units were used to assault Japanese positions on Pacific islands. Corpsmen at the battlefront first treated the wounded Marines, who were then transported to battalion aid stations on the beach. From there boats took them to medical facilities located on ships offshore.

At the peak of ground operations during the Tet Offensive in 1968, American troops received aeromedical support via 116 air ambulance detachments, each with five to seven UH-1E ("Huey") helicopters capable of transporting six to nine patients at a time. Each division had aeromedical helicopters organic to its medical detachment.[161] These medevac helicopters had trained medics aboard to provide in-flight advanced first aid to the casualty. The average medical evacuation flight from point of wounding to a hospital was only thirty-five minutes. The more seriously wounded usually reached a major surgical hospital within two hours of being wounded. Of the wounded who were still alive when they reached the hospital, 97.5 percent survived.[162]

The medical regulating officer controlled helicopter evacuation by designating assignments of medevac flights within his area of coverage. The call for a helicopter initially came from the combat unit's medic. Helicopters already in flight were diverted depending upon the seriousness of the wound. In planned battle operations, helicopters hovered near the site of the action, ready to land at a moment's notice. If no helicopter was in flight, machines of the aeromedical evacuation ambulances stood by on the ramp and upon receiving a call took to the air. Once on the landing zone (LZ), it took less than a minute to load the casualties and for the machine to become airborne again.

The medic aboard the helicopter contacted the radio controller, who had a direct "hot line" to the MRO. The MRO then designated the hospital destination depending upon the seriousness of the wound, the availability of expertise in a given hospital to treat the specific injury, and the time to transport the casualty to the hospital. Distance was always less important than time. If the helicopter commander questioned the decision to divert to a specific hospital, a physician was consulted by radio. The inbound helicopter then informed the receiving hospital of the number of patients aboard and their respective wounds; this information allowed the hospital to make any special necessary preparations. Usually within minutes of arrival, the patient was on the operating table.[163]

The medevac crews' heroism in landing their machines on "hot LZs" is testified to by the fact that in a two-year period 39 crew members were killed and 210 wounded while flying medical evacuation missions. They flew 13,004 missions in 1965, and they increased to 76,910 in 1966, to 85,804 in 1967, and peaked in 1969 at 206,229.[164] In addition to evacuating casualties, the medical helicopters also transported blood, supplies, and medical personnel throughout the medical evacuation system.

The Vietnam War saw the repair of vascular injuries become routine, and vascular surgeons were present at every major medical installation. The overall success rate of vascular surgery approached 75 percent by war's end. During World War II, division-level medical facilities used almost no whole blood, relying instead on stored plasma as the primary agent to prevent shock. In Vietnam, 14 percent of all blood transfusions were done at division level, mostly with whole blood that could be stored safely in a new Styrofoam blood box.[165] The forward units' liberal use of whole blood was a major factor in reducing death by shock. Further, medical personnel found that the blood types stamped on the soldiers' dog tags were incorrect in approximately10 percent of the cases, so blood typing became routine practice in surgical hospitals.[166] To reduce blood transfusion reactions, a decision was made in 1965 to send only type O universal donor blood to the war zone. Between 1967 and 1969, 364,900 blood transfusions were accomplished with less than a thousand reactions of all kinds.[167] For the first time in U.S. military history, military personnel, their dependents, and civilian employees at military installations donated free of charge every unit of whole blood used for casualties.[168]

The military introduced disease control programs early in the war, and these prevention programs did much to reduce troops lost to sickness. The major diseases affecting U.S. troops were malaria, viral hepatitis, diarrheal diseases, skin infections, fevers of undetermined origin, and venereal diseases. The average annual disease admission rate in Vietnam was 351 per 1,000 men compared with 611 per 1,000 in

Korea and 844 per 1,000 in the Pacific theater in World War II.[169] The encounter with a resistant strain of malaria resulted in a malaria rate of 26.7 percent, more than double the rate of 11.2 percent for Korea.[170]

NOTES

1. An excellent overview of the major contributions of military physicians in the early twentieth century is found in William H. Crosby, "The Golden Age of the Army Medical Corps: A Perspective from 1901," *Military Medicine* 148, no. 9 (September 1983): 707–11.
2. The racial theorists of this period argued that the slaughter of war was actually beneficial to the genetic health of the population because it weeded out "the unfit."
3. Rayne Kroger, *Good-bye Dolly Gray* (London: Cassell, 1960), 167.
4. Rice, "Evolution of the Military Medical Service," 149.
5. Peter Lovegrove, *Not Least in the Crusade: A Short History of the Royal Army Medical Corps* (Aldershot, UK: Gale and Polden, 1951), 26.
6. Redmond McLaughlin, *The Royal Army Medical Corps* (London: Leo Cooper, 1972), 22.
7. Lovegrove, *Not Least in the Crusade*, 27.
8. Ibid.
9. McLaughlin, *Royal Army Medical Corps*, 22.
10. Edward H. Benton, "British Surgery in the South African War: The Work of Major Frederick Porter," *Medical History* 21 (July 1977): 277.
11. Garrison, *Notes on the History*, 192.
12. Benton, "British Surgery," 277.
13. Fraser, "Doctor's Debt to the Soldier," 66.
14. Theodore James, "Gunshot Wounds of the South African War," *South African Medical Journal* 45 (October 1971): 1089.
15. Ibid., 1092.
16. Benton, "British Surgery," 280.
17. Lovegrove, *Not Least in the Crusade*, 26.
18. Ibid., 23.
19. McLaughlin, *Royal Army Medical Corps*, 23.
20. W. Charles Cockburn, "The Early History of Typhoid Vaccination," *Journal of the Royal Army Medical Corps* 101, no. 3 (July 1955): 174.
21. Stephen A. Pagaard, "Disease in the British Army in South Africa, 1899–1900," *Military Affairs* (April 1986): 74.
22. Ibid.
23. McLaughlin, *Royal Army Medical Corps*, 24.
24. Benenson, "Immunization and Military Medicine," 2.
25. Denis Warner and Peggy Warner, *The Tide at Sunrise: A History of the Russo-Japanese War, 1904–1905* (New York: Charterhouse, 1974), x.
26. Gurdjian, "Treatment of Penetrating Wounds,"164.
27. McGrew, *Encyclopedia of Medical History*, 104.
28. Gilbert W. Beebe, *Battle Casualties: Incidence, Mortality, and Logistic Considerations* (Springfield, IL: Charles C. Thomas, 1946), 77.
29. Warner and Warner, *Tide at Sunrise*, 351.
30. Ibid., 447–48.

31. McCord, "Scurvy as an Occupation Disease," 591.
32. McGrew, *Encyclopedia of Medical History*, 104.
33. Louis L. Seaman, *The Real Triumph of Japan, The Conquest of the Silent Foe* (New York: D. Appleton, 1906), 103. Seaman's report is that of an American military physician serving as an observer with the Japanese Army during the war. It represents the best and most complete work on the subject of Japanese military medicine during the Russo-Japanese War available in English. See also Jan K. Herman, "Dr. Rixey and the Medical Observations of the Russo-Japanese War," *The Grog: A Journal of Navy Medical History and Culture* 4 (Winter 2011): 4–10.
34. The Japanese military preventive medicine programs were so effective that during the war the Japanese Army suffered only 362 cases of smallpox with 35 deaths from the disease in an army of almost three-quarters of a million men, even though smallpox was endemic to Japan at this time. See Grissinger, "Development of Military Medicine," 347.
35. Seaman, *Real Triumph of Japan*, 223–25.
36. Ibid., 106–7. The surgeon general of the Japanese Navy believed that beriberi was caused by a nutritional deficiency and experimented with reducing the amount of rice in the sailor's diet while increasing the amount of other foods. His observations proved correct, and two years before the war the Japanese Navy had all but eliminated beriberi in its ranks. The Japanese Army, however, refused to accept the navy's success and stubbornly continued to feed its troops mostly on rice. The result was that 24 percent of the army's total disease casualties during the war were caused by beriberi. See Alan Hawk, "The Great Disease Enemy: Kak'ke (Beriberi), and the Imperial Japanese Army," *Military Medicine* 171, no. 4 (April 2006): 333–39.
37. Ibid., 336.
38. Ibid., 334.
39. Ibid.
40. For an interesting description of medical care in Japanese hospitals and hospital ships during this period, see Teresa Eden Richardson, *In Japanese Hospitals during Wartime: Fifteen Months with the Red Cross Society of Japan, April 1904–July 1905* (London: William Blackwood and Sons, 1905), 259–62. This work is one of the few accounts of Japanese military medicine available in English and was written by a nurse who served in Japanese military hospitals. The basic information source for many works on the Japanese Army in the war is British War Office Staff Study, *The Russo-Japanese War*, 6 vols. (London: His Majesty's Stationery Office, 1906–1908).
41. Seaman, *Real Triumph of Japan*, 123.
42. For an evaluation of British surgical doctrine as a consequence of the Boer War, see James, "Gunshot Wounds of the South African War," 1089–1094.
43. In General Kuroki's army at the battle of the Yalu River, 7,967 men were wounded: 6,753 by small arms fire, 1,073 by shellfire and hand grenades, and another 141 from bayonets. See Seaman, *Real Triumph of Japan*, 112.
44. Ibid., 125.
45. Garrison, *Notes on the History*, 193.
46. Ibid.
47. Seaman, *Real Triumph of Japan*, 125.
48. Ibid., 7.
49. Garrison, *Notes on the History*, 193.
50. Warner and Warner, *Tide at Sunrise*, 353.

51. Ibid., 365.
52. In collecting their dead for cremation, special medical teams cut the corpse's Adam's apple so that a small bone, the *nodobotoke*, or "little Buddha," could be retrieved from the body and sent home to relatives. According to Japanese tradition, the shape of the bone determined the future fate of the dead. If the bone was shaped in the image of a small Buddha, it meant that the person's next life would be one of happiness. If the bone was misshapen or shapeless, it indicated that the person's next life would be one of pain. The relatives deposited these bones at the temple of Tennoji in Osaka, where they were placed in a vault. After years of collection, the bones were retrieved, ground, and mixed into a paste, and a statue of Buddha was sculptured from the material.
53. Richardson, *In Japanese Hospitals*, 48.
54. Seaman, *Real Triumph of Japan*, 32.
55. Ibid., 60.
56. Ibid., 261.
57. Warner and Warner, *Tide at Sunrise*, 387.
58. Garrison, *Notes on the History*, 193.
59. Seaman, *Real Triumph of Japan*, 177.
60. Warner and Warner, *Tide at Sunrise*, 421.
61. Ibid., 390.
62. McCord, "Scurvy as an Occupational Disease," 591.
63. As a general rule, indirect fire is the greatest objective generator of psychiatric casualties. During the Crimean War, tremendous bombardments were common. It is likely that hundreds of psychiatric casualties resulted on all sides, but the lack of diagnostic tools to define psychiatric conditions meant that they were neither recorded nor treated outside the normal medical evacuation chain.
64. Gabriel, *Soviet Military Psychiatry*, 35–36. This work remains the only complete work on the history and development of Russian military psychiatry published in English.
65. This section on Russian military psychiatry is taken largely from Richard A. Gabriel's works *No More Heroes* and *The Painful Field*.
66. Aldea and Shaw, "Evolution of the Surgical Management," 561.
67. Ibid.
68. Anthony Bowlby, "The Hunterian Oration: On British Military Surgery in the Time of Hunter and the Great War," *Lancet* 1 (February 22, 1919): 288.
69. Aldea and Shaw, "Evolution of the Surgical Management," 561.
70. London, "An Example to Us All," 86.
71. Aldea and Shaw, "Evolution of the Surgical Management," 563.
72. Ibid.
73. McGrew, *Encyclopedia of Medical History*, 34.
74. Fraser, "Doctor's Debt to the Soldier," 71.
75. Aker et al., "Causes and Prevention," 923.
76. Stark, "Plastic Surgery in Wartime," 511.
77. Ibid.
78. Fulton, "Medicine, Warfare, and History," 483.
79. Grissinger, "Development of Military Medicine," 346.
80. Fulton, "Medicine, Warfare, and History," 483.
81. Grissinger, "Development of Military Medicine," 345.
82. Fraser, "Doctor's Debt to the Soldier," 72.

83. Garrison, *Notes on the History*, 196.
84. Ibid., 200.
85. Stanislas Kohn, *The Cost of The War to Russia: The Vital Statistics of European Russia during the World War, 1914–1917* (New Haven, CT: Yale University Press, 1932), 137.
86. McCord, "Scurvy as an Occupational Disease," 591.
87. Kohn, *Cost of the War to Russia*, 137.
88. P. M. Ashburn, *A History of the Medical Department of the United States Army* (New York: Houghton Mifflin, 1929), 334.
89. Sieur, "Tribulations of the Medical Corps," 224.
90. Ibid., 226.
91. Ibid., 225.
92. Ibid., 226.
93. Ibid.
94. Lovegrove, *Not Least in the Crusade*, 36.
95. Ibid.
96. McLaughlin, *Royal Army Medical Corps*, 38.
97. Bowlby, "On British Military Surgery," 289.
98. London, "An Example to Us All," 85.
99. Bowlby, "On British Military Surgery," 289.
100. McLaughlin, *Royal Army Medical Corps*, 54.
101. The field hospitals behind the lines at Ypres, for example, were struck by artillery fire with horrendous casualties. One of these hospitals was located in a place the soldiers called "Sanctuary Wood." The Germans deployed long-range guns and, probably by accident, shelled the hospital, causing high casualties among the already wounded.
102. Ashburn, *History of the Medical Department*," 347.
103. Garrison, *Notes on the History*, 200.
104. Ibid.
105. Ibid., 196.
106. Ashburn, *History of the Medical Department*, 215.
107. Garrison, *Notes on the History*, 197.
108. Ibid.
109. Ashburn, *History of the Medical Department*, 215.
110. The American rates of psychiatric casualties were no lower after psychiatric screening was introduced than they were before. Moreover, even though psychiatric testing was regularly used during the induction process in World War II, American psychiatric casualty rates during the war were actually higher than they had been in World War I.
111. Ashburn, *History of the Medical Department*, 306.
112. Ibid., 342.
113. Garrison, *Notes on the History*, 200.
114. Ashburn, *History of the Medical Department*, 325.
115. Ibid.
116. Ibid.
117. Rose C. Engelman and Robert J. T. Joy, *Two Hundred Years of Military Medicine* (Fort Dietrich, MD: Historical Section, U.S. Army Medical Department, 1975), 17.
118. Edward A. Strecker, "Military Psychiatry in World War I, 1917–1918," in Hall et al., *One Hundred Years of American Psychiatry*, 386.
119. Fraser, "Doctor's Debt to the Soldier," 68–70.

120. Ibid., 70.
121. Lovegrove, *Not Least in the Crusade*, 56.
122. Ibid., 57–58.
123. McLaughlin, *Royal Army Medical Corps*, 67.
124. Derby, "The Military Surgeon," 184.
125. McLaughlin, *Royal Army Medical Corps*, 64.
126. Ibid., 67.
127. McGrew, *Encyclopedia of Medical History*, 318.
128. Ibid., 249.
129. Fulton, "Medicine, Warfare, and History," 484.
130. Aldea and Shaw, "Evolution of the Surgical Management," 563.
131. McLaughlin, *Royal Army Medical Corps*, 87.
132. Beebe, *Battle Casualties*, 93.
133. Ibid., 22.
134. Ibid., 75.
135. Aldea and Shaw, "Evolution of the Surgical Management," 563.
136. See Charles M. Wiltse, *The U.S. Army in World War II* (Washington, DC: Military History Section, Department of the Army, 1963), appendix C, 602, for a description of the German military medical service.
137. Ibid., 603.
138. Ibid., 606.
139. Ibid., 607.
140. Ibid.
141. Ibid.
142. Frank A. Reister, *Battle Casualties and Medical Statistics: U.S. Army Experience in the Korean War* (Washington, DC: Office of the Surgeon General, 1973), 3.
143. Ibid., 16.
144. Ibid., 8.
145. Fulton, "Medicine, Warfare, and History," 484.
146. Reister, *Battle Casualties and Medical Statistics*, 83.
147. Albert E. Cowdrey, *The Medic's War* (Washington, DC: Center for Military History, Department of the Army, 1987), 151. See also Warner F. Bowers, "Evacuating the Wounded from Korea," *Army Information Digest* 5 (December 1950): 50.
148. Cowdrey, *The Medic's War*, 150.
149. Reister, *Battle Casualties and Medical Statistics*, 79–80.
150. Ibid.
151. Aldea and Shaw, "Evolution of the Surgical Management," 566.
152. Ibid., 565.
153. Ibid., 566.
154. Ibid.
155. Derby, "The Military Surgeon," 184.
156. Spurgeon Neel, *Medical Support of the U.S. Army in Vietnam, 1965–1970* (Washington, DC: Department of the Army, 1973), 50–51.
157. Aldea and Shaw, "Evolution of the Surgical Management," 566.
158. Neel, *Medical Support*, 56.
159. Ibid., 50–51.
160. Leonard D. Heaton et al., "Military Surgical Practices of the U.S. Army in Vietnam," *Cur-*

rent Problems in Surgery 3, no. 1 (November 1966): 3–4.

161. Medical evacuation helicopters were often called "medevacs." The term was derived from the radio call sign of one of the first evacuation helicopters used in the war. Its pilot, Maj. Charles L. Kelly, MSC, was killed on July 1, 1964, while trying to rescue casualties from a firefight.
162. Neel, *Medical Support*, 70.
163. Ibid., 74.
164. Ibid., 75.
165. Heaton et al., "Military Surgical Practices," 8.
166. Ben Eiseman, "Combat Casualty Management in Vietnam," *Journal of Trauma* 7, no. 1 (January 1967): 58.
167. Neel, *Medical Support*, 122.
168. Ibid., 127.
169. Ibid., 32.
170. Ibid.

7

THE TWENTY-FIRST CENTURY
Unconventional Warfare

The Soviet Union's dissolution in 1991 and the empire's transformation into a number of independent national states marked the end of the forty-three-year-long Cold War between the United States and the Soviet Union. Although these events greatly diminished the possibility of a major ground war in Europe, the superpowers' competition was replaced by a series of colonial-style military interventions carried out in pursuit of their respective political and economic interests. The Soviet Union intervened militarily in Afghanistan (1979–1989) and the new Russian state in Armenia, Georgia, Moldova, and Tajikistan. The United States sent military forces into Somalia, Iraq, Afghanistan, Grenada, El Salvador, Panama, and Bosnia-Herzegovina, among others. The military medical establishments of the Soviet and American armies were still configured for large-scale conventional wars when these interventions occurred. Both quickly discovered that the old methods of rescuing, transporting, and treating casualties were ill suited to the difficulties that the terrain, weapons, and wounds that insurgency warfare in unfamiliar bacteriological environments presented. Their attempts to adjust to these difficulties led to changes in how military medicine was delivered on the battlefield.

THE SOVIET-AFGHAN WAR

The Soviet Union had been the first state to recognize the newly created Afghan state in 1919 and, in return, the Afghans were the first country to recognize Vladimir Lenin's new Bolshevik regime. From 1920 to 1979, the Soviets were the Afghans' main suppliers of economic and military aid, investing heavily in dams, roads, railroads, schools, and irrigation systems. By 1978, the Soviets had trained almost the entire Afghan officer corps and had strong sympathies with the People's Democratic Party of Afghanistan, the country's Communist Party.[1] In October 1978, with the Afghan military's support, the party carried out a coup in Kabul. A widespread tribal revolt broke out in response to the communist reforms, which included equal rights and education for women, credit reform, and land redistribution. After more than a year of internal turmoil, the regime began to weaken as the popular revolt gained strength. On Christmas Day 1979, the Soviet Union sent military forces into Afghanistan to rescue the regime. Moscow expected its troops would encounter little resistance and planned to stay less than three years. They were there for nine years, one month, and eighteen days.

Within a month, the Soviets had deployed 750 tanks, 2,100 combat vehicles, and 80,000 troops to Afghanistan.[2] By the end of the year, the Soviets had deployed 300 combat helicopters, 130 fighter aircraft, and a few squadrons of heavy bombers in Turkmenistan, and from there they launched carpet-bombing strikes into Afghanistan.[3] The Soviets deployed their troops in a skeleton-like base network from which they launched "destroy and search" missions. They made no attempt to win the support of the mostly rural and illiterate population. Instead, the Soviets reprised the methods they had used in the collectivization operation in the Ukraine in 1937 and attempted to rip up Afghanistan by the roots as a prelude to reconstructing a new society.

The Soviets began to depopulate the countryside with airpower. Waves of Mi-24 Hind helicopter gunships attacked villages, then troops landed to probe the ruins for weapons and insurgents. Survivors were routinely shot. Fixed-wing aircraft laid mines in the narrow valleys, and gunships doused crops and orchards with napalm. The Soviets gunned down herds of goats and sheep from the air and sowed farmland with mines to prevent further cultivation. They dropped hundreds of thousands of "butterfly mines," essentially plastic bags filled with explosives, from aircraft over the country. Unable to be disarmed, the mine's explosive charge is specifically designed to be nonlethal but sufficient to cause traumatic amputation. The Soviets painted many of these mines in bright colors to attract and injure children.

By mid-1984, 3.5 million Afghanis had become refugees in Pakistan, another 1.5 million were displaced to Iran, and 2 million Afghanis became displaced persons in their own country. One analyst called the Soviet policy "migratory genocide."[4] The advantage of Soviet tactics from a medical perspective was that they minimized their ground forces' exposure to attack and kept their casualties low. The Soviets' brutal treatment of the Afghan population, however, angered the Muslim and Pashtun population in Pakistan. In short order, the Pakistani government formed an alliance of resistance groups, recruited fighters from the many Afghans living in refugee camps in Pakistan, provided arms and military training, and created a national insurgency movement to fight the Soviets. The Soviets found themselves mired in a guerrilla war that lasted nine years.

Over the course of almost a decade, 620,000 Soviet soldiers served in Afghanistan. Of these troops, 14,453 were killed or died from wounds, accidents, or disease, or 2.33 percent of the total force. Another 53,753, or 8.67 percent, were wounded or injured, the later mostly in vehicle accidents on poor-quality roads.[5] In the early days of the war, the mujahideen insurgents were armed mostly with rifles; however, as the war wore on, they acquired mortars, land mines, and high-velocity weapons, like rocket-propelled grenades and machine guns, from their Pakistani allies. These weapons changed the type of wounds that the Soviet soldiers suffered. Early in the war, soldiers suffered twice as many bullets wounds as shrapnel wounds. By the end of the war, however, the pattern had reversed, with 2.5 times as many Soviet soldiers wounded or killed by shrapnel than by bullets. The proportion of multiple and combination wounds also quadrupled over the course of the war.[6] The Soviets adjusted relatively well to these new medical circumstances. Their ratio of dead to wounded improved over the course of the war, going from one dead for every three wounded who survived to one for every five. Enforced wearing of flak jackets and the introduction of improved body armor changed the medical profile of wounds. Wounds to the chest, stomach, and pelvis declined while wounds to arms and legs increased. Despite the increased severity of their wounds from mines and homemade explosive devices, more wounded survived at the end of the war than they did in the beginning.

The Soviet war in Afghanistan was a conventional military operation, and its medical support structure was organized along conventional lines. Medical personnel were assigned at the maneuver company level and higher. A medic and assistant medic provided medical care in each company. A medical section consisting of a physician and physician's assistant provided initial medical treatment at the battalion level. Their task was to provide advanced first aid, stabilization, and preparation for evacuation. The first serious medical intervention for the wounded was available at the regimental medical post staffed by a medical platoon, which consisted of two or three doctors, a dentist, two physician assistants, a technician, a pharmacist, nurses, a cook, a radio operator, and some enlisted orderlies and drivers.[7] The post's mission was to serve as a dressing station and provide immediate surgery, transfusions, treatment for the lightly wounded, and preparation for evacuation of the more seriously wounded to the division medical battalion.

The division's medical battalion was the basic medical service unit. The battalion staffed and operated a field hospital with a capacity to deal with four hundred patients every twenty-four hours, conduct surgery, and run a sixty-bed recovery facility. The medical battalion had three or more surgeons, a therapist, a doctor of internal medicine, an epidemiologist, and a toxicologist.[8] Each Soviet division deployed to Afghanistan was accompanied by a medical battalion, and each of the separate motorized rifle brigades, air assault brigades, and motorized rifle regiments had a medical company attached to it to provide medical care. In addition, the Soviets deployed eight hospitals in Afghanistan and two others on the Soviet-Afghan border to handle the wounded and patients suffering from disease. Two of these hospitals—a five-hundred-bed central military hospital and a five-hundred-bed infectious disease hospital—were located in Kabul. Another five-hundred-bed infectious disease hospital was in Bagram, with a small facility located in Kunduz. Field hospitals of two-hundred-bed capacities were located in Puli-Khumri, Kandahar, and Shindand.[9]

The Soviet medical system was designed to treat the sick and wounded at the lowest possible combat echelon (platoon/company) and evacuate the most serious cases through the various echelons of treatment, holding the least wounded at the lowest level for their possible return to duty. The Soviets established a greater number of major hospitals than would have been expected for the size of their force because the number of wounded requiring intensive care was significantly higher than anticipated. This situation developed not only because of the changed nature of the insurgents' weapons but also because more wounded survived to reach medical treatment. The wounded owed their initial survival rate to the medical teams' ability to reach and transport them more quickly than they had in previous Soviet wars.

The Soviet medical establishment moved into Afghanistan planning to evacuate the majority of its sick and wounded by ground transport, as it had in its previous military expeditions. Afghanistan's harsh terrain and inadequate road network, the ambushing of medical convoys, and the frequent long distances between regimental staging areas and medical facilities forced the Soviets to turn to air evacuation as an alternative. From 1980 to 1988, the Soviet Army moved 68 percent of its wounded by air transport. It evacuated more than 25,000 casualties by helicopter during combat and moved more than 152,000 sick and wounded by air during some stage of medical treatment.[10] Soviet aircraft also transferred 40,000 patients between the military hospitals in-country, and another 78,000, or more than 40 percent, went to hospitals in the Soviet Union for treatment and recovery.[11]

The air evacuation system remained a work in progress until the end of the war. The primary Soviet medical evacuation helicopter, the Mi-8MB (Bisector), was too small and underpowered to carry more than a few patients at a time. It often could not reach the altitudes where troops were fighting, and seriously wounded soldiers in the high mountains could not often be evacuated and died where they fell. Troops carried the slightly wounded soldiers down the mountains to a location where the helicopters could reach them. Because the carrying party required security while transporting the wounded soldier, frequently fifteen men were occupied evacuating one wounded solider. The unit's only doctor or medic usually accompanied the wounded soldier, leaving the rest of the unit without medical support.

Official Soviet statistics state that 98 percent of the wounded received first aid during the first thirty minutes of being wounded, 90 percent were seen by a doctor within six hours, and 88 percent were in surgery within twelve hours.[12] These figures seem optimistic in light of the usual difficulties associated with locating the wounded at Afghan battle sites and with getting airborne transport to them. Without enough medical evacuation helicopters, the wounded often had to wait for attack or cargo helicopters, which did not carry medical teams, to become available and transport them to medical facilities. Many wounded soldiers died either waiting for medical transport or en route aboard attack and cargo helicopters because they were not stabilized before or during transport. Moreover, it seems likely that the Soviet medics did not always render the best quality first aid. One study revealed that 10 percent of the fatalities examined stemmed from errors in pre-hospital care, with 10.6 percent of these errors attributed to poor first aid treatment.[13]

Soviet authorities eventually realized that they had to reform the medical system, and prior to major military operations, they established special surgical and medical treatment teams to augment existing medical assets. These special surgical teams were integrated into the medical battalions that were then moved closer to the combat zone. The teams consisted of three thoracic-abdominal surgeons, a neurosurgeon, a rheumatologist, a heart surgeon, three anesthesiologists, five nurse anesthetists, two surgical nurses, five assistant surgical nurses, and two blood transfusion specialists. The division's senior medical officer formed the reinforced medical battalion into a triage group and a specialty surgical group that performed thoracic, abdominal, neurosurgical, trauma, vascular, and general surgery.[14] Casualties evacuated by air usually bypassed the company and battalion medical stations and were carried directly to the special surgical teams at the division.

The Soviets' effort in increasing the surgical and treatment capabilities of the medical facilities and moving them closer to the combat zone was successful. Soviet data note that in the specially supported combat operations, 90 percent of the wounded received first aid within thirty minutes of being wounded, and 88.3 percent were evacuated by helicopter to the reinforced medical battalion. Thirty-one percent of the wounded were in surgery within an hour and another 38.7 percent within two hours. Taken together, 92.4 percent of the wounded were in surgery within six hours of being wounded.[15] Using special surgical teams reduced fatalities among the moderately wounded from 4.3 percent to 2 percent over the course of two years.[16] Over the course of the war, the Soviet medical system in Afghanistan proved only slightly less effective in saving lives than the American system had been in Vietnam. The overall death-to-wounded ratio for the Soviets in Afghanistan was 1 to 3.6 compared to 1 to 5 for the American efforts in Vietnam.[17]

The one area where the Soviet military medical system failed miserably was in preventing infectious disease. Of the 620,000 soldiers who served in Afghanistan, 469,685 were hospitalized for wounds or disease. This is an astonishing figure. Fully 75.76 percent of the Soviet force was hospitalized, with 11.4 percent for wounds and an amazing 415,932 soldiers, or 88.56 percent, for serious diseases. The latter included 115,308 cases of infectious hepatitis and 31,080 cases of typhoid fever.[18] Another 233,554 cases were distributed among those who contracted plague, malaria, cholera, diphtheria, meningitis, heart disease, shigellosis (infectious dysentery), amoebic dysentery, rheumatism, heat stroke, pneumonia, typhus, and paratyphus.[19] A substantial number of hospitalizations reflected a high incidence of combined infections, such as typhoid and infectious hepatitis, typhoid and amebiasis, and infectious hepatitis A and acute dysentery.[20] The Soviet experience with disease in Afghanistan was nothing short of a medical disaster.

The effect of disease on Soviet combat power was substantial. At any given time, more than a quarter of the total force (the Fortieth Army) was unavailable for combat due to disease. From October through December 1981, the entire Fifth Motorized Rifle Division was rendered combat ineffective when more than three thousand of its troops were stricken with hepatitis. The sick included the division commander, four regimental commanders, and most of the division's staff. Every year a third of the entire Fortieth Army was stricken with some form of infectious disease.[21]

The Soviet Army was fully equipped with preventive medicine teams, vector control teams, and water purification units, but they were never able to control the spread of infectious disease. The causes of disease infection were the lack of sufficient supplies of clean drinking water, the failure to enforce basic field sanitation practices, the failure of unit cooks to wash their hands after defecation, an infestation of lice and rodents, a nutritionally insufficient diet, and the failure to provide soldiers with regular changes of underwear and uniforms. In short, the Soviets suffered from the same causes that had plagued armies throughout history and had previously afflicted Russian armies in the Crimean War, the 1905 Russo-Japanese War, World War I, and World War II. It wasn't so much Soviet military medicine that failed in Afghanistan as it was the traditional Russian disregard for basic field hygiene.

The most prevalent disease among Soviet troops was infectious hepatitis, accounting for almost half of all disease hospitalizations. The disease is highly infectious and spread through the fecal-oral route, usually because an infected person failed to wash his hands. The incubation period in Afghanistan was thirty-seven days, and recovery took six to eight weeks with relapses. Most significant was that almost three-quarters (74 percent) of the cases were contracted in Soviet base camps, where one would expect that the best sanitation practices would have been enforced. Instead, the disease proliferated where it could have been best prevented.

Soviet field hygiene was terrible. Garbage dumps were often collocated within the base camps, and garbage collection was poor. Field latrines and flush toilets were installed in some base camps, but Soviet soldiers often did not use them and relieved themselves close to the camps' living and dining areas. Troops often did not wash their hands after relieving themselves and paid little attention to washing their mess kits. A soldier was entitled to one bath or shower a week in the base camp, but he seldom washed in the field. A major source of infection was the unit cooks. Because of their poor personal hygiene, they became a primary cause of disease infection for the troops. A Soviet study of unit cooks found a considerable number infected with shigellosis, typhus, *E. coli*, and salmonella.[22] Only a few sick cooks could contaminate an entire unit.

The Soviet soldier's field rations proved nutritionally inadequate. Units in field outposts often had nothing more to eat than "dry" rations, which were similar to the old U.S. Army C ration and held a can of meat with some crackers, jam, and a tea bag or two cans of meat mixed with oatmeal and a can of vegetables or fruit. The lack of nutritionally balanced meals coupled with the harsh climate, high altitudes, and an average combat load of seventy pounds quickly reduced the resistance of many Soviet soldiers to illness, especially when they sought to supplement their meager rations with local meat and vegetables, which carried a range of pathogens. The Soviet logistics system was unable to provide its troops with adequate supplies of clean water, so soldiers often drank from the local springs and wells. Water in Afghanistan has a high bacteriological content to which the locals are mostly immune. The local water often carried typhus and amoebic dysentery that infected Soviet troops.

Soviet positions were often marked by an accumulation of refuse that were rife with rats and disease. Stagnant pools of water in discarded ration cans served as breeding grounds for malaria-carrying mosquitos. The Soviet soldier was entitled to three sets of underwear that were supposed to be changed weekly; however, in practice, the soldier often received only one set that he wore for months at a time. This unhygienic practice and the failure to wash bedding regularly led to an infestation of lice. The resulting epidemics of typhus crippled the combat units' ability to fight.

The lack of a professional career noncommissioned officer (NCO) corps also contributed to the Soviets' failure to control infectious diseases. The Soviet NCO was a conscript who first attended a six-month training course to serve as an NCO; however, these conscript NCOs had no effective practical or moral authority over their fellow conscripts with whom they identified and sympathized. As with the average Soviet conscript, the NCO looked forward to being released from service as soon as possible. Soviet NCOs were little help to their platoon leaders in enforcing discipline and military standards, and complete responsibility fell upon the young lieutenant commanding the unit. Thus, in addition to his primary responsibilities for training, maintenance, and combat duty, the platoon leader personally had to ensure that his troops were free of lice, washed their hands, drank clean water, disposed of their trash properly, and dug and used latrines. Without professional NCOs to help him, the Soviet platoon leader often failed to perform all of his duties adequately. One result was a breakdown in field sanitation.

The Soviet military medical system in Afghanistan functioned relatively well when it came to dealing with the wounded, but it became overwhelmed when handling large numbers of diseased and sick soldiers. Apparently the Soviets grossly underestimated the amount of medical support their army would require to treat casualties and disease simultaneously. The Soviet solution was to evacuate large numbers of sick and wounded to military hospitals in the Soviet Union and Warsaw Pact countries to relieve overcrowded hospitals in-country. In Afghanistan, meanwhile, the Soviets' infectious disease hospitals and rehabilitation center for recovering disease patients were constantly filled with patients, and evacuating the sick out of the country became the norm.[23] The army constantly shipped replacements into the theater of operations to compensate for the large amount of manpower lost to disease. After the war, media reports indicated that significant numbers of Soviet troops who had fought in Afghanistan also had acquired an addiction to the cheap opiates available there. Soviet officials, however, have not released any statistics on drug abuse by Soviet troops, and no evidence suggests that it affected the fighting ability of the Soviet Army as a whole.

POST-USSR RUSSIAN OPERATIONS

An analysis of Soviet military operations since the Afghanistan war suggests that the Russian ground forces made few reforms to their medical support system after their experience in Afghanistan. In 1988, the Soviet Army was sent to Armenia to provide earthquake relief. Their lack of a good diet, field sanitation, and clean clothing resulted in high rates of disease and illness; consequently, the rescuers had to be rescued themselves. In 1989, a Soviet air assault regiment, an airborne regiment, and a motorized rifle regiment were sent to Tbilisi, Georgia, to put down rioting. The troops deployed with only a single change of underwear.

In 1992, the Russian Fourteenth Army engaged in combat in Tiraspol, Moldova. The lack of clean water and an abundance of disease-contaminated cooks once again led to an outbreak of disease. Only the brevity of the deployment kept events from getting medically out of hand. In 1992, the Russian 201st Motorized Rifle Division deployed to the border region between Afghanistan and Tajikistan to help guard the newly independent republic's border against mujahideen infiltration. Once again the Russian medical establishment failed to provide sanitary mess halls, field messes, and adequate clean water for drinking. Within weeks, viral hepatitis, intestinal infections, and malaria had rendered the division combat ineffective as hospital wards filled with sick soldiers.[24]

The Russian medical experience in Chechnya (1994–1996) was not much different than it had been in Afghanistan or in its other post-Afghanistan military operations. In two years, the Russians suffered 4,739 dead and 13,108 wounded.[25] The Chechnya war was primarily a conflict fought in urban zones and produced different types of casualties than those suffered in Afghanistan. The majority of Soviets killed in Chechnya were victims of sniper fire and had been hit in the head or upper chest. While the normal ratio of wounded to dead is roughly three or four to one, this ratio was reversed in the Chechnya fighting, which saw three killed for every one wounded.[26] This type of combat confronted the Soviet medical system with new challenges. Snipers and the willingness of Chechnya insurgents to shoot down medical evacuation helicopters forced the Russians to rely on armored personnel carriers (BTR-80) as ambulances and other ground transport to reach and transport their casualties. The Russians seem to have anticipated the unique nature of the urban combat they would face in Chechnya, and weeks before the invasion they established and trained special emergency medical treatment detachments that deployed with the army.[27] In addition, each maneuver company was reinforced with a physician's assistant, and each maneuver battalion received an additional doctor and ambulance section. On balance, the Russian medical system performed about as well as it had in Afghanistan when dealing with combat casualties.

The Russians' medical performance in dealing with infectious disease, however, was as dismal as it had been in Afghanistan.[28] The same causes that had plagued the Russians in Afghanistan—a nutritionally inadequate diet; a lack of clean drinking water, clean clothing, and bathing facilities; poor hygiene among unit cooks; and generally poor field hygiene by the troops—plagued them again in Chechnya. Acute viral hepatitis and cholera were epidemic among Russian troops, and units were frequently rendered combat ineffective during outbreaks of disease. Throughout the war, the Russian Ministry of Defense could barely maintain its combat field units in Chechnya at 60 percent because of disease.[29]

THE U.S. WARS IN IRAQ AND AFGHANISTAN

The American military has been engaged almost continually in combat operations from 1990 to 2012. During this period, the United States conducted combat operations in Iraq (1990–1991), Somalia (1992–1993), Iraq again (2003–2012), and Afghanistan (2001–2012). American casualties in all of these conflicts were light by historical standards. In the Gulf War (1990–1991), 382 soldiers died, but only 147 of them, or 38.5 percent, were killed in combat. In Somalia, 31 American soldiers were killed and less than 200 wounded. Nine years of insurgency warfare in Iraq has cost 3,480 deaths by hostile fire and 31,931 wounded; 928 soldiers died in accidents or by disease. During ten years of war in Afghanistan, U.S. forces have suffered 1,227 dead, 11,411 wounded, and 253 dead due to disease and nonhostile causes.[30] Of the

5,684 soldiers in Iraq and Afghanistan who suffered major limb injuries, 862 underwent amputation. The injured-to-amputation rate for both wars was 7.4 percent, or approximately the same as in Vietnam (8.3 percent).[31] The traumatic limb injuries that casualties in Iraq and Afghanistan have suffered often were far worse than those seen in Vietnam, however, as they combine penetrating, blunt, and burn injuries with contamination by shrapnel, dirt, clothing, and even bone.[32]

From a medical perspective, U.S. casualties have been generally light, and in only a few battles, such as Mogadishu (1993) and Fallujah (2003), was the immediate casualty stream even moderately heavy. Field medical facilities have never been overwhelmed by the volume of casualties similar to those that occurred occasionally during Vietnam and commonly in Korea and World War II. In World War II, 22.8 percent of the wounded died; in Vietnam the figure was 16.5 percent. Taking the Iraq and Afghanistan Wars together, 8.8 percent of the wounded died.[33] The performance of the medical disease control teams and the troops' general field hygiene were excellent in all wars. In Somalia, for example, where the endemic disease and contagion profiles are high, the health of American troops remained excellent. The weekly disease and non-battle injury rate was approximately 11.5 percent, with only 0.5 percent requiring hospitalization.[34] Only seventy-two cases of malaria were recorded, and problems with diarrhea and heat stroke were minimal.[35] Excellent diet, field hygiene, clean water, mosquito and rat control, and a program of disease surveillance were responsible for these outcomes.

Until after the Gulf War, the U.S. Army was medically configured to deal with casualties that were expected to occur in a conventional large-scale conflict. The emphasis on conventional conflict was evident in the training and equipment of American troops in the Gulf War for operations in the chemical and biological environments that U.S. commanders believed they would face. They issued troops were chemical suits and gave them atropine syringes for use in reversing the effects of some chemical weapons. Medical teams were outfitted with chemical suits, and decontamination facilities were placed near medical service points. All of these practices had been developed earlier during the Cold War when the United States expected to fight a conventional war against the Soviets in Europe.

In 1998, the U.S. military undertook a study and reevaluated its military medical practices, taking into consideration its experience in its most recent conflicts. In 2007 it resulted in the Tactical Combat Casualty Care program, which instituted a number of changes in the medical structure and practices for treating casualties in the tactical environment of guerrilla war. Casualty statistics revealed that the most common killers of the wounded were shock and bleeding, as they had been since time immemorial. Renewed emphasis was placed on stopping bleeding quickly and reversing blood loss, and the guidelines called for improving the training and equipment of combat medics to accomplish these goals. The military also recognized that some individuals who are not medics should be trained in additional medical skills beyond those that all soldiers were trained to have. The military instituted the Combat Lifesaver Program in which selected soldiers were trained in four basic skills to keep a wounded man alive: conducting a needle thoracostomy (an operation in which a responder makes an incision in the chest wall and maintains the opening for drainage of fluid or abnormal accumulation of air; heretofore performed only by surgeons but now by field medics), starting an intravenous (IV) line, performing fluid resuscitation, and using traction splinting.[36] American soldiers were issued improved first aid kits that contained combat gauze, a tourniquet, and a nasopharyngeal airway for stopping hemorrhage and inadequate airway difficulties, both of which are frequent causes of death on the battlefield.

The initial stimulus for reexamining field medical practices came from the American experience in the Battle of Mogadishu. That engagement involved 170 soldiers in a fifteen-hour urban battle with guerrillas in which 100 American troops were wounded and 14 died on the battlefield. Another 4 died later in hospital. Experience in Iraq and Afghanistan also showed that besides producing more serious injuries than did previous wars, these wars were wounding more soldiers relative to the number killed in action. Paradoxically, although the overall casualty rates were low, the number of wounded that required medical attention was relatively high compared to other wars. In World War II, the U.S. military suffered 1.6 wounded for every man killed; in Vietnam, 2.8 wounded for each man killed; and in Iraq and Afghanistan, 16 servicepeople wounded for each soldier killed.[37] These experiences led to major changes in U.S. military medical practice and the incorporation of new medical technologies for treating the wounded. Among the most important new practices was the extensive use of the tourniquet.

American armies have used the tourniquet since at least the Civil War and did so extensively in World War I. However, it acquired a reputation as being dangerous when misuse (overtightening) caused tissue damage or when the time lapse between initial application and the casualty reaching a medical facility where the tourniquet could be safely removed was too long to prevent necrosis of the limb. The tourniquet consequently fell out of use. Nonetheless, the tourniquet was especially critical for blast injuries where damage to the extremities caused massive bleeding. A severed femoral artery, for example, will cause a person to bleed to death in seven minutes. At the start of the Gulf War, U.S. combat medics had no longer been trained in the use of the tourniquet and did not carry them in their medical kits.

The experience in Mogadishu led to the rediscovery of the tourniquet as in important life-saving device. The tourniquet stops bleeding quickly before shock can set in, and it helps stabilize the casualty for further treatment or evacuation. Newly designed tourniquets equalize the force distributed across the pressure strap to prevent tissue damage. The new models used in Iraq and Afghanistan can be tightened with one hand to prevent overtightening, and even the wounded soldier can apply it with only one hand. Equally important, the ability to reach and transport casualties quickly to nearby medical facilities where the tourniquet can be removed has done much to reduce necrotic damage to injured limbs, an important factor in saving the limb from amputation. Today every American soldier carries a tourniquet in his or her medical pack before going out on a dangerous mission, and medics carry a half dozen for immediate use. Soldiers have also come to appreciate the value of the device and commonly place tourniquets loosely around their arms and legs for quick use in the event that they are wounded. The military is also experimenting with incorporating gas-powered tourniquets into battle uniforms that inflate automatically when the soldier is wounded. Using the tourniquet in Iraq and Afghanistan has saved an estimated two thousand lives.[38]

The focus on preventing shock has also led to changes in the medical assessment of casualties. Since World War II, medics had been trained to keep the casualty's blood pressure up and to administer intravenous fluids to prevent shock. The IV bottle hung from a pole became part of the standard tableau of military medical treatment through Vietnam. This procedure continued to be recommended even though the medical community had recognized during the war that raising blood pressure was dangerous and caused clots to dislodge and start bleeding again. Medics in Iraq and Afghanistan are now trained to assess the casualty's blood pressure by pulse and not to worry about low blood pressure, because a wounded soldier can tolerate lower blood pressure with beneficial results. Gone, too, is the IV bottle. Medics now carry a capped catheter that can be used to push fluids into a vein if the soldier goes into severe shock.[39]

The widespread use of the Kevlar flak jacket has greatly reduced bullet wounds to the chest and thorax, and many of the casualties now present with wounds to the neck, groin, and abdomen, locations were the tourniquet cannot be used. An army study of "potentially survivable" wounded in Iraq who reached medical help showed that 80 percent died of hemorrhage, 70 percent of the time from wounds in locations where the tourniquet could not be used to stop bleeding.[40] The army searched for effective hemostatic agents to treat these wounds, and in 2007 approved the use of two such agents, QuikClot and HemCon, to be carried by combat medics. Since then, a new technology called Combat Gauze has come into use. Combat Gauze is a fabric bandage impregnated with kaolin, a powdered clay that stimulates blood-clotting. It has proved more effective than other clot-forming powders and granules, which often blew away or were washed away by the bleeding. Combat Gauze has a shelf life of thirty-six months, making it easy to store and transport.

The almost magical power of whole blood to revive trauma patients had been recognized as early as World War I, but once scientists learned to separate blood's components—red cells, plasma, and platelets—which were easier to store and had a longer shelf life than whole blood, the use of whole blood for transfusions fell out of use. Instead, physicians used IV fluid mixed with red blood cells, but in many cases this led to more extensive bleeding. During the second battle of Fallujah, Iraq (2004), no blood bank was available, and dozens of casualties were treated on the battlefield with whole blood drawn from fellow troops. All of the transfused casualties survived to be evacuated. This experience led the army to conduct a study in the Baghdad hospital and found that casualties who received whole blood had a survival rate nearly nine times greater than those who had been transfused with red blood cells and IV fluid.[41] In addition to restoring clotting, whole blood reduces the risk of acute respiratory failure, a condition first recognized in the Korean War and treated in Vietnam as "Da Nang lung," as well as multiple organ failure. Standard practice is now to transfuse whole blood to the wounded whenever possible and to use blood that is less than twenty-one days old, before its components decay.[42]

The Tactical Combat Casualty Care program also recommended the use of prophylactic antibiotics and that medics be equipped to apply broad-spectrum antibiotics immediately to the wounded. In Mogadishu, the delayed evacuation of casualties often resulted in rapid infection of battle wounds due to contamination by dirt, shrapnel, clothing, and the general bacteria in the area. Infected wounds also became a problem in Iraq. Casualties evacuated to stateside hospitals from Iraq often presented with wounds infected by a multidrug-resistant *Acinetobacter baumannii* infection.

Combat medics also are now equipped with more effective pain-controlling analgesics for battlefield use. Morphine and fentanyl, the traditional analgesics, are cardiorespiratory depressants and potentially dangerous. New drugs, such as intranasal or IV ketamine, that don't depress one's breathing or heart beat are now in use.

Both the Afghanistan and Iraq Wars initially produced high rates of blinding injuries. Soldiers had been issued eye protection goggles but refused to wear them because soldiers thought "they look like something a Florida senior citizen would wear."[43] The military bowed to fashion and issued new Wiley-brand ballistic eye wear, and the rate of eye injuries decreased markedly in both operational theaters.

In both theaters, the military evacuated casualties from the battlefield mostly via medevac helicopters whose onboard medical teams were trained to prevent shock, stop bleeding, and stabilize the soldier being transported to a medical facility. In Vietnam, only 2.4 percent of the wounded who were alive when they reached a field hospital died of their wounds. This statistic indicated that most deaths occurred before the wounded soldier made it to surgical care; thus, experience emphasizes reducing bleeding and shock to keep the soldier alive on the battlefield and in the transport helicopter. In a fundamental departure from U.S. medical practice in previous wars, another innovation was to move surgical teams and facilities closer to the battle area and make them more mobile to shorten the time between the soldier's being wounded and his receiving surgical care.[44] The result has been that a medevac helicopter and medic reached most wounded in Iraq and Afghanistan within forty minutes of their being wounded.

It is estimated that the U.S. Army has only 120 general surgeons on active duty and a similar number in the reserves.[45] The army has strived to keep thirty to fifty general surgeons and ten to fifteen orthopedic surgeons in each theater of war. Most of the surgeons serve in forward surgical teams (FSTs) consisting of twenty people: three general surgeons, one orthopedic surgeon, two nurse anesthetists, three nurses, and a collection of medics and other support personnel. Each FST is equipped to move directly behind the troops and can set up a functioning surgical hospital with four ventilator-equipped beds and two operating tables within an hour. The team travels in six of its own Humvees and carries three lightweight deployable rapid assembly shelters (known as a DRASH) that can be attached to one another to form a medical facility of nine hundred square feet. Supplies to resuscitate and operate on the wounded come in five backpacks: an intensive care unit pack, a surgical-technician pack, an anesthesia pack, a general surgery pack, and an orthopedic pack. These packs contain sterile instruments, anesthesia equipment, medicines, drapes, gowns, catheters, and a handheld unit that allows clinicians to obtain a hemogram and measure electrolytes or blood gases using only a single drop of blood. The FST also carries a small ultrasound machine, portable monitors, transport ventilators, an oxygen concentrator, twenty units of packed red cells, and six roll-up stretchers with litter stands. The FST has sufficient supplies to perform surgery on as many as thirty wounded soldiers. They are not equipped, however, for providing more than six hours of postoperative intensive care.[46]

The surgical strategy of the FST is to stabilize and control the patient's damage and not to undertake definitive repair unless it can be done quickly. The goal is to stop bleeding, prevent shock, and control contamination without allowing the patient to lose body temperature or become coalgulopathic, a condition in which the blood's ability to clot is impaired. The surgeons try to limit surgery to two hours or less, and then the unit ships the patient to a combat support hospital (CSH), the next level of care. For this approach to be successful, however, the military must have control of the airspace and major roadways and have established the next level hospital.

The CSH is equipped with 248 beds, six operating tables, some specialty surgical services, and radiology and laboratory facilities. These hospitals are mobile and arrive in modular units by air, tractor trailer, or ship. They can be set up to function fully within twenty-four to forty-eight hours. Even at the CHS, the goal is not definitive repair except, again, when it can be done quickly. The maximum stay is intended to be no longer than three days. Any soldier who requires more care is transferred to a level-four hospital. There again, if treatment is expected to take more than thirty days, the wounded soldier is transferred to a medical facility in the United States. The system required some retraining of the surgeons who, instead of transferring their patients, had the caregiver's tendency to keep them at whatever level they were being treated. In the early days of the Iraq War, it took an average of eight days for a wounded soldier to move from the battlefield to a stateside hospital. The travel time is now less than four days. During the Vietnam War, it took a wounded soldier forty-five days to make the journey home.[47]

The Iraq and Afghanistan Wars have become notorious for the number of soldiers suffering brain damage from explosive devices. Fully 20 percent of the wounded have suffered some form of brain trauma.[48] If the full spectrum of brain injuries are considered, thousands of soldiers may be suffering from brain injuries who have gone undiagnosed. Brig. Gen. Stephen Xenakis, a psychiatrist with the Psychiatric Institute in Washington, D.C., has observed that beyond the thousand or so cases of major brain trauma (fractured skulls, penetration, etc.), thousands of soldiers have suffered concussions, some temporary loss of consciousness, memory, hearing, and so on, from blasts that would produce mild brain injury. "But you also have literally hundreds of thousands of troops who've been exposed to blast, maybe repeatedly. We don't know the long-term effect on these soldiers. That's the big worry."[49]

Of great concern are the 30 percent of the soldiers who have developed Post-Traumatic Stress Disorder (PTSD) within a few months of returning home from the combat theaters. The symptoms of PTSD are remarkably similar to those associated with mild brain injury: confusion, depression, irritability, rage, and fatigue. When PTSD was first diagnosed during World War I, doctors called it "shell shock" and thought it was caused by explosive concussion that produced micro-bleeding in the brain. Russian and German neurologists performed dozens of autopsies in search of the physical evidence of micro-damage with little success. As a consequence, American and British military psychiatrists rejected the biological explanations of the Russians and Germans, opting for then popular Freudian psychological explanations. Now, it turns out the Russians and Germans might have been right all along.

To explain the high rates of PTSD among American soldiers, psychiatrists have turned to a new theory regarding its cause that bears a strong resemblance to the original shell shock explanations of World War I. The new theory suggests that the overpressure from an explosive shock wave traveling thousands of feet per second creates microscopic gas bubbles in the brain that then pop, leaving tiny cavities that never heal. The result is minor brain damage that produces PTSD's symptoms and is similar to the minor brain damage acquired through other causes.[50] The great fear is that these injuries may have affected tens of thousands or hundreds of thousands of soldiers who were exposed to blasts but were never counted among the wounded because they did not show any immediate symptoms of injury. Prior to the Afghanistan and Iraq Wars, the Pentagon had greatly reduced its research funding for brain injury by almost 50 percent. In 2007, however, the military reversed its decision and once more began to budget money for brain research. In addition, all returning soldiers are screened after three to six months for previously unnoticed brain injury.[51] In 2002, 200,000 American soldiers sought mental health counseling for post-traumatic stress–related disorders. In 2011, the number of soldiers who actually received treatment or counseling from behavioral health specialists increased to 280,000.[52]

Beyond the advances in treating brain injuries, the U.S. military has made great strides in developing prosthetic limbs for amputees and has greatly funded surgical trials to deal with the facial disfigurement that explosive devices often cause. In many cases, surgeons can now repair or replace entire faces. Most recently, surgeons have succeeded in transplanting forearms and hands. Once more the terrible human costs of war have produced significant medical advances from which the larger population may benefit.

NOTES

1. Stephen Tanner, *Afghanistan: A Military History from Alexander the Great to the War against the Taliban* (New York: Da Capo Press, 2009), 228.
2. Ibid.
3. Ibid., 248.
4. Ibid., 255.
5. Lester W. Grau and William A. Jorgensen, "Handling the Wounded in a Counter-Guerrilla War: The Soviet-Russian Experience in Afghanistan and Chechnya," *Army Medical Department Journal*, January–February 1998, 2, citing official Russian statistics in G. F. Krivosheev, "The Secret Seal Is Removed," *Voyenizdat*, 1993, 401–5.
6. Grau and Jorgensen, "Handling the Wounded," 2, citing Soviet source: E. A. Nechaev, A. K. Tutokhel, A. I. Gritsanov, and I. D. Kosachev, "Medical Support of the 40th Army: Facts and Figures," *Military Medical Journal*, August 1991, 4.
7. Soviet Studies Research Center, *The Sustainability of the Soviet Army in Battle* (The Hague: SHAPE Technical Center: September, 1986): 286–96.
8. Department of the U.S. Army, *FM-100-2-2: The Soviet Army Specialized Warfare and Rear Area Support* (Washington, DC: U.S. Government Printing Office, 1984), 13–21.
9. V. D. Kurvshinskiy, "Technical Service and Repair of Medical Equipment in the Course of Military Activity," *Military Medical Journal*, 1992, 42–44.
10. I. M. Chizh and N. I. Makarov, "The Experience of Medical Support to Local Wars and the Problems of Air Evacuation of the Sick and Wounded," *Military Medical Journal*, January 1993, 23.
11. Ibid.
12. Grau and Jorgensen, "Handling the Wounded," 8.
13. Ibid.
14. Yuri Nemytin, "Special Medical Aid to the Wounded in Afghanistan," *Military Medical Journal*, January 1991, 17.
15. Grau and Jorgensen, "Handling the Wounded," 8.
16. Ibid.
17. Ibid., 2.
18. Lester W. Grau and William A. Jorgensen, "Medical Support in a Counter-Guerrilla War: Epidemiological Lessons Learned in the Soviet-Afghan War," *U. S. Army Medical Department Journal*, May–June 1998, 2.
19. Ibid.
20. I. V. Sinopal'nikov, "Medical Losses of Soviet Troops during the War in Afghanistan: Medical Losses from Infectious Diseases," *Military Medical Journal*, September 2000), 4–11.
21. Grau and Jorgensen, "Medical Support," 3, citing E. A. Nechaev, "Medical Rehabilitation of Veterans of Wars and Local Conflicts," *Military Medical Journal*, February 1994, 5.
22. Ibid., 7.

23. Yuri Nemytin and V. V. Boldyrev, "Rehabilitation Management of Infectious Patients in Overcrowded Hospitals," *Military Medical Journal*, April–May 1992, 38–39.
24. Lester W. Grau and William A. Jorgensen, "Viral Hepatitis and the Russian War in Chechnya," *U S. Army Medical Department Journal*, May–June 1997, 2.
25. *The Russian Weekly*, February 21, 2003, 1.
26. N. N. Novichkov et al., *The Russian Armed Forces in the Chechnyan Conflict* (Moscow: Holweg-Infoglobe-Trivola, 1995), 133.
27. Ibid., 18.
28. Grau and Jorgensen, "Viral Hepatitis," 1–5, for a good overview of the health problems confronting the Russian Army there.
29. Ibid., 2.
30. Casualty figures are up to date as of June 2011.
31. L. G. Stansbury et al., "Amputations in U.S. Military Personnel in Afghanistan and Iraq," *Journal of Orthopedic Trauma* 22, no. 1 (2008): 43–46.
32. Owen Dyer, "The Iraq War and the Military Medicine Sea Change," *National Review of Medicine* 4, no. 8 (April 2007).
33. David Brown, "U.S. Military Medics Use Old and New Techniques to Save Wounded in Afghanistan," *Washington Post*, November 1, 2010.
34. Lester W. Grau and William A. Jorgensen, "Beaten by the Bugs: The Soviet-Afghan War Experience," *Military Review* 77, no. 6 (November–December 1997): 5.
35. Ibid.
36. Frank K. Butler Jr., "Tactical Combat Casualty Care 2007: Evolving Concepts and Battlefield Experience," *Military Medicine* 172 (November 2007): 11.
37. Dyer, "The Iraq War and Military Medicine," 1.
38. Brown, "U.S. Military Medics."
39. Ibid.
40. Ibid.
41. Ibid.
42. Ibid.
43. Gawande, "Casualties of War."
44. Ibid.
45. Ibid.
46. Ibid.
47. Ibid.
48. Deborah White, "Iraq War Facts: Results and Statistics as of April 26, 2011," Ask.com.
49. Dyer, "Iraq War and Military Medicine," 1.
50. Ibid.
51. Ibid.
52. Greg Jaffe, "Departing General Favors Ending Ban on Women in Battle," *Boston Globe*, February 5, 2012.

8

SOME THOUGHTS ON WAR

Not a single major military establishment in the world is without a military medical service. The connection between civilian and military medical establishments in highly industrialized societies is now symbiotic, with advances in one being quickly adopted by the other. The paralysis once engendered by the separation of the civilian and military establishments, closely paralleled in the tension between the physician and surgeon, is gone. Gone, too, is the dependence upon the brilliance of a few people, often military doctors, for medical advances. The search for new medical technologies is so highly organized and requires so many organizational resources that individual genius is unlikely to be productive unless linked with large research facilities. Even then, it is more likely that medical advances will be the product of research teams than of brilliant individuals.

The impact of military medicine on casualty survival rates has been dramatic. It is noteworthy that almost 65 percent of the wounded receive only minor injuries and 20 percent of soldiers struck by enemy weapons are killed outright; thus, only 35 percent of the wounded require medical attention to survive. Undoubtedly battlefield medicine has had an enormous impact on survival rates and on the fighting ability of modern armies.

It is wise to remember, however, that the military surgeon's role has not changed much since he first appeared in ancient Sumer. His task is still to rescue as many salvageable bodies as possible from the carnage, treat them quickly, and return them to the battlefield so that the carnage may continue until, finally, one side's will gives way. To accomplish this task, some practical realities remain historical constants. The first is that only 35 percent of the wounded in any given battle require serious medical attention to survive their wounds. As body armor recently has become a normal item of military equipment for the first time in almost five hundred years, the number of wounded requiring serious medical intervention to survive has declined by yet another 6 percent. The second constant is that regardless of the increasing destructiveness of modern weapons, the ratio of dead to wounded has remained almost unchanged for five hundred years. Third, although disease causes far fewer deaths than it used to, disease-related infirmities still account for the highest percentage of temporary manpower loss in campaigns. Together, the challenges confronting the military physician have remained remarkably similar throughout history.

What has changed, of course, are the conditions under which the military physician must apply his or her skill. Three factors have altered these conditions: the dispersion of combat forces over far greater areas, the increased rates of destruction of locally engaged forces made possible by increases in the rates of fire and lethality of modern weaponry, and the greatly increased vulnerability of combat medical assets on the high-mobility battlefield. While the challenges to the military physician have remained essentially unchanged, the nature of modern war has greatly transformed the medical practitioner's ability to meet them.

The increased ability of weapons to acquire targets at longer ranges and to destroy them with greater certainty has necessarily dispersed combat forces. In World War II, the probability of a tank round hitting another tank on the first attempt was less than 10 percent, and then only if the tank was shooting from a stationary position. Today, the probability of a moving tank getting a first-round hit is almost 98 percent. Smart bombs and other precision-guided munitions, including guided artillery rounds, have made the modern battlefield a terribly lethal place. The tactician's only solution when facing exponential increases in firepower, accuracy, and lethality is to disperse forces over wider areas and rely upon increased mobility to avoid being killed.

One consequence of dispersion is that troops spread over very wide areas make it almost impossible to locate casualties. Unlike earlier wars of fixed lines and relatively shallow zones of operation, the modern conventional battlefield vastly complicates military medical teams' efforts to determine the location, number, and severity of casualties and to react in time. The dispersion of casualties, first brought about by the introduction of gunpowder weapons and then by the adoption of linear tactics, has reached far greater proportions than anyone imagined even twenty years ago. In future wars, it may take much longer to locate and reach casualties for treatment.

Despite the best efforts of medical teams, wounded men will remain untreated for many hours and even days. Many who would have been saved in earlier wars are likely to die. Those who survive until medical help reaches them are likely to present with infected wounds that will greatly complicate treatment and recovery.

Increased firepower and lethality of modern weapons cause very high rates of destruction and wounding when employed in compact battle areas. Dispersion, after all, only works so long as one is avoiding contact or moving toward the battle engagement. At some point the forces must concentrate at the *schwerpunkt* (focal point) and the battle against contending forces joined. The loss of life and equipment in these engagements will probably be quite high for both attacker and defender, with kill and wound rates rising past 60 percent. It is unlikely that any medical service will be able to handle the sudden flood of the casualty stream under these conditions. In the case of a successful attack, the victor might be able to move rear area medical assets to the battlefield in time to treat some of the wounded. In the defender's case, however, once his battle area is penetrated and the attack continued to his rear, his available medical assets are likely to be destroyed or crippled in a battle of annihilation. Iraqi forces faced this scenario in the Gulf War in 1991 and again in 2003. A defeated enemy, furthermore, can expect little in the way of medical help from a victor already overburdened by its own casualties.

The swirling nature of modern tactics requiring mobility and deep penetration coupled with the presence of precision-guided munitions and air capability on both sides means that medical assets will be extremely vulnerable to planned or accidental destruction. A division commander, for example, currently possesses the capacity to exert lethal force as far as sixty miles into the interior of the enemy front. Any medical assets close enough to deal with frontline casualties are within the zone of destruction and vulnerable to attack. Since a critical factor in keeping most wounded alive is that they be reached quickly, stabilized, and then evacuated for further treatment, how this lifesaving effort might be accomplished in a modern war is unclear. The old standbys of motor ambulance, wheeled or tracked vehicles, and the helicopter are all extremely vulnerable when they venture close to the forward edge of the battle area where casualties are expected to be concentrated. Motorized transport survived well enough in World War II and Korea because the weapons used in these conflicts were so inaccurate. In the U.S. military's efforts in Vietnam, Iraq, and Afghanistan, the helicopter survived well enough as an evacuation vehicle because the U.S. military enjoyed complete air superiority to suppress enemy fire at the evacuation point. In future wars, these conditions are not likely to obtain.

The professionally staffed and well-equipped medical services of modern armies are apt to face considerable difficulties in delivering medical care to the soldier on the battlefield. Again, too, the danger is that armies plan for the next war as though they are refighting the last one. In Iraq, for example, had the Iraqi Army not lost its will to fight and its air force not been destroyed *before* the ground battle began, the U.S. Army's medical assets would have been vulnerable to attack, especially from chemical munitions delivered by air, artillery, and barrage rockets. As partial consolation, current statistics show that for every three soldiers wounded only one will require serious medical intervention to save his life. The key to survival may be in increasing the medical training in traumatic first aid for all soldiers so that they will be able to stop bleeding and prevent shock. It is also probable that high-intensity conflicts will be relatively short affairs, and perhaps planners should not give too much thought to returning the wounded to the battle as they might not have time to make much difference in its outcome. Increasing the soldiers' medical training so that they can act as trained medical resources on the spot may make the most difference in saving lives. The idea is not a new one. In both ancient Greece and Rome, soldiers relied primarily on each other rather than on an organized military medical service to treat their wounds.

Fortunately, since the 1970s no nation has yet fought a modern, high-intensity, conventional war in which both sides were well equipped and had the stomach for a fight. The closest example to this type of conflict was the Israeli-Arab War in 1973. In that war, the Israelis lost almost half of their ground forces to death, wounds, and injury and almost as much of their equipment in less than twenty days of sustained combat. The loss ratios for the forces of the engaged Arab states were even greater. While both sides tried desperately to provide what medical support they could, the nature of modern battle made it difficult, and thousands died of their wounds. In the case of the Iraqi-U.S. conflict of 1991, the Iraqis quit fighting within hours of the ground attack, and in the 2003 war they quit within two weeks. In the few places where Iraqi Army units chose to stand, the superior firepower, accuracy, and lethality of American weapons destroyed them within hours. While no official death rates have been released for the Iraqi Army, senior American combat commanders suggested publicly that as many as a hundred thousand Iraq combatants were killed or wounded in less than a hundred hours of combat. Under these lethal conditions, it is extremely unlikely that the Iraqi military medical service could have done much to stem the tide of death that swept over its army.

The advances in the conduct of war have proceeded so rapidly that the military medical services can never really catch up and realistically provide the kind of survival assistance that the modern soldier has come to expect. Certainly this state of affairs has already been reached in other areas of the military arts. Training exercises conducted by the U.S. Army at the National Training Center at Fort Irwin, California, reveal time and again that against a relatively equally matched enemy, even the victor can expect little more than a Pyhrric victory in intense engagements. Military psychiatrists suggest that under those conditions, manpower loss from psychiatric collapse is likely to surpass the number of men killed by enemy fire. At the extreme, of course, no one really expects to survive a battle in which tactical nuclear weapons are used.

Maybe the destructiveness of war has indeed exceeded our wildest expectations, and only foolish stubbornness motivates us to fend off the horror of war with the delusion that we can salvage the human wreckage so that life can go on after the battle. Yet, precisely this belief makes the conduct of war seem a plausible means for resolving national conflicts. No soldier who truly thought he was going to die would venture upon the battlefield unless he was insane. The paradox is that having striven for more than six millennia to find ways to relieve the suffering and pain of the wounded, we have finally achieved the goal, only to have it snatched from our grasp by the terrible power of modern weaponry. Even so, who among us is willing to suggest that the search for saving the wreckage of war ought to end?

BIBLIOGRAPHY

Abbott, S. L. "A Report on the Quality of Ambulance Service as Observed in 1862." *New York State Journal of Medicine* 82, no. 3 (March 1982): 393–94.

Adams, G. W. "Confederate Medicine." *Journal of Southern History* 6 (1940): 149–57.

Adamson, P. B. "The Military Surgeon: His Place in History." *Journal of the Royal Army Medical Corps* 128 (1982): 43–50.

Agnew, J. B. "The Great War That Almost Was: The Crimea, 1853–1856." *Parameters* 3, no. 1 (1973): 46–57.

Aker, Frank, Dawn Schroeder, and Robert Baycar. "Cause and Prevention of Maxillofacial War Wounds: A Historical Review." *Military Medicine* 148, no. 12 (December 1983): 921–27.

Aldea, Peter, and William Shaw. "The Evolution of the Surgical Management of Severe Lower Extremity Trauma." *Clinics in Plastic Surgery* 13, no. 4 (October 1968): 549–69.

Aldrete, J. Antonio, G. Manuel Marron, and A. J. Wright. "The First Administration of Anesthesia in Military Surgery: On Occasion of the Mexican-American War." *Anesthesiology* 61, no. 5 (November 1984): 585–88.

Alexander, John T. "Medical Developments in Petrine Russia." *Canadian-American Slavic Studies* 8, no. 2 (Summer 1974): 198–221.

Allison, R. S. *Sea Diseases: The Story of the Great National Experiment in Preventive Medicine in the Royal Navy.* London: John Bale, 1943.

Anderson, Donald Lee, and Godfrey Tryggve Anderson. "Nostalgia and Malingering in the Military during the Civil War." *Perspectives in Biology and Medicine* 28, no. 1 (Autumn 1984): 156–66.

Appell, Rodney A. "Medical Aspects of the Confederacy." *Our Medical Heritage* 73, no. 6 (June 1980): 784–86.

Applegate, Howard Lewis. "Effect of the American Revolution on American Medicine." *Military Medicine*, July 1961, 551–53.

———. "The Need for Further Study in the Medical History of the American Revolutionary Army." *Military Medicine,* August 1961, 616–18.

———. "Preventive Medicine in the American Revolutionary Army." *Military Medicine* 126 (May 1961): 379–81.

Ashburn, P. M. *A History of the Medical Department of the United States Army.* New York: Houghton Mifflin, 1929.

Atkins, J. *The Naval Surgeon, or a Practical System of Surgery.* London: J. Hodges, 1732.

Baylen, Joseph O., and Alan Conway, eds. *Soldier-Surgeon: The Crimean War Letters of Dr. Douglas A. Reid, 1855–1856.* Knoxville: University of Tennessee Press, 1968.
Bayne-Jones, Stanhope. *The Evolution of Preventive Medicine in the U.S. Army, 1607–1939.* Washington, DC: U.S. Government Printing Office, 1968.
Beebe, Gilbert W. *Battle Casualties: Incidence, Mortality, and Logistic Considerations.* Springfield, IL: Charles C. Thomas, 1946.
Bell, W. J. "A Portrait of the Colonial Physician." *Bulletin of the History of Medicine* 44 (1970): 497–506.
Benenson, Abram S. "Immunization and Military Medicine." *Clinical Infectious Diseases* 6, no. 1 (January–February 1984): 1–12.
Benton, Edward H. "British Surgery in the South African War: The Work of Major Frederick Porter." *Medical History* 21, no. 3 (July 1977): 275–90.
Billings, John Shaw. "Medical Reminiscences of the Civil War." *Transactions of the College of Physicians of Philadelphia.* 3rd series, no. 27 (1905): 115–16.
Blaisdell, F. William. "Medical Advances during the Civil War." *Archives of Surgery* 123, no. 9 (September 1988): 1045–50.
Blanco, Richard L. "The Development of British Military Medicine, 1793–1814." *Military Affairs* 38, no. 1 (February 1974): 4–10.
———. "James McGrigor and the Army Medical Department." *History Today* 21 (1971): 132–40.
———. "Reform and Wellington's Post-Waterloo Army." *Military Affairs* 29 (1965): 123–31.
———. *Wellington's Surgeon General: Sir James McGrigor.* Durham, NC: Duke University Press, 1974.
Bouchier, Ian. "Some Experiences of Ship's Surgeons during the Early Days of Sperm Whale Fishery." *British Medical Journal* 285 (December 1982): 18–25.
Bowers, Warner F. "Evacuating the Wounded from Korea." *Army Information Digest* 5 (December 1950): 49–51.
Bowlby, Anthony. "The Hunterian Oration: On British Military Surgery in the Time of Hunter and the Great War." *Lancet* 1 (February 22, 1919): 285–90.
Breedon, James O. "Andersonville: A Southern Surgeon's Story." *Bulletin of the History of Medicine* 67, no. 4 (July–August 1971): 317–43.
———. "A Medical History of the Later Stages of the Atlanta Campaign." *Journal of Southern History* 35, no. 1 (1969): 31–69.
Brewer, Lyman A. "Baron Dominique Jean Larrey (1766–1842): Father of Modern Military Surgery, Innovator, Humanist." *Journal of Thoracic Cardiovascular Surgery* 92, no. 6 (December 1986): 1096–98.
———. "Respiration and Respiratory Treatment: A Historical Overview." *American Journal of Surgery* 138, no. 3 (September 1979): 342–54.
Brodman, Estelle, and Elizabeth B. Carrick. "American Military Medicine in the Mid-Nineteenth Century: The Experience of Alexander H. Hoff, M.D." *Bulletin of the History of Medicine* 64 (Spring 1990): 63–78.
Brooks, Stewart. *Civil War Medicine.* Springfield, IL: Charles C. Thomas, 1966.
Brown, A. J. "The Surgery of Albucasis." *Surgery, Gynecology, and Obstetrics* 39 (1924): 423–29.
———. "The Surgery of Hieronymus Braunschwig." *Surgery, Gynecology, and Obstetrics* 38 (1924): 131–39.
Brown, David. "U.S. Military Medics Use Old and New Techniques to Save Wounded in Afghanistan." *Washington Post,* November 1, 2010.
Burns, Stanley B. "Early Medical Photography in America: Civil War Medical Photography." *New York State Journal of Medicine* 80, no. 9 (August 1980): 1444–69.
Butler, Frank K., Jr. "Tactical Combat Casualty Care 2007: Evolving Concepts and Battlefield Experience." *Military Medicine* 172 (November 2007): 1–11.

Calhoun, J. T. "Nostalgia as a Disease of Field Service." *Medical Surgical Reporter* 11 (February 27, 1864): 130–32.

Calkins, Beverly M. "Florence Nightingale: On Feeding an Army." *American Journal of Clinical Nutrition* 50 (1989): 1260–65.

Campbell, R. M. "History in Relation to Some Principles and Practices of Confederate Surgeons." *Virginia Medical Monthly* 94 (1967): 600–608.

Cantlie, Neil A. *A History of the Army Medical Department.* London: Churchill-Livingstone, 1974.

Cash, Philip. "Medical Men at the Siege of Boston." *Memoirs of the American Philosophical Society* (Philadelphia) 98 (1973): 53–62.

Chamberlain, Weston P. "History of Military Medicine and Its Contributions to Science." *Boston Medical and Surgical Journal* (April 1917): 235–49.

Chandler, David G. "The Egyptian Campaign of 1801." *History Today* 11 (1962): 117–23.

Chevalier, A. G. "Hygienic Problems of the Napoleonic Armies." *Ciba Symposium* 3 (1941–1942): 974–80.

———. "Physicians of the French Revolution." *Ciba Symposium* 3 (1941–1942): 964–74.

Chizh, I. M., and N. I. Makarov. "The Experience of Medical Support to Local Wars and the Problems of Air Evacuation of the Sick and Wounded." *Military Medical Journal,* January 1993, 22–30.

Churchill, Edward D. "Military Surgery." In *Textbook of Surgery by American Authors,* edited by Frederick Christopher, 153–54. Philadelphia: Saunders, 1945.

Cockburn, W. Charles. "The Early History of Typhoid Vaccination." *Journal of the Royal Army Medical Corps* 101, no. 3 (July 1955): 171–85.

Cohen, William A. "What Price Body Armor?" *Ordnance,* May–June 1973, 490–93.

Collins, H. P. "The Crimea: The Fateful Weeks." *Army Quarterly* 71 (1955): 86–96.

Courtwright, David T. "Opiate Addiction as a Consequence of the Civil War." *Civil War History* 24, no. 2 (1978): 101–11.

Cowdrey, Albert E. *The Medic's War.* Washington, DC: Center for Military History, Department of the Army, 1987.

Cozen, Lewis N. "Military Orthopedic Surgery." *Clinical Orthopaedics and Related Research* 200 (November 1985): 50–53.

Crew, F. A. E. *History of the Second World War: The Army Medical Services.* Vol. 2, *Campaigns.* London: Her Majesty's Stationery Office, 1957.

Crissey, John Thorne, and Lawrence Charles Parish. "Wound Healing: Development of the Basic Concepts." *Clinics in Dermatology* 2, no. 3 (July–September 1984): 1–7.

Crosby, William H. "The Golden Age of the Army Medical Corps: A Perspective from 1901." *Military Medicine* 148, no. 9 (September 1983): 707–11.

Crummer, Le Roy. "Joseph Schmidt: Barber Surgeon." *American Journal of Surgery* 4 (February 1928): 236–41.

Crumplin, M. K. H. "Surgery at Waterloo." *Journal of the Royal Society of Medicine* 81, no. 1 (January 1988): 38–42.

———. "Vascular Problems at the Battle of Waterloo." *European Journal of Vascular Surgery* 1 (April 1987): 137–42.

Cunningham, H. H. "The Confederate Medical Officer in the Field." *Bulletin of the New York Academy of Medicine* 34, no. 7 (July 1958): 461–84.

———. *Doctors in Gray: The Confederate Medical Service.* Baton Rouge: Louisiana State University Press, 1958.

Curtis, Edward E. *The Organization of the British Army in the American Revolution.* New Haven, CT: Yale University Press, 1926.

Cushman, Paul, Jr. "Amos Evans, M.D.: Surgeon on the USS *Constitution* in the War of 1812." *New York State Journal of Medicine* 80, no. 11 (October 1980): 1753–56.

———. "Naval Surgery in the War of 1812." *New York State Journal of Medicine* 72, no. 14 (July 1972): 1881–87.
Da Costa, J. Chalmers. "Baron Larrey: A Sketch." *Bulletin of Johns Hopkins Hospital* 17 (July 1906): 195–215.
Dammann, Gordon E. "Dental Care during the Civil War." *Illinois Dental Journal*, January–February 1984, 12–17.
Davidson, J. T., and S. Cotev. "Anesthesia in the Yom Kippur War." *Annals of the Royal College of Surgeons* 56, no. 6 (June 1975): 304–11.
Davis, David B. "Medicine in the Canadian Campaign of the Revolutionary War." *Bulletin of the History of Medicine* 44, no. 5 (September–October 1970): 460–71.
Davis, J. S. "Plastic Surgery in World War I and World War II." *Plastic Reconstructive Surgery* 1 (1946): 255–61.
Defense Intelligence Agency. "Medical Organization." *Handbook on the Soviet Armed Forces*. Washington, DC: Directorate of Intelligence Research, Defense Intelligence Agency, February 1978, 7–9.
Department of the U.S. Army. *Field Manual 8-15: Medical Service in Divisions, Separate Brigades, and the Armored Cavalry Regiment*. Washington, DC: Department of the Army, September 1972.
———. *Field Manual 54-9: Corps Support Command*. Washington, DC: Department of the Army, 1976.
———. *Field Manual 100-2-2: The Soviet Army Specialized Warfare and Rear Area Support*. Washington, DC: U.S. Government Printing Office, 1984.
Derby, A. Campbell. "The Military Surgeon—Not Least in the Crusade." *Canadian Journal of Surgery* 28, no. 2 (1985): 183–86.
Deutsch, Albert. "Military Psychiatry: The Civil War." In Hall et al., *One Hundred Years of American Psychiatry*, 367–84.
———. "Military Psychiatry: World War II, 1941–1943." In Hall et al. *One Hundred Years of American Psychiatry*, 419–41.
Dibble, J. H. *Napoleon's Surgeon*. London: Heinemann Medical Books, 1970.
Diffenbaugh, Willis G. "Military Surgery in the Civil War." *Military Medicine* 130 (1965): 490–96.
Donchin, Yoel, M. Wiener, M. Grande, and Shamay Cotev. "Military Medicine: Trauma Anesthesia and Critical Care on the Battlefield." *Overview of Trauma Anesthesia and Critical Care* 6, no. 1 (January 1990): 185–202.
Donnelly, C. "The Soviet Attitude toward Stress in Battle." *Journal of the Royal Army Medical Corps* 128 (1982): 72–78.
Dunbar, R. G. "The Introduction of the Practice of Vaccination in Napoleonic France." *Bulletin of the History of Medicine* 10 (1941): 633–50.
Dunbar-Miller, R. A. "Alcohol and the Fighting Man: An Historical Review." *Journal of the Royal Army Medical Corps*. vol. 2 (June 1984): 117–121.
Duncan, L. C. "Medical History of General Scott's Campaign to the City of Mexico in 1847." *U.S. Army Medical Services Bulletin* 50 (1939): 61–117.
Dupuy, R. Ernest, and Trevor N. Dupuy. *The Encyclopedia of Military History*. New York: Harper & Row, 1968.
Dupuy, Trevor N. *Attrition: Forecasting Battle Casualties and Equipment Losses in Modern War*. Fairfax, VA: HERO Books, 1990.
———. *The Evolution of Weapons and Warfare*. New York: Bobbs-Merrill, 1980.
———. *Numbers, Predictions, and War*. New York: Bobbs-Merrill, 1979.
Dyer, Owen. "The Iraq War and the Military Medicine Sea Change." *National Review of Medicine* 4, no. 8 (April 2007): 1–5.
Eakins, W. A. "Thomas Crawford: Regimental Medical Officer in the Crimea, 1855." *Ulster Medical Journal* 51, no. 1 (1982): 46–51.

Eckert, William G. "History of the U.S. Army Graves Registration Service: 1917–1950s." *American Journal of Forensic Medicine and Pathology* 4, no. 3 (September 1983): 231–43.

Eichner, L. G. "The Military Practice of Medicine during the Revolutionary War." Lecture presented at the Tredyffrin Easttown History Society, Pennsylvania, October 2003.

Eiseman, Ben. "Combat Casualty Management in Vietnam." *Journal of Trauma* 7, no. 1 (January 1967): 53–63.

———. "The Next War: A Prescription." *U.S. Naval Institute Proceedings* 101 (1975): 33–40.

———. "Planning for Future Combat Casualty Care." *U.S. Naval Institute Proceedings* 105 (1979): 117–119.

Essame, H. "A Redcoat Surgeon's Account of 1776: From an Unpublished Diary of a Young British Surgeon in the American Colonies." *Military Review* 42 (1962): 66–78.

Estes, J. Worth. "Naval Medicine in the Age of Sail: The Voyage of the New York." *Bulletin of the History of Medicine* 56 (1961): 238–53.

Evatt, G. J. H. *Army Medical Organization.* Allahabad, India: Pioneer Press, 1877.

Eve, Paul F. "Remarks on the Statistics of Amputation." *Southern Medical and Surgical Journal* 2 (1846): 465–69.

Feibel, Robert M. "What Happened at Walcheren: The Primary Medical Sources." *Bulletin of the History of Medicine* 42 (1968): 62–72.

Foltz, Charles. *Surgeon of the Seas: The Life of Surgeon General Jonathan M. Foltz.* Indianapolis: Bobbs-Merrill, 1931.

Forrest, Robert D. "Development of Wound Therapy from the Dark Ages to the Present." *Journal of the Royal Society of Medicine* 75 (April 1982): 268–73.

Foster, Walter. "The Hospital Scandals in South Africa." *The Contemporary Review*, 1900, 12–14.

Fraser, Ian. "The Doctor's Debt to the Soldier." Mitchiner Memorial Lecture. Royal Army Medical College, June 8, 1971, 60–75.

———. "Penicillin: Early Trials on War Casualties." *British Medical Journal* 289 (1984): 1723–25.

Freeman, Frank R. "Administration of the Medical Department of the Confederate States Army, 1861–1865." *Southern States Medical Journal* 80, no. 5 (May 1987): 630–37.

———. "The Health of the American Slave Examined by Means of Union Army Medical Statistics." *Journal of the National Medical Association* 77, no. 1 (1985): 49–52.

Fulton, John F. "Medicine, Warfare, and History." *Journal of the American Medical Association* 153, no. 5 (October 1953): 177–82.

Gabriel, Richard A. "The History of Armaments." In *Italian Encyclopedia of Social Sciences*, 347–68. Rome: Marchesi Grafiche Editoriali, 1990.

———. *Military Psychiatry: A Comparative Perspective.* Westport, CT: Greenwood Press, 1986.

———. *No More Heroes: Madness and Psychiatry in War.* New York: Hill and Wang, 1987.

———. *Operation Peace for Galilee: The Israeli-PLO War in Lebanon.* New York: Hill and Wang, 1984.

———. *The Painful Field: The Psychiatric Dimension of Modern War.* Westport, CT: Greenwood Press, 1988.

———. *Soviet Military Psychiatry: The Theory and Practice of Coping with Battle Stress.* Westport, CT: Greenwood Press, 1986.

Gabriel, Richard A., and Karen S. Metz. *From Sumer to Rome: The Military Capabilities of Ancient Armies.* Westport, CT: Greenwood Press, 1991.

Garrison, Fielding. *Introduction to the History of Medicine.* London: W. B. Saunders, 1967.

———. *Notes on the History of Military Medicine.* Washington, DC: Association of Military Surgeons, 1922.

———. "The Statistics of the Austro-Prussian ('7 Weeks') War, 1866, as a Measure of Sanitary Efficiency in Campaign." *Military Surgeon* 41 (1917): 711–17.
Gawande, Atul. "Casualties of War: Military Care for the Wounded from Iraq and Afghanistan." *New England Journal of Medicine*, December 9, 2004, 3–6.
Giao, Manuel. "British Surgeons in the Portuguese Army during the Peninsular War." *Journal of the Royal Army Medical Corps* 62 (1934): 299–303.
Gihon, Albert L. "Transportation of Casualties in the Navy." *The Grog Ration* 3, no. 6 (November–December 2008): 6–9.
Gillett, Mary C. *The Army Medical Department, 1775–1818.* Washington, DC: The Center of Military History, U.S. Army, 1981.
Ginzberg, Eli, John Herma, and Sol W. Ginsburg. *Psychiatry and Military Manpower Policy: A Reappraisal of the Experience in World War II.* New York: Columbia University, King's Crown Press, 1953.
Gladstone, W. "Medical Photography in the Civil War." *Photographica* 9, no. 11 (February 1979): 11–22.
Glass, Albert J. "Army Psychiatry before World War II." In Hall et al., *One Hundred Years of American Psychiatry*, 211–24.
Gouldner, René M. "A Surgeon of Napoleon." *The Medical Herald,* February 1930, 43–47.
Grau, Lester W., and William A. Jorgensen. "Beaten by the Bugs: The Soviet-Afghan War Experience." *Military Review* 77, no. 6 (November–December 1997): 5–14.
———. "Handling the Wounded in a Counter-Guerrilla War: The Soviet-Russian Experience in Afghanistan and Chechnya." *Army Medical Department Journal,* January–February 1998, 2–10.
———. "Medical Support in a Counter-Guerrilla War: Epidemiological Lessons Learned in the Soviet-Afghan War." *U.S. Army Medical Department Journal,* May–June 1998, 2–11.
———. "Viral Hepatitis and the Russian War in Chechnya." *U.S. Army Medical Department Journal,* May–June 1997, 1–9.
Great Britain War Office, General Staff. *The Russo-Japanese War.* 6 vols. London: War Office Study, His Majesty's Stationery Office, 1906–1908.
Greenbaum, Louis S. "'Measure of Civilization': The Hospital Thought of Jacques Tenon on the Eve of the French Revolution." *Bulletin of the History of Medicine* 49 (1975): 43–56.
———. "Science, Medicine, Religion: Three Views of Health Care in France on the Eve of the French Revolution." *Studies in Eighteenth-Century Culture* 10 (1981): 373–91.
Griffenhagen, George B. *Drug Supplies in the American Revolution.* Washington, DC: U.S. National Museum Bulletin, 1961.
Grissinger, Jay W. "The Development of Military Medicine." *New York Academy of Medicine* 3, no. 5 (May 1927): 301–56.
Gubbins, Launcelotte. "The Life and Work of Jean Dominique, First Baron Larrey." *Journal of the Royal Army Medical Corps* 22 (1914): 186–98.
Gurdjian, E. Stephen. "The Treatment of Penetrating Wounds of the Brain Sustained in Warfare." *Journal of Neurosurgery* 39 (February 1974): 157–66.
Hall, C. R. "Caring for the Confederate Soldier." *Medical Life,* 1935, 445–51.
Hall, J. K., G. Zilboorg, and H. A. Bunker, eds. *One Hundred Years of American Psychiatry.* New York: Columbia University Press, 1944.
Halperin, George. "Nikolai Ivanovich Pirogov: Surgeon, Anatomist, Educator." *Bulletin of the History of Medicine* 30, no. 4 (July–August 1956): 347–55.
Halsted, W. S. "Ligature and Suture Material." *Journal of the American Medical Association* 60 (1913): 1120–24.
Hardy, J. D., and E. F. Du Bois. "The Technique of Measuring Radiation and Convection." *Journal of Nutrition* 15 (1938): 466–73.

Harrison, J. A. B. "Military Medicine in the United Kingdom: Similarities and Differences with Respect to the United States and Other NATO Countries." *Military Medicine* 145, no. 6 (June 1980): 288–92.
Hargreaves, Reginald. "Ally of Defeat." *The Practitioner* 202 (May 1960): 713–18.
———. "The Long Road to Military Hygiene." *The Practitioner* 196 (March 1966): 339–447.
Harland, Kathleen. "A Short History of Queen Alexandra's Royal Naval Nursing Service." *Journal of the Royal Naval Medical Service* 70, no. 2 (Summer 1984): 59–65.
Harstad, Peter. "Billy Yank through the Eyes of the Medical Examiner." *Rendezvous* 1 (Spring 1966): 37–51.
Hart, A. G. *The Surgeon and the Hospital in the Civil War.* Boston: Military Historical Society of Massachusetts, Boston Papers, April 1902, 230–85.
Harvey, S. C. "The History of Hemostasis." *Annals of Medical History* 1 (1929): 129–35.
Hawk, Alan. "The Great Disease Enemy, Kak'ke (Beriberi), and the Imperial Japanese Army." *Military Medicine* 171, no. 4 (2006): 333–39.
Heaton, Leonard D., and Joe M. Blumberg. "Lt. Colonel Joseph J. Woodward (1833–1884): U.S. Army Pathologist-Researcher-Photomicroscopist." *Military Medicine* 131, no. 6 (June 1966): 530–38.
Heaton, Leonard D., Carl Hughes, Harold Rosegay, George Fisher, and Robert E. Feighny. "Military Surgical Practices of the U.S. Army in Vietnam." *Current Problems in Surgery* 3, no. 1 (November 1966): 1–58.
Heizmann, Charles L. "Military Sanitation in the Sixteenth, Seventeenth, and Eighteenth Centuries." *Annals of Medical History* 1 (1917–1918): 281–300.
Herman, Jan K. "Dr. Rixey and the Medical Observations of the Russo-Japanese War." *The Grog: A Journal of Navy Medical History and Culture* 4 (Winter 2011): 4–10.
———. "Occupational Hazards Aboard the Ironclad Fleet." *The Grog Ration* 5, no. 3 (May–June 2010): 2–7.
Hibbertt, Charles. "Report on Russian Wounded Admitted to Canacao Hospital, June, 1905." BUMED General Correspondence Files. Letter # 9778. Washington, DC.
Hopkinson, D. A. W., and T. K. Marshall. "Firearm Injuries." *British Journal of Surgery* 54, no. 4 (May 1967): 344–53.
Howard, M. *The Franco-Prussian War.* London: Collins, 1967.
Howell, H. A. L. "The British Medical Arrangements during the Waterloo Campaign." *Proceedings of the Royal Society of Medicine* 17 (1923): 39–50.
———. "The Story of the Army Surgeon and the Care of the Sick and Wounded in the British Army, from 1715 to 1748." *Journal of the Royal Army Medical Corps* 22 (1914): 320–34, 445–71, 643–58.
Howie, William B. "Medical Education in 18th Century Hospitals." *Scottish Society of the History of Medicine.* 1970.
Hume, Edgar Erskine. "Chimborazo Hospital: America's Largest Military Hospital." *Military Surgeon* 75 (1934): 256–61.
———. "The Days Gone By: Military Medicine in the Eighteenth Century." *Military Surgeon*, October 1929, 561–76.
———. "The Precepts of Military Hygiene of the Prince of Ligne." *Military Surgeon*, October 1929, 61–76.
Humphreys, H. F. "The Medical Organization for Cavalry." *Journal of the Royal Army Medical Corps* 44 (1924): 431–39.
Irey, Thomas R. "Soldiering, Suffering, and Dying in the Mexican War." *Journal of the West* 11, no. 2 (1972): 285–93.
Iveson, J. D. "History of the Navy Nurse." *Nursing Mirror* 153, no. 1 (1981): 22–24.
Jackson, Robert. *A System of Arrangement and Discipline for the Medical Department of the Armies.* London: J. Murray, 1805.

James, Theodore. "Gunshot Wounds of the South African War." *South African Medical Journal* 45 (October 1971): 1089–94.

Janis, J. "Observations upon Losses of Confederate Armies from Battle Wounds and Disease." *Richmond and Louisville Medical Journal* 8 (1869): 339–451.

Jensen, Joseph E. "Napoleonic Medicine." *Maryland State Medical Journal.* July 1981, 66–68.

Johns, Frank S., and Anne Page Johns. "Chimborazo Hospital and J. B. McCaw, Surgeon in Chief." *Virginia Magazine of History and Biography* 62 (1954): 1–16.

Jones, Colin. *The Charitable Imperative: Hospitals and Nursing in Ancien Régime and Revolutionary France.* London: Routledge, 1989.

Jones, J. "Medical Corps of the Confederate Army and Navy." *Atlanta Medical and Surgical Journal* 7 (1891): 339.

Kalisch, Philip A., and Beatrice J. Kalisch. "Untrained but Undaunted: The Women Nurses of the Blue and the Gray." *Nursing Forum* 15, no. 1 (1976): 6–33.

Kampmeier, Rudolph. "Veneral Disease in the U.S. Army, 1775–1900." *Sexually Transmitted Disease* 9 (April–June, 1982): 100–103.

Keegan, John. *The Face of Battle.* New York: Viking, 1977.

Keen, W. W. "Surgical Reminiscences of the Civil War." *Transactions of the College of Physicians of Philadelphia.* 3rd series, no. 27 (1905): 109–15.

Keene, W., S. Mitchell, and G. Morehouse. "On Malingering, Especially in Regard to Simulation of Diseases of the Nervous System." *American Journal of Medical Science* 48 reprint (1964): 367–94.

Kempthorne, G. A. "The American War, 1812–1814." *Journal of the Royal Army Medical Corps* 62 (1934): 139–40.

———. "The Army Medical Service at Home and Abroad, 1803–1808." *Journal of the Royal Army Medical Corps.* August and September 1933, 144–46, 223–32.

———. "The Army Medical Services, 1816–1825." *Journal of the Royal Army Medical Corps* 60 (1933): 299–310.

———. "The Egyptian Campaign of 1801." *Journal of the Royal Army Medical Corps* 55 (1930): 217–30.

———. "The Medical Department in the Crimea." *Journal of the Royal Army Medical Corps* 53, no. 55 (August 1929): 131–46.

———. "The Medical Department of Wellington's Army." *Journal of the Royal Army Medical Corps,* February–March 1930, 212–25.

———. "Notes on the History of the Medical Staff Corps and the Army Hospital Corps, 1854–1898." *Journal of the Royal Army Medical Corps* 51 (October 1928): 265–77.

———. "The Walcheren Expedition and the Reform of the Medical Board." *Journal of the Royal Army Medical Corps* 62 (1934): 133–38.

———. "The Waterloo Campaign." *Journal of the Royal Army Medical Corps* 60 (1933): 52–59.

Kennedy, Paul. *The Rise and Fall of the Great Powers.* New York: Random House, 1987.

King, Joseph E. "Shoulder Straps for Aesculapius: The Vicksburg Campaign in 1863." *Military Surgeon* 114 (1954): 216–21.

Kirkup, J. R. "The History and Evolution of Surgical Instruments." *Annals of the Royal College of Surgeons of England* 63 (1981): 279–85.

Kohn, Stanislas. *The Cost of the War to Russia: The Vital Statistics of European Russia during the World War, 1914–1917.* New Haven, CT: Yale University Press, 1932.

Kopperman, Paul E. "Medical Services in the British Army, 1742–1783." *Journal of the History of Medicine and Allied Sciences* 34, no. 4 (October 1979): 430–55.

Krivosheev, G. F. "The Secret Seal Is Removed." *Voyenizdat,* 1993, 401–5.

Kruger, Rayne. *Good-bye Dolly Gray: The Story of the Boer War.* London: Cassell, 1960.

Kurvshinskiy, V. D. "Technical Service and Repair of Medical Equipment in the Course of Military Activity." *Military Medical Journal,* 1992, 41–45.

Lada, John, ed. *Medical Statistics in World War II.* Washington, DC: Office of the Surgeon General, Department of the Army, 1975.

Laffont, Robert. *The Ancient Art of Warfare.* 2 vols. London: Crescent Press, 1966.

Lane, J. E. "Jean François Coste, Chief Physician of French Expeditionary Forces in the American Revolution." *Americana* 22 (1928): 2–10.

Langley, Harold. "Notes on Psychiatric Care in the Early Navy, 1830–1865." *The Grog Ration*, September–October 2007, 5–6.

Lankford, Nelson D. "The Victorian Medical Profession and Military Practice: Army Doctors and National Origins." *Bulletin of the History of Medicine* 54 (1980): 511–28.

Larrey, Dominique Jean. *Memoirs of Military Surgery and Campaigns of the French Armies.* Translated by R. W. Hill Baltimore: J. Cushing, 1814.

Lawson, Robert. "Amputations through the Ages." *Australian–New Zealand Journal of Surgery* 42, no. 3 (February 1973): 222–30.

Lee, Charles O. "The Shakers as Pioneers in the American Herb and Drug Industry." *American Journal of Pharmacy* 132 (May 1960): 178–84.

Lewin, Walpole, and Myles Gibson. "Missile Head Wounds in the Korean Campaign." *British Journal of Surgery* 43 (1956): 628–32.

Lewis, J. "Exemption from Military Service on Account of Loss of Teeth." *American Dental Association Transactions,* July 1985, 164–69.

Liddell, J. "On the Medical Preparations for Naval Action, and on the Casualties at the Battle of Navarino." *Medical Times and Gazette* 1 (1854): 312–14.

Lindskog, Gustaf E. "Some Historical Aspects of Thoracic Trauma." *Journal of Thoracic and Cardiovascular Surgery* 42 (1961): 1–11.

Link, Kenneth. "Potomac Fever: The Hazards of Camp Life." *Vermont History* 51, no. 2 (1983): 69–88.

Lister, Joseph. "An Address on the Catgut Ligature." *British Medical Journal* 1 (1881): 183–84.

Liston, Robert. "Four Cases of Amputation by R. Liston, Illustrating His Mode of Operating after Treatment." *British Annals of Medical Pharmacy* 1 (1837): 518–22.

Logue, Daniel C. "Treating the Wounded aboard the USS *Monitor,* 1862." *U.S. Navy Medicine* 73, no. 1 (1982): 4–5.

London, P. S. "An Example to Us All: The Military Approach to the Care of the Injured." *Journal of the Royal Army Medical Corps* 134 (1988): 81–90.

Longmore, Sir Thomas. *A Treatise on the Transportation of Sick and Wounded Troops.* London: Her Majesty's Stationery Office, 1866.

Love, Albert G. *War Casualties.* Carlisle, PA: Medical Field Service School, 1931.

Lovegrove, Peter. *Not Least in the Crusade: A Short History of the Royal Army Medical Corps.* Aldershot, UK: Gale and Polden, 1951.

MacCormac, Sir. W. "The Wounded in the Present War." *Lancet,* 1900, 13–18.

Macleod, George H. B. *Notes on the Surgery of the War in the Crimea, with Remarks on the Treatment of Gunshot Wounds.* London: J. Churchill, 1858.

Manucy, Albert. *Artillery through the Ages.* Washington, DC: U.S. Government Printing Office, 1985.

Marsh, A. R. "A Short but Distant War: The Falklands Campaign." *Journal of the Royal Society of Medicine* 76 (November 1983): 972–82.

Marshall, M. L. "Medicine in the Confederacy." *Bulletin of the Medical Library Association* 30 (1942): 279–91.

Martin, Sylvia. "The Australian Army Hospitals." *The Lamp* 37, no. 5 (1980): 53–58.

Matheson, J. M. "Comments on the Medical Aspects of the Battle of Waterloo, 1815." *Medical History* 10 (1966): 204–7.

Mayerhoff, Max. "A Short History of Ophthalmia during the Egyptian Campaign of 1798–1807." *British Journal of Ophthalmology* 16 (1933): 129–52.

McConaghy, Lorraine. "Medicine aboard the *Decatur*, 1854–1859." *The Grog Ration* 1, no. 4 (November–December 2006): 1–4.

McCord, Carey P. "Scurvy as an Occupational Disease: Scurvy in the World's Armies." *Journal of Occupational Medicine* 13, no. 12 (December 1971): 586–92.

McGreevy, Patrick S. "Surgeons at the Battle of Little Big Horn." *Surgery, Gynecology, and Obstetrics* 140 (May 1975): 774–80.

McGrew, Roderick E. *Encyclopedia of Medical History.* New York: McGraw-Hill, 1985.

McLaughlin, Redmond. *The Royal Army Medical Corps.* London: Leo Cooper, 1972.

"Medical Management and Operations." *Fundamentals of Tactical Logistics Manual.* Fort Leavenworth, KS: U.S. Army Command and General Staff College, July 1980, 7-1 to 7-31.

Meid, P., and J. M. Yinling. *U.S. Marine Operations in Korea, 1950–1953.* Vol. 5, *Operations in West Korea.* Washington: DC: Historical Division of the Headquarters, U.S. Marine Corps, 1954.

Middleton, William Shainline. "Medicine at Valley Forge." *Annals of Medical History* 3, no. 6 (November 1941): 461–86.

Millar, W. M. "'Plain Remarks'—America's First Manual of Surgery." *American Journal of Surgery* 26 (1934): 599–611.

Mitchell, Silas Weir. "The Medical Department of the Civil War." *Journal of the American Medical Association* 66 (1914): 1445–50.

Moffat, W. C. "British Forces Casualties in Northern Ireland." *Journal of the Royal Army Medical Corps* 112 (1976): 3–8.

Murray, Eleanor M. "The Medical Department of the Revolution." *Bulletin of Fort Ticonderoga Museum* 3, no. 8 (1949): 106–8.

Napier, W. F. P. "War in the Peninsula and in the South of France from 1807 to 1814." *Journal of the Royal Army Medical Corps* 16 (1911): 103–11.

NATO. *Emergency War Surgery, NATO Handbook.* Washington, DC: U.S. Government Printing Office, 1958.

Nechaev, E. A., A. K. Tutokhel, A. I. Gritsanov, and I. D. Kosachev. "Medical Support of the 40th Army: Facts and Figures." *Military Medical Journal,* August 1991, 3–11.

Neel, Spurgeon. *Medical Support of the U.S. Army in Vietnam, 1965–1970.* Washington, DC: Department of the Army, Government Printing Office, 1973.

Nemytin, Yuri. "Special Medical Aid to the Wounded in Afghanistan." *Military Medical Journal,* January 1991, 14–19.

Nemytin, Yuri, and V. V. Boldyrev. "Rehabilitation Management of Infectious Patients in Overcrowded Hospitals." *Military Medical Journal,* April–May 1992, 37–41.

Niebyl, Peter H. "The English Bloodletting Revolution, or Modern Medicine before 1850." *Bulletin of the History of Medicine* 51 (1977): 464–83.

Nightingale, Florence. *Army Sanitation Administration and the Reforms under the Late Lord Herbert.* London: McCorquodale and Company, 1862.

———. "Military Hospitals and Nursing." *American Medical Times.* May 11, 1861, 306–7.

———. *Mortality of the British Army at Home and Abroad and during the Russian War, as Compared with the Mortality of the Civilian Population in England.* London: Harrison and Sons, 1858.

Novichkov, N. N., V. Ya. Snnegovsky, A. G. Sokolov, and V. Yu. Shvarev. *The Russian Armed Forces in the Chechen Conflict.* Moscow: Holwege-Infoglobe-Trivola, 1995.

Olch, Peter D. "Medicine in the Indian-Fighting Army, 1866–1890." *Journal of the West* 21, no. 3 (1982): 32–41.

Oliver, John Rathbone. "The Renaissance." *International Clinics* 1 (March 1928): 239–62.

Oman, C. W. *The Art of War in the Middle Ages.* Ithaca, NY: Cornell University Press, 1982.

Overholser, Winfred. "Dorothea Dix: A Note." *Bulletin of the History of Medicine* 9 (1941): 210–16.

Owen, W. C. "The Legislative and Administrative History of the Medical Department of the United States Army during the Revolutionary Period." *Annals of Medical History* 1, no. 1 (1917): 13–38.

Pagaard, Stephen A. "Disease in the British Army in South Africa, 1899–1900." *Military Affairs,* April 1986, 71–76.

Patton, M. A. "An Early Case of Battle Hysteria." *British Journal of Psychiatry* 138 (February 1981): 182–83.

Pinkham, Barbara M. "The U.S. Sanitary Commission and Its Impact on Civil War Medicine." *Medical Record News* 47 (August 1976): 70–75.

Porter, J. B. "Medical and Surgical Notes of Campaigns in the War with Mexico during the Year 1845." *American Journal of Medical Science* 23 (1852): 13–27.

———. "Medical and Surgical Notes of the Campaigns in the War with Mexico during the Year 1846." *American Journal of Medical Science* 24 (1852): 13–30.

———. "Medical and Surgical Notes of the Campaigns in the War with Mexico during the Year 1847." *American Journal of Medical Science* 25 (1852): 25–42.

———. "Medical and Surgical Notes of the Campaigns in the War with Mexico during the Year 1848." *American Journal of Medical Science* 26 (1852): 297–333.

———. "Medical and Surgical Notes of the Campaigns in the War with Mexico during the Year 1848." *American Journal of Medical Science* 35 (1852): 347–52.

Quinones, Mark A. "Drug Abuse during the Civil War, 1861–1865." *International Journal of the Addictions* 10 (1975): 1019–26.

Ramer, Samuel. "Who Was the Russian Feldsher?" *Bulletin of the History of Medicine* 50, no. 2 (1976): 213–25.

Raymond, Edward A. "American Doctors in the Crimean War." *Connecticut Medicine* 38, no. 7 (July 1974): 373–76.

Reasoner, M. A. "The Development of the Medical Supply Service." *Military Surgeon* 63, no. 1 (July 1928): 1–21.

Rees, John Rawlings. *The Shaping of Psychiatry by War.* New York: Norton, 1945.

Reid, Robert L. "The British Crimean Medical Disaster: Ineptness or Inevitability?" *Military Medicine* 140 (June 1975): 420–26.

Reister, Frank A. *Battle Casualties and Medical Statistics: U.S. Army Experience in the Korean War.* Washington, DC: Office of the Surgeon General, 1973.

Rice, G. H. "The Evolution of the Military Medical Service from 1854 to 1914." *Journal of the Royal Army Medical Corps* 135, no. 3 (1989): 147–50.

Richardson, F. M. "Wellington, Napoleon, and the Medical Services." *Journal of the Royal Army Medical Corps* 131, no. 1 (1985): 9–15.

Richardson, Teresa Eden. *In Japanese Hospitals during Wartime: Fifteen Months with the Red Cross Society of Japan, April 1904–July 1905.* London: William Blackwood and Sons, 1905.

Riley, Harris D. "Medicine in the Confederacy." *Military Medicine* 118 (1956): 144–53.

Roddis, L. H. "Naval Medicine in the Early Days of Our Republic." *Journal of the History of Medicine* 16 (1961): 104–9.

———. *A Short History of Nautical Medicine.* New York: Hoeber, 1940.

Roemer, Milton L. "History of the Effects of Warfare on Medicine." *Annals of Medical History.* 3rd series, vol. 4 (1942): 189–209.

Rogers, Blair O. "Surgery in the Revolutionary War: Contributions of John Jones, M.D. (1729–1791)." *Plastic and Reconstructive Surgery* 49 (January 1972): 1–13.

Rosen, George. "Health, Medical Care, and Social Policy in the French Revolution." *Bulletin of the History of Medicine* 30 (1956): 124–49.

———. "Nostalgia: A 'Forgotten' Psychological Disorder." *Psychological Medicine* 5 (1975): 340–54.

Rush, Benjamin. "Directions for Preserving the Health of the Soldier." *Military Surgeon* 22 (1908): 183–90.

Ryerson, G. Sterling. "Medical and Surgical Experiences in the South African War." *The Canadian Practitioner,* October 1900, 3–17.

Sandos, James A. "Prostitution and Drugs: The U.S. Army on the Mexican-American Border: 1916–1917." *Pacific Historical Review* 49, no. 4 (November 1980): 621–45.

"Sanitary Officers in the Field." *British Medical Journal* 1 (1901): 89–96.

Schwartz, Aaron M. "The Historical Development of Methods of Hemostasis." *Surgery* 44, no. 3 (September 1958): 604–10.

Seaman, Louis J. *The Real Triumph of Japan, The Conquest of the Silent Foe.* New York: D. Appleton, 1906.

Shepard, John A. "The Smart of the Knife: Early Anesthesia in the Services." *Journal of the Royal Army Medical Corps* 131, no. 2 (June 1985): 109–15.

Sieur, Hercule. "Tribulations of the Medical Corps of the French Army from Its Origins to Our Own Time." *Military Surgeon* 64, no. 6 (June 1929): 210–28, 843–56.

Sigerist, Henry E. "Ambroise Paré's Onion Treatment of Burns." *Bulletin of the History of Medicine* 15, no. 2 (February 1944): 43–149.

———. "War and Medicine." *Journal of Laboratory and Clinical Medicine* 28, no. 5 (February 1943): 531–38.

Sinopal'nikov, I. V. "Medical Losses of Soviet Troops during the War in Afghanistan: Medical Losses from Infectious Diseases." *Military Medical Journal* 321, no. 9 (September 2000): 4–10.

Skinner, George A. "Influence of Epidemic Disease on Military Operations in the History of the Western Hemisphere." *Military Surgeon* 69, no. 6 (December 1931): 579–95.

Smart, William R. E. "On the Medical Services of the Navy and Army from the Accession of Henry VIII to the Restoration." *British Medical Journal* 1 (1874): 168–69, 199–200, 228–29, 264–66.

Smith, Fred L. *A Short History of the Royal Army Medical Corps.* Aldershot, UK: Gale and Polden, 1946.

Smith, G. P. "On Military Medical Practice in the East." *Lancet* 1 (1855): 648–51.

Smith, John David. "Kentucky Civil War Recruits." *Medical History* 24, no. 2 (April 1980): 185–96.

Soviet Studies Research Center. *The Sustainability of the Soviet Army in Battle.* The Hague: SHAPE Technical Center, 1986.

Spear, Raymond. *Report on the Russian Medical and Sanitary Features of the Russo-Japanese War to the Surgeon General, U.S. Navy.* Washington, DC: U.S. Government Printing Office, 1906.

Stansbury, L. G., S. J. Lallis, J. G. Branstetter, M. R. Bagg, and J. B. Holcomb. "Amputations in U.S. Military Personnel in Afghanistan and Iraq." *Journal of Orthopedic Trauma* 22, no. 1 (2008): 43–46.

Stark, Richard B. "The History of Plastic Surgery in Wartime." *Clinics in Plastic Surgery* 2, no. 4 (October 1975): 509–16.

———. "Surgeons and Surgical Care of the Confederate States Army." *Virginia Medical Monthly* 87 (1960): 230–41.

Steiner, Meir, and Micha Neumann. "Traumatic Neurosis and Social Support in the Yom Kippur War." *Military Medicine,* December 1978, 866–74.

Steinfeld, Jesse L. "Southern Medicine in the Civil War." *Southern Medical Journal* 73, no. 4 (April 1980): 497–98.

Sternberg, George M. *Sanitary Lessons of the War.* Washington, DC: Byron Adams, 1912.

Stevens, H. E. R. "The Influence of War on the Craft of Surgery." *Journal of the Royal Army Medical Corps* 62 (1934): 40–46.

Stevenson, Lloyd G. "Notes on the Relation of Military Service to Licensing in the History of the British Army." *Bulletin of the History of Medicine* 27 (1953): 420–27.

Stewart, Miller J. *Moving the Wounded: Litters, Cacolets & Ambulance Wagons, U.S. Army, 1776–1876.* Johnstown, CO: Old Army Press, 1979.

Stillé, Charles J. *The History of the United States Sanitary Commission.* Philadelphia: J. B. Lippincott, 1866.

Stimson, Byron. "Scurvy in the Civil War." *Civil War Times* 5 (August 1966): 20–24.

Stookey, Byron. *A History of Colonial Medical Education: In the Province of New York, with Its Subsequent Development, 1767–1830.* Springfield, IL: Charles C. Thomas, 1962.

Stout, S. H. "Reminiscences of the Medical Officers of the Confederate Army of the Department of Tennessee." *St. Louis Medical and Surgical Journal* 64 (1893): 228–29.

———. "Some Facts on the History of the Organization of the Medical Services of the Confederate Armies and Hospitals." *Southern Practitioner* 23 (1901): 159–51.

Strecker, Edward A. "Military Psychiatry in World War I, 1917–1918." In Hall et al., *One Hundred Years of American Psychiatry*, 385–416.

"Surgery before Anesthetics." *Journal of the Missouri Medical Association* 32 (1935): 169–75.

Swain, Valentine A. J. "The Franco-Prussian War, 1870–1871: Voluntary Aid for the Wounded and Sick." *British Medical Journal* 29, no. 3 (August 1970): 511–14.

Sweetman, John. "The Crimean War and the Foundation of the Medical Staff Corps." *Journal for the Society for Army Historical Research* 53, no. 214 (1975): 113–19.

Tanner, Stephen. *Afghanistan: A Military History from Alexander the Great to the War against the Taliban.* New York: Da Capo Press, 2009.

Taylor, Blaine. "Some Medical-Historical Aspects of the Later Napoleonic Wars, 1812–1815." *Maryland State Medical Journal*, December 1978, 24–31.

Taylor, Charles R. *Medical Support of the Soviet Ground Forces.* Washington, DC: Soviet/Warsaw Pact Division, Defense Intelligence Agency, March 1979.

Teodorico, dei Borgognoni. *Theodoric: The Surgery of Theodoric.* 2 vols. Translated by E. Campbell and J. Colton. New York: Appleton-Century-Crofts, 1955–60.

Thompson, C. J. S. "The Evolution and Development of Surgical Instruments." *British Journal of Surgery* 97 (1937): 4–9.

Thompson, J. *Report on Observations Made in British Military Hospitals in Belgium after the Battle of Waterloo.* Edinburgh, UK: Blackwood, 1816.

Thoresby, F. P., and H. M. Darlow. "The Mechanisms of Primary Infection of Bullet Wounds." *British Journal of Surgery* 54 (1967): 359–69.

Trueta, J. "Reflections on the Past and Present Treatment of War Wounds and Fractures." *Military Medicine* 141 (1976): 255–369.

U.S. Army Intelligence and Threat Analysis Center. "Medical Evacuation and Treatment." *Soviet Army Operations.* Arlington, VA: Department of the Army, April 1978, 3–13.

U.S. Surgeon General's Office. *Medical and Surgical History of the War of the Rebellion.* 6 vols. Washington, DC: U.S. Government Printing Office, 1870–1888.

Van Rensselaer-Hoff, John. "Resume of the History of the Medical Department of the U.S. Army from 1775 to the Beginning of the Spanish-American War." *Military Surgeon* 10 (1901–1902): 347–98.

Vess, David M. "The Collapse and Revival of Medical Education in France: A Consequence of Revolution and War." *History of Education Quarterly* 7 (1967): 71–92.

———. "French Military Medicine during the Revolution." PhD diss., University of Alabama, 1965.

Wagner, Robert, and Benjamin Slivko. "History of Nonpenetrating Chest Trauma and Its

Treatment." *Minnesota Medical Journal* 37, no. 4 (April 1988): 297–304.
Wangensteen, Owen H., Jacqueline Smith, and Sarah D. Wangensteen. "Some Highlights in the History of Amputation Reflecting Lessons in Wound Healing." *Bulletin of the History of Medicine* 41, no. 2 (March–April 1967): 97–131.
Wangensteen, Owen H., and Sarah D. Wangensteen. *The Rise of Surgery: From Empiric Craft to Scientific Discipline.* New York: Dawson, 1978.
Wangensteen, Owen H., Sarah D. Wangensteen, and Charles F. Klinger. "Wound Management of Ambroise Paré and Dominique Larrey: Great French Military Surgeons of the 16th and 19th Centuries." *Bulletin of the History of Medicine* 65, no. 3 (May–June 1973): 207–34.
Ward, Geoffrey C. *The Civil War: An Illustrated History.* New York: Knopf, 1990.
Warner, Denis, and Peggy Warner. *The Tide at Sunrise: A History of the Russo-Japanese War, 1904–1905.* New York: Charterhouse, 1974.
Watson, William N. "An Edinburgh Surgeon of the Crimean War: Patrick Heron Watson." *Medical History* 10 (1966): 166–76.
Weir, Robert F. "Remarks on the Gunshot Wounds of the Civil War." *New York State Journal of Medicine* 82, no. 3 (March 1982): 391–93.
Wells, T. S. "Remarks on the Results of Inhalation of Ether in 106 Cases." *London Medical Gazette* 40 (1847): 547–49.
West, Charles G. H. "A Short History of the Management of Penetrating Missile Injuries to the Head." *Surgical Neurology* 16, no. 2 (August 1981): 145–49.
Wiese, E. Robert. "Larrey: Napoleon's Chief Surgeon." *Annals of Medical History* 1 (July 1929): 435–50.
Wiltse, Charles M. *The U.S. Army in World War II.* Washington, DC: Military History Section, Department of the Army, 1963.
Winter, J. M. "Military Fitness and Civilian Health in Britain during the First World War." *Journal of Contemporary History* 15 (1980): 211–44.
Wolfe, Edwin P. "The Genesis of the Medical Department of the United States Army." *Bulletin of the New York Academy of Medicine* 5 (September 1929): 823–44.
Wood, Casey. "A Few Civil War Hospitals." *Military Surgeon* 42 (May 1918): 539–48.
Wooden, Allen C. "Dr. Jean François Coste and the French Army in the American Revolution." *Delaware Medical Journal* 48, no. 7 (July 1976): 397–404.
———. "The Wounds and Weapons of the Revolutionary War from 1775 to 1783." *Delaware Medical Journal* 44, no. 3 (March 1972): 59–65.
Woodward, Theodore E. "The Public's Debt to Military Medicine." *Military Medicine* 146 (March 1981): 168–73.
Wrench, E. M. "Midland Branch: The Lessons of the Crimean War." *British Medical Journal,* July 1899, 205–6.
Young, James. "A Short History of English Military Surgery and Some Famous Military Surgeons." *Journal of the Royal Army Medical Corps* 21 (1913): 484–89.
Young, Peter Alexander. "The Army Medical Staff: Its Past Services and Its Present Needs." *Edinburgh Medical Journal* 4 (1898): 11–20.
Zellem, Ronald T. "Wounded by Bayonet, Ball, and Bacteria: Medicine and Neurosurgery in the American Civil War." *Neurosurgery* 17, no. 5 (1988): 850–60.

INDEX

Printed in the USA
CPSIA information can be obtained
at www.ICGtesting.com
LVHW041126071223
765754LV00001B/59

9 781612 348223